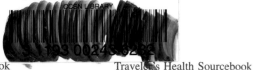

Injury & Trauma Sourcebook

Learning Disabil

Leukemia Sour

Liver Disorders

Lung Disorders

Medical Tests S

Men's Health C

Edition

Mental Health Disorders Sourcebook, 3rd
Edition

Mental Retardation Sourcebook

Movement Disorders Sourcebook

Multiple Sclerosis Sourcebook

Muscular Dystrophy Sourcebook

Obesity Sourcebook

Osteoporosis Sourcebook

Pain Sourcebook, 3rd Edition

Pediatric Cancer Sourcebook

Physical & Mental Issues in Aging
Sourcebook

Podiatry Sourcebook, 2nd Edition

Pregnancy & Birth Sourcebook, 2nd
Edition

Prostate Cancer Sourcebook

Prostate & Urological Disorders Sourcebook

Reconstructive & Cosmetic Surgery
Sourcebook

Rehabilitation Sourcebook

Respiratory Disorders Sourcebook, 2nd
Edition

Sexually Transmitted Diseases Sourcebook,
3rd Edition

Sleep Disorders Sourcebook, 2nd Edition

Smoking Concerns Sourcebook

Sports Injuries Sourcebook, 3rd Edition

Stress-Related Disorders Sourcebook, 2nd
Edition

Stroke Sourcebook, 2nd Edition

Surgery Sourcebook, 2nd Edition

Thyroid Disorders Sourcebook

Transplantation Sourcebook

Travelers Health Sourcebook

Diseases &

k, 2nd Edition

ns Sourcebook, 2nd

ty Sourcebook

ebook

**Learning
disabilities
sourcebook**

JUN 1 5 2009

D0428645

Alcohol Information

Allergy Information for Teens

Asthma Information for Teens

Body Information for Teens

Cancer Information for Teens

Complementary & Alternative
Medicine Information for Teens

Diabetes Information for Teens

Diet Information for Teens, 2nd Edition

Drug Information for Teens, 2nd Edition

Eating Disorders Information for Teens

Fitness Information for Teens, 2nd
Edition

Learning Disabilities Information for
Teens

Mental Health Information for Teens,
2nd Edition

Pregnancy Information for Teens

Sexual Health Information for Teens,
2nd Edition

Skin Health Information for Teens

Sleep Information for Teens

Sports Injuries Information for Teens,
2nd Edition

Stress Information for Teens

Suicide Information for Teens

Tobacco Information for Teens

Learning Disabilities

SOURCEBOOK

Third Edition

Health Reference Series

Third Edition

Learning Disabilities
SOURCEBOOK

Basic Consumer Health Information about Dyslexia, Auditory and Visual Processing Disorders, Communication Disorders, Dyscalculia, Dysgraphia, and Other Conditions That Impede Learning, Including Attention Deficit/Hyperactivity Disorder, Autism Spectrum Disorders, Hearing and Visual Impairments, Chromosome-Based Disorders, and Brain Injury

Along with Facts about Brain Function, Assessment, Therapy and Remediation, Accommodations, Assistive Technology, Legal Protections, and Tips about Family Life, School Transitions, and Employment Strategies, a Glossary of Related Terms, and Directories of Additional Resources

Edited by
Joyce Brennfleck Shannon

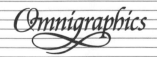
Omnigraphics

P.O. Box 31-1640, Detroit, MI 48231

Bibliographic Note

Because this page cannot legibly accommodate all the copyright notices, the Bibliographic Note portion of the Preface constitutes an extension of the copyright notice.

Edited by Joyce Brennfleck Shannon

Health Reference Series

Karen Bellenir, *Managing Editor*
David A. Cooke, M.D., *Medical Consultant*
Elizabeth Collins, *Research and Permissions Coordinator*
Cherry Edwards, *Permissions Assistant*
EdIndex, Services for Publishers, *Indexers*

* * *

Omnigraphics, Inc.

Matthew P. Barbour, *Senior Vice President*
Kevin M. Hayes, *Operations Manager*

* * *

Peter E. Ruffner, *Publisher*

Copyright © 2009 Omnigraphics, Inc.

ISBN 978-0-7808-1039-6

Library of Congress Cataloging-in-Publication Data

Learning disabilities sourcebook : basic consumer health information about dyslexia, auditory and visual processing disorders, communication disorders, dyscalculia, dysgraphia, and other conditions that impede learning, including attention deficit/hyperactivity disorder, autism spectrum disorders, hearing and visual impairments, chromosome-based disorders, and brain injury; along with facts about brain function, assessment, therapy and remediation, accommodations, assistive technology, legal protections, and tips about family life, school transitions, and employment strategies, a glossary of related terms, and directories of additional resources / edited by Joyce Brennfleck Shannon. -- 3rd ed.
  p. cm. -- (Health reference series)
  Includes bibliographical references and index.
  Summary: "Provides basic consumer health information about various learning disabilities, with facts about diagnosis, instructional approaches, legal and financial issues, and with coping tips. Includes index, glossary of related terms, and other resources"--Provided by publisher.
  ISBN 978-0-7808-1039-6 (hardcover : alk. paper) 1. Learning disabilities--United States--Handbooks, manuals, etc. 2. Learning disabled children--Education--United States--Handbooks, manuals, etc. 3. Learning disabled--Education--United States--Handbooks, manuals, etc. 4. Learning disabilities--United States--Diagnosis--Handbooks, manuals, etc. I. Shannon, Joyce Brennfleck.
  LC4705.L434 2008
  371.90973--dc22

                                                                        2008043262

Printed in the United States

Table of Contents

Visit www.healthreferenceseries.com to view *A Contents Guide to the Health Reference Series*, a listing of more than 14,000 topics and the volumes in which they are covered.

Part III: Specific Learning Disabilities

Part IV: Other Health Conditions That Impede Learning

Part V: Assessment, Accommodations, and Therapies for Learning Disabilities

Part VI: Legal and Financial Information for Individuals with Learning Disabilities

Part VII: Living with a Learning Disability

Part VIII: Additional Help and Information

Preface

About This Book

The U.S. Department of Education reports that as many as one out of every five Americans has a learning disability. Learning disabilities make it difficult to learn to read, write, listen, speak, reason, or do math. They occur because of problems in how the brain receives and processes information. Early intervention services help many children avoid the stigma of failure; however, identifying learning disabilities can be difficult. While there is no cure for learning disabilities, research has identified effective learning strategies. In fact, with help, most children and adults with learning disabilities are able to accomplish their educational and career goals.

Learning Disabilities Sourcebook, Third Edition provides updated information about specific learning disabilities and other conditions that make learning difficult. These include dyslexia, dyscalculia, dysgraphia, auditory and visual processing, communication disorders, attention deficit/hyperactivity disorder, autism spectrum disorders, hearing and visual impairments, and brain injury. Current research on brain processes and function is described, along with facts about evidence-based therapy, instructional strategies, and federal education laws. Tips for building social skills and family relationships, making transitions from school to work, and dealing with financial issues are also provided, along with a glossary of related terms and directories of additional resources.

How to Use This Book

This book is divided into parts and chapters. Parts focus on broad areas of interest. Chapters are devoted to single topics within a part.

Part I: Introduction to Learning Disabilities provides an overview of learning disabilities. Facts are included about signs and definitions of learning disabilities and perceptions, expectations, and outcomes. The part concludes with a chapter in which a mother shares ten things she wishes she had known about learning disabilities as her child struggled.

Part II: The Brain and Learning Disabilities explains the basic brain functions involved in learning. Facts about neuropsychological evaluation are presented, and the impact of executive function and brain maturity on learning is discussed. The part also includes findings from recent brain imaging studies.

Part III: Specific Learning Disabilities provides detailed information about the learning disabilities defined under the Individuals with Disabilities Education Act, including auditory and visual processing disorders, speech and language disorders, dyscalculia, dysgraphia, dyslexia, and nonverbal learning disorder.

Part IV: Other Health Conditions That Impede Learning describes various impairments and disorders that impact learning. These include attention deficit/hyperactivity disorder in children and adults, chromosome-based disorders, emotional/behavioral disorders, fetal alcohol syndrome and other mental retardation, Gerstmann syndrome, hearing impairment, pervasive development disorders (autism spectrum and Asperger syndrome disorders), traumatic brain injury, and visual impairment.

Part V: Assessment, Accommodations, and Therapies for Learning Disabilities describes the tools and strategies used for the determination and remediation of learning disorders. Tools for remediation include the use of speech and language therapy, reading instruction, the strategic instruction model, multisensory teaching, and assistive technology. A chapter on the principles of effective instruction for adults with learning disabilities is also included.

Part VI: Legal and Financial Information for Individuals with Learning Disabilities presents information about services for students in preschool and public and private schools mandated by the No Child Left Behind Act and the Individuals with Disabilities Education Act. Alternate assessments, modified academic achievement standards, and summary of performance reports are described. The impact of the American Disabilities Act is also discussed, and facts are presented about special needs trusts and scholarships for students with disabilities.

Part VII: Living with a Learning Disability gives practical advice for individuals and families. Suggestions for coping with a learning disability, building self-esteem and social competence, and recognizing and stopping bullying are presented. Tips are also offered for helping a person with difficult behaviors and for transitioning from school to work.

Part VIII: Additional Help and Information provides a glossary of terms related to learning disabilities and directories for help in finding local resources, literacy materials, and further information about learning disabilities.

Bibliographic Note

This volume contains documents and excerpts from publications issued by the following U.S. government agencies: Centers for Disease Control and Prevention (CDC); Health Resources and Services Administration (HRSA); National Dissemination Center for Children with Disabilities (NICHCY); National Institute for Literacy; National Institute of Biomedical Imaging and Bioengineering (NIBIB); National Institute of Mental Health (NIMH); National Institute of Neurological Disorders and Stroke (NINDS); National Institute on Deafness and Other Communication Disorders (NIDCD); National Institutes of Health (NIH); National Library of Medicine, Genetics Home Reference; National Research Center on Learning Disabilities; U.S. Department of Education; and the U.S. Department of Labor.

In addition, this volume contains copyrighted documents from the following individuals and organizations: A.D.A.M., Inc.; American Art Therapy Association; American Psychological Association (APA); Ernest Bordini; Dale S. Brown; Children and Adults with Attention-Deficit/Hyperactivity Disorder (CHADD); Colorado Department of Education; EyeCare America; FinAid Page, L.L.C.; Fisher Landau Center for the Treatment of Learning Disabilities; GreatSchools; Job Accommodation Network (JAN); LDinfo Publishing; Learning Disabilities Association of America; National Center for Learning Disabilities;

National Center on Educational Outcomes; National Fragile X Foundation; National Joint Committee on Learning Disabilities; Nemours Foundation; Neuropsychology Central; New York University Child Study Center; North Dakota Department of Public Instruction; Organisation for Economic Co-operation and Development; PACER Center Inc.; Performance Learning Systems; David Pitonyak; Smart Kids with LD; University of Michigan Health System; and the University of Washington Office of News and Information.

Acknowledgements

In addition to the listed organizations, agencies, and individuals who have contributed to this *Sourcebook*, special thanks go to managing editor Karen Bellenir, research and permissions coordinator Liz Collins, and document engineer Bruce Bellenir for their help and support.

About the Health Reference Series

The *Health Reference Series* is designed to provide basic medical information for patients, families, caregivers, and the general public. Each volume takes a particular topic and provides comprehensive coverage. This is especially important for people who may be dealing with a newly diagnosed disease or a chronic disorder in themselves or in a family member. People looking for preventive guidance, information about disease warning signs, medical statistics, and risk factors for health problems will also find answers to their questions in the *Health Reference Series*. The *Series*, however, is not intended to serve as a tool for diagnosing illness, in prescribing treatments, or as a substitute for the physician/patient relationship. All people concerned about medical symptoms or the possibility of disease are encouraged to seek professional care from an appropriate health care provider.

A Note about Spelling and Style

Health Reference Series editors use *Stedman's Medical Dictionary* as an authority for questions related to the spelling of medical terms and the *Chicago Manual of Style* for questions related to grammatical structures, punctuation, and other editorial concerns. Consistent adherence is not always possible, however, because the individual volumes within the *Series* include many documents from a wide variety of different producers and copyright holders, and the editor's primary goal is to present material from each source as accurately as is possible following the terms specified by each document's producer. This sometimes means that information in different chapters or sections may follow other guidelines and alternate spelling authorities. For example, occasionally a copyright holder may require that eponymous terms be shown in possessive forms (Crohn's disease *vs.* Crohn disease) or that British spelling norms be retained (leukaemia *vs.* leukemia).

Locating Information within the Health Reference Series

The *Health Reference Series* contains a wealth of information about a wide variety of medical topics. Ensuring easy access to all the fact sheets, research reports, in-depth discussions, and other material contained within the individual books of the *Series* remains one of our highest priorities. As the *Series* continues to grow in size and scope, however, locating the precise information needed by a reader may become more challenging.

A *Contents Guide to the Health Reference Series* was developed to direct readers to the specific volumes that address their concerns. It presents an extensive list of diseases, treatments, and other topics of general interest compiled from the Tables of Contents and major index headings. To access *A Contents Guide to the Health Reference Series*, visit www.healthreferenceseries.com.

Medical Consultant

Medical consultation services are provided to the *Health Reference Series* editors by David A. Cooke, M.D. Dr. Cooke is a graduate of Brandeis University, and he received his M.D. degree from the University of Michigan. He completed residency training at the University of Wisconsin Hospital and Clinics. He is board-certified in Internal Medicine. Dr. Cooke currently works as part of the University of Michigan Health System and practices in Brighton, MI. In his free time, he enjoys writing, science fiction, and spending time with his family.

Our Advisory Board

We would like to thank the following board members for providing guidance to the development of this *Series*:

- Dr. Lynda Baker, Associate Professor of Library and Information Science, Wayne State University, Detroit, MI

- Nancy Bulgarelli, William Beaumont Hospital Library, Royal Oak, MI

- Karen Imarisio, Bloomfield Township Public Library, Bloomfield Township, MI

- Karen Morgan, Mardigian Library, University of Michigan-Dearborn, Dearborn, MI

- Rosemary Orlando, St. Clair Shores Public Library, St. Clair Shores, MI

Health Reference Series *Update Policy*

The inaugural book in the *Health Reference Series* was the first edition of *Cancer Sourcebook* published in 1989. Since then, the *Series* has been enthusiastically received by librarians and in the medical community. In order to maintain the standard of providing high-quality health information for the layperson the editorial staff at Omnigraphics felt it was necessary to implement a policy of updating volumes when warranted.

Medical researchers have been making tremendous strides, and it is the purpose of the *Health Reference Series* to stay current with the most recent advances. Each decision to update a volume is made on an individual basis. Some of the considerations include how much new information is available and the feedback we receive from people who use the books. If there is a topic you would like to see added to the update list, or an area of medical concern you feel has not been adequately addressed, please write to:

Editor
Health Reference Series
Omnigraphics, Inc.
P.O. Box 31-1640
Detroit, MI 48231-1640
E-mail: editorial@omnigraphics.com

Part One

Introduction to Learning Disabilities

Chapter 1

Learning Disabilities: An Overview

Learning Disabilities

Noah felt like he was always hitting the books. While his friends were meeting for pickup soccer games after school, he was back home in his room reading and rereading the same material. But no matter how hard Noah studied, he had difficulty remembering things and his grades stayed average. Meanwhile, his friend Sean, who never seemed to study, always aced tests. It didn't seem fair.

Because Noah was so frustrated, his dad and teachers made an appointment with the school psychologist. She diagnosed Noah with a learning disability. Although Noah felt relieved to know what was going on, he was also worried. He didn't like the "disability" label. And he was concerned about what it might mean for his future. Would he be able to go to college and study engineering as he'd hoped?

This chapter includes text from: "Learning Disabilities," March 2007, reprinted with permission from www.kidshealth.org. Copyright © 2007 The Nemours Foundation. This information was provided by KidsHealth, one of the largest resources online for medically reviewed health information written for parents, kids, and teens. For more articles like this one, visit www.KidsHealth.org, or www.TeensHealth.org. Also included is an excerpt titled "Learning Disability Defined and Tips for Parents and Teachers," from "Learning Disabilities (Fact Sheet 7)," National Dissemination Center for Children with Disabilities (NICHCY), January 2004.

What Are Learning Disabilities?

For someone diagnosed with a learning disability, it can seem scary at first. But a learning disability doesn't have anything to do with a person's intelligence—after all, such successful people as Walt Disney, Alexander Graham Bell, and Winston Churchill all had learning disabilities.

Learning disabilities are problems that affect the brain's ability to receive, process, analyze, or store information. These problems can make it difficult for a student to learn as quickly as someone who isn't affected by learning disabilities. There are many kinds of learning disabilities. Most students affected by learning disabilities have more than one kind. Certain kinds of learning disabilities can interfere with a person's ability to concentrate or focus and can cause someone's mind to wander too much. Other learning disabilities can make it difficult for a student to read, write, spell, or solve math problems.

The way our brains process information is extremely complex—it's no wonder things can get messed up sometimes. Take the simple act of looking at a picture, for example: Our brains not only have to form the lines into an image, they also have to recognize what the image stands for, relate that image to other facts stored in our memories, and then store this new information. It's the same thing with speech—we have to recognize the words, interpret the meaning, and figure out the significance of the statement to us. Many of these activities take place in separate parts of the brain, and it's up to our minds to link them all together.

If, like Noah, you've been diagnosed with a learning disability, you're not alone. Nearly four million school-age children and teens have learning disabilities, and at least 20% of them have a type of disorder that makes it difficult to focus.

What Are the Signs of Learning Disabilities?

You can't tell by looking that a person has a learning disability, which can make learning disabilities hard to diagnose. Learning disabilities typically first show up when a person has difficulty speaking, reading, writing, figuring out a math problem, communicating with a parent, or paying attention in class. Some kids' learning disabilities are diagnosed in grade school when a parent or a teacher notices a kid can't follow directions for a game or is struggling to do work he or she should be able to do easily. But other kids develop sophisticated ways of covering up their learning issues, so learning disabilities don't show up until the teen years when schoolwork—and life—gets more complicated.

4

Most learning disabilities fall into one of two categories: verbal and nonverbal.

People with verbal learning disabilities have difficulty with words, both spoken and written. The most common and best-known verbal learning disability is dyslexia, which causes people to have trouble recognizing or processing letters and the sounds associated with them. For this reason, people with dyslexia have trouble with reading and writing tasks or assignments.

Some people with verbal learning disabilities may be able to read or write just fine but they have trouble with other aspects of language. For example, they may be able to sound out a sentence or paragraph perfectly, making them good readers, but they can't relate to the words in ways that will allow them to make sense of what they're reading (such as forming a picture of a thing or situation). And some people have trouble with the act of writing as their brains struggle to control the many things that go into it—from moving their hand to form letter shapes to remembering the correct grammar rules involved in writing down a sentence.

People with nonverbal learning disabilities may have difficulty processing what they see. They may have trouble making sense of visual details like numbers on a blackboard. Someone with a nonverbal learning disability may confuse the plus sign with the sign for division, for example. Some abstract concepts like fractions may be difficult to master for people with nonverbal learning disabilities.

A behavioral condition called attention deficit hyperactivity disorder (ADHD) is often associated with learning disabilities because people with ADHD may also have a hard time focusing enough to learn and study. Students with ADHD are often easily distracted and have trouble concentrating. They may also be excessively active or have trouble controlling their impulses.

What Causes Them?

No one's exactly sure what causes learning disabilities. But researchers do have some theories as to why they develop. They include:

- **Genetic influences:** Experts have noticed that learning disabilities tend to run in families and they think that heredity may play a role. However, researchers are still debating whether learning disabilities are, in fact, genetic, or if they show up in families because kids learn and model what their parents do.

- **Brain development:** Some experts think that learning disabilities can be traced to brain development, both before and after birth. For this reason, problems such as low birth weight, lack of oxygen, or premature birth may have something to do with learning disabilities. Young children who receive head injuries may also be at risk of developing learning disabilities.

- **Environmental impacts:** Infants and young children are susceptible to environmental toxins (poisons). For example, you may have heard how lead (which may be found in some old homes in the form of lead paint or lead water pipes) is sometimes thought to contribute to learning disabilities. Poor nutrition early in life may also lead to learning disabilities later in life.

How Do You Know If You Have a Learning Disability?

Just because you have trouble studying for a test doesn't mean you have a learning disability. There are as many learning styles as there are individuals. For example, some people learn by doing and practicing, others learn by listening (such as in class), and others prefer to read material. Some people are just naturally slower readers or learners than others, but they still perform well for their age and abilities. Sometimes, what seems to be a learning disability is simply a delay in development; the person will eventually catch up with—and perhaps even surpass—his or her peers.

But many people with learning disabilities struggle for a long time before someone realizes that there's a reason they're having so much trouble learning. For most people in their teen years, the first telltale sign of most learning disabilities occurs when they notice that there's a disconnect between how much they studied for a test and how well they performed. Or it may just be a feeling a person has that something isn't right. If you're worried, don't hesitate to share your thoughts with a parent or a teacher.

The first step in diagnosing a learning disability is ruling out vision or hearing problems. A person may then work with a psychologist or learning specialist who will use specific tests to help diagnose the disability. Often, these can help pinpoint that person's learning strengths and weaknesses in addition to revealing a particular learning disability.

Coping with a Learning Disability

Although a diagnosis of a learning disability can feel upsetting, it's actually the first step in resolving the condition. Once an expert has pinpointed a person's particular problem, he or she can then follow strategies or take medicines to help cope with the disability. And taking steps to manage the disability can often help restore a student's self-esteem and confidence.

Some students who have been diagnosed with a learning disability work with a special teacher or tutor for a few hours a week to learn special study skills, note-taking strategies, or organizational techniques that can help them compensate for their learning disability. If you've been diagnosed with a learning disability, you may need support just for the subjects that give you the most trouble. Your school may have a special classroom with a teacher who is trained to help students overcome learning problems.

Some schools develop what is called an Individualized Education Program (or IEP), which helps define a person's learning strengths and weaknesses and make a plan for the learning activities that will help the student do his or her best in school. A student's IEP might include some regular time with a tutor or in a specialized classroom for a certain subject, or the use of some special equipment to help with learning, such as books on tape or laptop computers for students who have dyslexia.

Medication is often prescribed to help students with ADHD. There are several medicines on the market today to help improve a student's attention span and ability to focus and to help control impulses and other hyperactive behavior.

There's no cure for a learning disability. And you don't outgrow it. But it's never too late to get help. Most people with learning disabilities learn to adapt to their learning differences, and they learn strategies that help them accomplish their goals and dreams.

Learning Disability Defined and Tips for Parents and Teachers

Individuals with Disabilities Education Act (IDEA) Definition of "Learning Disability"

Our nation's special education law, the Individuals with Disabilities Education Act, defines a specific learning disability as: "... a disorder in one or more of the basic psychological processes involved in understanding or in using language, spoken or written, that may manifest itself in an imperfect ability to listen, think, speak, read, write, spell, or do mathematical calculations, including conditions such as perceptual disabilities, brain injury, minimal brain dysfunction, dyslexia, and developmental aphasia."

However, learning disabilities do not include, "...learning problems that are primarily the result of visual, hearing, or motor disabilities, of mental retardation, of emotional disturbance, or of environmental, cultural, or economic disadvantage." 34 Code of Federal Regulations §300.7(c)(10)

Tips for Parents

- Learn about LD. The more you know, the more you can help yourself and your child.

- Praise your child when he or she does well. Children with LD are often very good at a variety of things. Find out what your child really enjoys doing, such as dancing, playing soccer, or working with computers. Give your child plenty of opportunities to pursue his or her strengths and talents.

- Find out the ways your child learns best. Does he or she learn by hands-on practice, looking, or listening? Help your child learn through his or her areas of strength.

- Let your child help with household chores. These can build self-confidence and concrete skills. Keep instructions simple, break down tasks into smaller steps, and reward your child's efforts with praise.

- Make homework a priority. Learn how to help your child be a success at homework.

- Pay attention to your child's mental health (and your own). Be open to counseling, which can help your child deal with frustration, feel better about himself or herself, and learn more about social skills.

- Talk to other parents whose children have learning disabilities. Parents can share practical advice and emotional support. Call NICHCY (800-695-0285) and ask how to find parent groups near you and the parent training and information (PTI) center in your state.

- Meet with school personnel and help develop an educational plan to address your child's needs. Plan what accommodations your child needs, and don't forget to talk about assistive technology.

- Establish a positive working relationship with your child's teacher. Through regular communication, exchange information about your child's progress at home and at school.

Tips for Teachers

- Learn as much as you can about the different types of learning disabilities.

- Seize the opportunity to make an enormous difference in this student's life. Find out and emphasize the student's strengths and interests. Give the student positive feedback and lots of opportunities for practice.

- Review the student's evaluation records to identify specifically where the student has trouble. Talk to specialists in your school (such as the special education teacher) about methods for teaching this student. Provide instruction and accommodations to address the student's special needs. Examples include:

  - breaking tasks into smaller steps, and giving directions verbally and in writing;

  - giving the student more time to finish schoolwork or take tests;

  - letting the student with reading problems use audiobooks;

  - letting the student with listening difficulties borrow notes from a classmate or use a tape or digital recorder; and,

  - letting the student with writing difficulties use a computer with specialized software that spell checks, grammar checks, or recognizes speech.

- Learn about the different testing modifications that can really help a student with learning disability show what he or she has learned.

- Teach organizational skills, study skills, and learning strategies. These help all students but are particularly helpful to those with a learning disability.

- Work with the students' parents to create an educational plan tailored to meet the student's needs.

- Establish a positive working relationship with the student's parents. Through regular communication, exchange information about the student's progress at school.

Chapter 2

Facts about Learning Disabilities

Chapter Contents

Section 2.1

Children with Disabilities in the Public Schools

This section includes: "LD at a Glance: A Quick Look," Copyright © 2008 by the National Center for Learning Disabilities, Inc. All rights reserved. Used with permission. Also included is additional text from "The Condition of Education 2008: Indicator 8—Children and Youth with Disabilities in Public Schools," by M. Planty, W. Hussar, T. Snyder, S. Provasnik, G. Kena, R. Dinkes, A. KewalRamani, and J. Kemp. National Center for Education Statistics, Institute of Education Sciences, U.S. Department of Education, 2008.

LD at a Glance: A Quick Look

What you should know about learning disabilities (LD):

- LDs are specific neurological disorders that affect the brain's ability to store, process, or communicate information.

- "Specific learning disability" (SLD) is the term used in the federal law for any LD.

- LDs can affect different aspects of learning and functioning—see the Table 2.1 for specific types of learning disabilities and related disorders.

- LDs can be compensated for and even overcome through alternate ways of learning, accommodations, and modifications.

- According to the U.S. Department of Education, LDs affect approximately 5% of all children enrolled in public schools.

- LDs can occur with other disorders (AD/HD, information processing disorders).

- LDs are not the same as mental retardation, autism, deafness, blindness, behavioral disorders, or laziness.

- LDs are not the result of economic disadvantage, environmental factors, or cultural differences.

The Condition of Education 2008

The Individuals with Disabilities Education Act (IDEA), first enacted in 1975, mandates that children and youth ages 3–21 with disabilities be provided a free and appropriate public school education. Data collection activities to monitor compliance with IDEA began in 1976.

Table 2.1. LD Terminology

Disability	Area of difficulty	Symptoms include trouble with	Example
Dyslexia	Processing language	Reading, writing, and spelling	Letters and words may be written or pronounced backwards
Dyscalculia	Math skills	Computation, remembering math facts, concepts of time and money	Difficulty learning to count by 2s, 3s, 4s
Dysgraphia	Written expression	Handwriting, spelling, composition	Illegible handwriting, difficulty organizing ideas
Dyspraxia	Fine motor skills	Coordination, manual dexterity	Trouble with scissors, buttons, drawing
Information Processing Disorders			
Auditory Processing Disorder	Interpreting auditory information	Language development, reading	Difficulty anticipating how a speaker will end a sentence
Visual Processing Disorder	Interpreting visual information	Reading, writing, and math	Difficulty distinguishing letters like "h" and "n"
Other Related Disorders			
Attention deficit hyperactivity disorder (AD/HD)	Concentration and focus	Over-activity, distractibility, and impulsivity	Can't sit still, loses interest quickly

The number and percentage of children and youth ages 3–21 receiving special education services increased nearly every year since the inception of IDEA until 2004–05 (see Table 2.2). However, the number and percentage declined between 2004–05 and 2006–07. In 1976–77, some 3.7 million children and youth were served under IDEA, representing five percent of all children and youth ages 3–21. By 2006–07, some 6.7 million children and youth received IDEA services, corresponding to about nine percent of all children and youth ages 3–21. Among students served under IDEA in 2006–07, about one percent were American Indian/Alaska Native, two percent were Asian/Pacific Islander, 17 percent were Hispanic, 20 percent were Black, and 59 percent were White. Since 1980–81 a larger percentage of children and youth ages 3–21 have received special education services

Table 2.2. Percentage of children and youth ages 3–21 served under the Individuals with Disabilities Education Act (IDEA) by disability: Selected years, 1976–77 through 2006–07

Disability	1976 –77	1980 –81	1990 –91	1995 –96	2000 –01	2004 –05	2005 –06	2006 –07
All disabilities	8.3	10.1	11.4	12.4	13.3	13.8	13.8	13.5
Specific learning disabilities [1]	1.8	3.6	5.2	5.8	6.1	5.7	5.6	5.4
Speech or language impairments	2.9	2.9	2.4	2.3	3.0	3.0	3.0	3.0
Mental retardation	2.2	2.0	1.3	1.3	1.3	1.2	1.1	1.1
Emotional disturbance	0.6	0.8	0.9	1.0	1.0	1.0	1.0	0.9
Hearing impairments	0.2	0.2	0.1	0.1	0.2	0.2	0.2	0.2
Orthopedic impairments	0.2	0.1	0.1	0.1	0.2	0.2	0.1	0.1
Other health impairments	0.3	0.2	0.1	0.3	0.6	1.1	1.2	1.2
Visual impairments	0.1	0.1	0.1	0.1	0.1	0.1	0.1	0.1
Multiple disabilities	—	0.2	0.2	0.2	0.3	0.3	0.3	0.3
Deaf-blindness	—	#	#	#	#	#	#	#
Autism	—	—	—	0.1	0.2	0.4	0.5	0.5
Traumatic brain injury	—	—	—	#	#	#	0.1	0.1

for specific learning disabilities than for any other disabilities. A specific learning disability is a disorder of one or more of the basic psychological processes involved in understanding or in using language, spoken or written, that may manifest itself in an imperfect ability to listen, think, speak, read, write, spell, or to do mathematical calculations. This includes conditions such as perceptual disabilities, brain injury, minimal brain dysfunction, dyslexia, and developmental aphasia. The percentage of children and youth ages 3–21 receiving special education services for a specific learning disability was three percentage points higher in 2006–07 than in 1976–77 (five percent versus two percent). In comparison, the prevalence of speech or language impairments remained fairly constant, with variations of less than one percentage point during this period.

Table 2.2. continued

Disability	1976 –77	1980 –81	1990 –91	1995 –96	2000 –01	2004 –05	2005 –06	2006 –07
Developmental delay	—	—	—	—	0.4	0.7	0.7	0.7
Preschool-age with disability [2]	t	t	0.9	1.2	t	t	t	t

— Not available.
t Not applicable.
Rounds to zero.

[1] A disorder in one or more of the basic psychological processes involved in understanding or in using language, spoken or written, that may manifest itself in an imperfect ability to listen, think, speak, read, write, spell, or to do mathematical calculations, including conditions such as perceptual disabilities, brain injury, minimal brain dysfunction, dyslexia, and developmental aphasia.

[2] Beginning in 1976, data were collected for preschool-aged children by disability type; those data are combined in this table with data for youth ages 6–21. However, the 1986 Amendments to the Education of the Handicapped Act (now known as IDEA) mandated that data not be collected by disability for students ages 3–5. Accordingly, those data are reported as a separate row for years 1990–91 through 1999–2000. Beginning in 2000–01, states were again required to report preschool children by disability.

Note: Detail may not sum to totals because of rounding. Special education services through the Individuals with Disabilities Education Act (IDEA) are available for eligible youth identified by a team of qualified professionals as having a disability that adversely affects academic performance and as in need of special education and related services. The total includes youth receiving special education services through IDEA in early education centers and elementary and secondary schools in the 50 states and the District of Columbia and in Bureau of Indian Affairs (BIA) schools through 1993–94. Beginning in 1994–95, estimates exclude BIA schools.

Source: U.S. Department of Education, Office of Special Education and Rehabilitative Services (OSERS), Office of Special Education Programs (OSEP), Data Analysis System (DANS), 1976–2006. Retrieved November 29, 2007, from https://www.ideadata.org/arc_toc8.asp#partbCC and https://www.ideadata.org/docs/PartBTrendData/B1.xls.

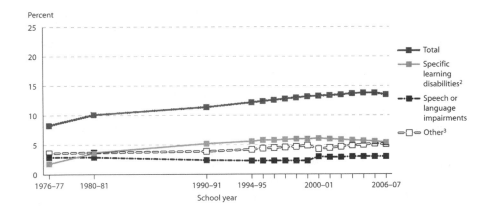

Figure 2.1. *Students with Disabilities: Percentage of children and youth ages 3–21 in early education centers or public schools receiving services under the Individuals with Disabilities Education Act (IDEA), by primary disability type: Selected years, 1976–1977 through 2006–2007.*

Section 2.2

Academic Achievement and Functional Performance of Youth with Learning Disabilities

Excerpted from "An Overview of Findings from Wave 2 of the National Longitudinal Transition Study–2 (NLTS2)," by M. Wagner, L. Newman, R. Cameto, P. Levine, and N. Garza. National Center for Special Education Research (NCSER), U.S. Department of Education, August 2006.

Academic Achievement

A considerable gap in achievement in language arts, mathematics, science, and social studies exists between youth with disabilities and their peers in the general population.

- Direct assessment results are reported as standard scores which for the general population of youth have a mean of 100 and a standard deviation of 15. In the general population, 50 percent of youth score at the mean of 100 or above and 50 percent score below. In contrast to this distribution for the general population, from 77 percent to 86 percent of youth with disabilities have standard scores below the mean across subtests.

- In the general population, about two percent of youth have standard scores that are more than two standard deviations below the mean (below 70). Among youth with disabilities represented by those who participated in the direct assessment, from 14 percent to 27 percent score more than two standard deviations below the mean across subtests.

- Youth with disabilities have the greatest difficulty with understanding what they read; the mean passage comprehension standard score of 79 is significantly lower than any of the other scores.

- Vocabulary, as measured by the use of synonyms and antonyms, appears to pose the fewest challenges, with a mean standard score of 87, significantly higher than all other scores.

- Despite the low scores overall, on each measure, some youth with disabilities have scores above the mean; across the measures, from 12–23 percent score above the mean of 100.

Factors Related to Academic Achievement

National Longitudinal Transition Study–2 (NLTS2) findings reinforce the fact that the academic achievement of youth with disabilities in reading, mathematics, science, and social studies is related to a complex array of factors that characterize youth, their households, and their school experiences. Multivariate analyses demonstrate that several individual factors differentiate youth on the basis of their academic achievement.

- The achievement of youth in several disability categories varies across the academic domains assessed. For example, youth with visual impairments outscore those with learning disabilities (the largest disability category, whose scores dominate the score for youth with disabilities as a whole) on three measures, but are similar on the other three, independent of other differences between them. Youth with hearing impairments score significantly higher than those with learning disabilities on mathematics calculation but significantly lower on science and social studies content knowledge.

- Youth in the categories of mental retardation and multiple disabilities consistently record significantly lower performance scores than youth with learning disabilities across the achievement measures.

- Independent of the nature of their disabilities, having higher functional cognitive skills relates consistently to higher academic achievement. Higher scores on the majority of subtests also are recorded for youth whose disabilities were not manifested until they were older and are reported to affect fewer functional domains.

Some demographic and household characteristics also are significantly related to academic achievement, independent of disability-related factors.

- Boys with disabilities score higher than girls with disabilities on mathematics calculation and problem-solving subtests as well as on science and social studies content knowledge subtests, with differences of three or four standard score points.

- White youth with disabilities score from 7–13 standard score points higher on all academic achievement measures than African American or Hispanic youth with disabilities or those with other racial/ethnic backgrounds.

- Youth with disabilities from low-income households ($25,000 in annual income or less) have lower average standard scores in all domains relative to youth from moderate income households, independent of racial/ethnic and other differences between them. Differences range from 3–5 standard score points.

- Given similar disability, functional, and demographic characteristics, youth with disabilities score from 4–6 standard score points higher with each successively higher level of parental expectations regarding their future enrollment in postsecondary school.

Few school experiences of youth with disabilities show statistically significant relationships with youth's academic achievement; students' grades and school mobility and having ever been retained at grade level are not significantly related to academic achievement, independent of other factors considered in the analyses. Two exceptions are:

- higher absenteeism is associated with lower scores on both mathematics subtests; and,

- having had disciplinary problems at school is associated with lower mathematics calculation scores.

In addition, using some kinds of accommodations during the assessment relates to some measures of academic performance, but not in a consistent direction.

- Controlling for other factors, using a calculator provides a 3- or 4-point advantage on the mathematics subtests.

- Using American Sign Language or a sign language interpreter and taking breaks during a session or needing multiple sessions to complete the assessment are associated with lower scores on some subtests.

Abilities of Youth Reported on the Functional Rating

Youth for whom a functional rating was completed were assessed on four clusters of functional skills (motor skills, social interaction and communication, personal living skills, and community living skills) and on an overall measure of independence.

- Average standard scores for youth with disabilities across the measures range from 43 to 57, compared with a mean of 100 for the general population.

- From 22–38 percent of youth with disabilities across subtests have scores that are more than six standard deviations below the mean.

- Across measures, from 11–15 percent of youth represented by those with a functional rating have scores above the mean for the general population.

- Youth are significantly less likely to score more than six standard deviations below the mean on personal living skills (22 percent) than on community living skills (38 percent) or the measure of broad independence (37 percent).

- The few youth with learning disabilities, speech or other health impairments, emotional disturbances, or traumatic brain injuries who have a functional rating together scored higher on the overall measure of broad independence than youth in other disability categories, with a mean of 90.

- The next highest-ranking mean score on the broad independence measure (53) was for youth with hearing impairments; it significantly surpassed the mean scores of all other categories, which ranged from 10–23.

- About two-thirds or more of youth with autism, multiple disabilities, visual or orthopedic impairments, or deaf-blindness score more than six standard deviations below the mean on the measure of broad independence.

- Only one statistically significant difference across functional performance measures is apparent in the mean standard scores of youth with disabilities who differ in gender, age, household income, or racial/ethnic background, favoring boys over girls on the motor skills measure (60 versus 42). Although there were some differences in the percentage of youth in particular standard deviation categories, no consistent patterns were apparent.

Section 2.3

Transitions: The First Few Years after High School

Excerpted from "An Overview of Findings from Wave 2 of the National Longitudinal Transition Study–2 (NLTS2)," by M. Wagner, L. Newman, R. Cameto, P. Levine, and N. Garza. National Center for Special Education Research (NCSER), U.S. Department of Education, August 2006.

Early Post-School Experiences of Youth with Disabilities

Data collected from youth and/or their parents are the source of information about the experiences of youth with disabilities in the first few years after leaving high school. Interview data are available for approximately 1,200 youth.

High School Leaving Status

By the time of the Wave–2 parent/youth interviews in 2003, 28 percent of youth with disabilities who had been in secondary school in the 2000–01 school year were no longer in high school. Although some youth had been out of high school as much as two years, the majority had been out of school from a few weeks to a little more than a year. Seventy-two percent of these 15- through 19-year-old youth had completed high school by graduating or receiving some kind of certificate of completion; 28 percent of these youth had not finished high school. The most common reasons reported for dropping out of school are dislike of school (36 percent) and poor relationships with teachers and students (17 percent).

- The vast majority of youth with visual or hearing impairments (95 percent and 90 percent) completed high school, as did more than 85 percent of out-of-school youth with autism or orthopedic impairments.

- The majority of youth with disabilities—those in the categories of learning disability, mental retardation, speech or other health impairment, or traumatic brain injury—have school completion rates of 72 percent to 79 percent.

21

- The school completion rate for youth with emotional disturbances (56 percent) is lower than the rate for all other categories, with the exception of youth with multiple disabilities or mental retardation.

- Youth with disabilities from households with annual incomes of more than $50,000 are significantly more likely to complete high school than those from households with incomes of $25,000 or less (82 percent versus 64 percent). There are no significant differences in school completion rates between youth who differ in gender or race/ethnicity.

Engagement in School, Work, or Preparation for Work

Up to two years after leaving high school, almost eight in ten out-of-school youth with disabilities have been engaged in postsecondary education, paid employment, or training to prepare them for employment. Employment is the sole mode of engagement in the community for about half of out-of-school youth with disabilities, four percent have attended postsecondary school without working or participating in job training, and about one-fifth have both gone to school and worked since leaving high school.

Postsecondary Education Participation

- About three in ten out-of-school youth with disabilities have been enrolled in some kind of postsecondary school since leaving high school, with one in five attending a postsecondary school at the time of the Wave–2 interview. This rate of current enrollment is about half that of their peers in the general population (41 percent).

- One-fifth of youth with disabilities have enrolled in two-year or community colleges since high school, and ten percent were attending such schools at the time of the interview, a participation rate similar to that of youth in the general population (12 percent).

- Since leaving high school, nine percent of youth with disabilities have attended a four-year college, with six percent doing so when interviewed. Youth in the general population are about four and one-half times as likely as youth with disabilities to be currently taking courses in four-year colleges (28 percent).

- About five percent of youth with disabilities attend post-secondary vocational, business, or technical schools within two years of leaving high school.

Multivariate analyses indicate that several youth and household characteristics and experiences are associated with a higher probability of having enrolled in two- or four-year colleges, including having a visual impairment or higher functional cognitive skills, being female, having a better educated head of household, progressing to the next grade level each year in school, and graduating from high school. Only having attention deficit disorder or attention deficit/hyperactivity disorder (ADD or AD/HD) is associated with the likelihood of enrolling in a postsecondary vocational, business, or technical school.

The experiences of postsecondary students with disabilities include the following:

- Almost three-fourths of postsecondary students with disabilities go to school full-time, and about eight in ten are enrolled steadily, rather than attending school intermittently.

- About half of postsecondary students with disabilities report that they do not consider themselves to have a disability, and another seven percent acknowledge a disability but have not informed their schools of it. Forty percent of postsecondary students with disabilities have informed their schools of their disabilities, and 35 percent receive accommodations, the large majority (88 percent) of those whose schools are aware of their disabilities.

Employment after High School

- About seven in ten out-of-school youth with disabilities have worked for pay at some time since leaving high school, and more than 40 percent were employed at the time of the Wave–2 interview. This rate is substantially below the 63 percent employment rate among same-age out-of-school youth in the general population.

- Since the Wave–1 interview, when youth were still in high school, out-of-school youth with disabilities have experienced an overall increase in the average number of hours they work per week, reaching 29 hours in Wave–2, and a nearly 20-percentage-point increase (to 40 percent) in those working full-time.

- Wages earned by out-of-school youth with disabilities increased an average of $1.30 since they were in high school two years previously, to $7.30 per hour. This results in a significant drop in the percentage of youth with disabilities working for less than minimum wage and a 25-percentage-point increase (to 41 percent) in the proportion of youth earning more than $7.00 per hour. However, receiving benefits as part of a total compensation package is not common; about one-third of out-of-school youth with disabilities receive any benefits (for example, paid vacation or sick leave, health insurance, or retirement benefits).

- Reliance on typically low-paying personal-care jobs (for example, child care), has decreased markedly among girls with disabilities—six percent of girls work in such jobs in Wave–2. At the same time, there has been an increase in jobs in the trades (for example, carpentry, plumbing) among boys—28 percent of boys hold these kinds of jobs up to two years after leaving high school.

- Eighty-four percent of working out-of-school youth report having employers who are unaware of their disabilities. Among those who report their employers are aware of their disabilities, 25 percent are receiving workplace accommodations; they constitute four percent of working youth with disabilities.

- Most working youth with disabilities have positive feelings about their employment experiences. Four in ten say they like their current job or liked their most recent job "very much," three-fourths believe their current or most recent job has put their education to good use and that they are well paid, and two-thirds believe they have opportunities for advancement. Among youth employed more than six months, about 60 percent report being promoted, taking on more responsibility, or receiving a pay increase.

Emerging Independence

- Up to two years after high school, about three-quarters of youth with disabilities still are living with their parents, a significant decline from two years earlier and a similar rate to that of the general population of youth (75 percent).

- There has been a significant increase in the proportion of age-eligible youth who have driving privileges; two-thirds can drive, whereas fewer than half could do so two years earlier.

- About 12 percent of out-of-school youth are living with a spouse or roommate outside of their parents' home in Wave–2; two-thirds of youth in this living arrangement are reported to have annual incomes of $5,000 or less.

- About one in ten out-of-school youth with disabilities participated in government benefit programs during high school, and participation has changed little during the first two post-school years.

- Personal financial management tools are being used by more youth with disabilities; about one-third have personal checking accounts, and almost one in five have a credit card or charge account in their own name, significantly more youth than two years earlier.

- Eight percent of out-of-school youth with disabilities are reported to have had or fathered a child by Wave–2, a rate of parenting similar to that for the general population (11 percent).

Leisure Activities, Social Involvement, and Citizenship

- Passive uses of leisure time, such as watching television or videos and listening to music, have declined in the two years since youth with disabilities left high school, as has communicating by computer. Whereas in Wave–1, 46 percent and 36 percent, respectively, reported these as their most common leisure activities, rates are 16 percent and 15 percent in Wave–2.

- Participation in organized community groups and in volunteer or community service activities also has declined. In Wave–2, 28 percent of out-of-school youth with disabilities belong to organized community groups, and a similar share take part in volunteer activities, down from about 46 percent pursuing each activity in Wave–1.

- In contrast, out-of-school youth with disabilities are seeing friends more often than they were two years earlier. Just over half of youth with disabilities report seeing friends at least weekly outside of organized groups and any school they may attend, an increase from about one-third of youth two years earlier.

- Almost two-thirds of youth with disabilities who are 18 or older are registered to vote, a rate similar to that for the general population of youth (approximately 60 percent).

- When they have been out of secondary school up to two years, about half of youth with disabilities have been stopped by police for other than a traffic violation, and 16 percent have spent a night in jail, both significant increases in a two-year period. Almost three in ten have been arrested at least once, and one in five are on probation or parole. These rates of arrest and being on probation or parole have not increased significantly since leaving high school, and the arrest rate is not significantly different from that of peers in the general population (23 percent).

Results Associated with Dropping-Out of School

Whether youth with disabilities complete high school is associated with a variety of differences in experiences in their early post-school years.

- Dropouts are significantly less likely to be engaged in school, work, or preparation for work shortly after high school than are those who complete school; 69 percent of dropouts have been engaged in these activities, compared with 86 percent of those who complete school.

- The form of post-school engagement undertaken by dropouts is unlikely to include postsecondary education.

- The rate of holding a paid job since high school among both dropouts and those who complete school is about 85 percent. However, dropouts with disabilities tend to work more hours per week (an average of 34 versus 27 for those who complete high school).

- Dropouts are more likely to support independent households and children than are those who complete school. More than one-fourth of dropouts with disabilities (27 percent) are living independently with a spouse or partner, compared with seven percent of those who complete school; 19 percent of dropouts are parenting, rates of independent living and parenting that are more than four times those of youth with disabilities who completed high school (3 percent).

- Dropouts are less likely than those who complete school to have a driver's license (51 percent versus 73 percent), a checking account (16 percent versus 39 percent), or to be registered to vote (48 percent versus 69 percent).

- More than one-third of dropouts with disabilities have spent a night in jail, three times the rate of youth with disabilities who finished high school. Controlling for other differences between them, dropouts are ten percentage points more likely to have been arrested than youth with disabilities who finished high school.

Disability Differences across Outcome Domains

Youth who differ in their disability category demonstrate different patterns of early post-school experiences.

Youth with Learning Disabilities or Other Health Impairments

- About three-fourths of out-of-school youth with learning disabilities or other health impairments have completed high school, almost all of those with a regular diploma.

- Among out-of-school youth with learning disabilities or other health impairments, 87 percent and 78 percent, respectively, have been engaged in school, work, or preparation for work since leaving high school, and about 45 percent were currently employed at the time of the Wave–2 interview.

- Among youth with learning disabilities or other health impairments, 27 percent and 33 percent, respectively, were expected by their parents definitely to go on to postsecondary education after high school, and 33 percent and 37 percent of the two groups have done so within two years of leaving high school. Enrollment in two-year colleges is most common (22 percent and 31 percent).

- Youth with learning disabilities or other health impairments have experienced among the broadest changes in their leisure-time and friendship pursuits, with significant reductions in passive leisure activities. For example, 45 percent and 47 percent of the two groups, respectively, indicated watching television was a primary leisure activity in Wave–1, rates that dropped by 33 and 31 percentage points in Wave–2. They also experienced increases in seeing friends at least weekly; approximately one-third of the two groups reported this frequency of seeing friends in Wave–1, whereas 56 percent of youth with learning disabilities and 47 percent of youth with other health impairments do so in Wave–2.

- Although these two groups of youth are among the most likely to be registered to vote (about 70 percent), they also have experienced 20- and 28-percentage-point declines, respectively, in participation in organized groups, from Wave–1 rates of 48 percent and 54 percent. Volunteer activities also are less common; there have been 20- and 25- percentage-point decreases from Wave–1 rates of 47 percent and 56 percent.

- Youth in these categories are second only to youth with emotional disturbances in the likelihood of being involved with the criminal justice system (for example, 50 percent and 52 percent, respectively, have been arrested), and those with other health impairments show the only significant increase in arrest rates in the two years between Wave–1 and Wave–2 (19 percentage points), reaching a rate of 35 percent.

Youth with Emotional Disturbances

- Youth with emotional disturbances are the most likely youth with disabilities to be out of secondary school at Wave–2 (36 percent), with 44 percent of those leaving school without finishing, the highest dropout rate of any disability category. Those who have emotional disturbances and complete school are also among the least likely to be reported by parents to have graduated with a regular diploma (86 percent).

- Thirty-five percent of youth with emotional disturbances no longer live with parents, the largest of any category of youth with disabilities, and they are the only group to show a significant increase in the likelihood of living in other arrangements (from less than 1–6 percent), including in criminal justice or mental health facilities, under legal guardianship, in foster care, or homeless.

- Youth in this category have experienced the largest increase in their rate of parenting; 11 percent of youth with emotional disturbances report having had or fathered a child, a 10-percentage-point increase from Wave–1.

- One-third of these youth have not found a way to become engaged in their community since leaving high school; for those who have, employment is the usual mode of engagement. Although more than six in ten youth with emotional disturbances have been employed at some time since leaving high school, only about half as many were working at the time of the Wave–2 interview.

- About one in five youth with emotional disturbances have been enrolled in any kind of postsecondary education since leaving high school.

- Youth with emotional disturbances are among the most likely to see friends often (52 percent report doing so at least weekly), yet they are among the least likely to take part in organized community groups (22 percent) or volunteer activities (20 percent) or to be registered to vote (52 percent).

- More than three-fourths have been stopped by police other than for a traffic violation, 58 percent have been arrested at least once, and 43 percent have been on probation or parole. These rates have not changed significantly since Wave–1.

Youth with Hearing or Visual Impairments

- Ninety percent or more of youth with hearing or visual impairments finish high school, virtually all reportedly with a regular diploma.

- Youth with hearing or visual impairments are more than twice as likely as youth with disabilities as a whole to have enrolled in a postsecondary school; about two-thirds have done so up to two years after high school. Further, they are the most likely to attend a four-year college or university; about four in ten have enrolled in such schools, a rate four times that of youth with disabilities as a whole.

- Unlike youth with disabilities as a whole, youth with these sensory impairments show no significant decline over time in their participation in organized community groups or volunteer activities; almost twice as many of them volunteer (47 percent of each group), compared with youth with disabilities as a whole. They are as likely to be registered to vote (64 percent and 62 percent) as any other category of youth with disabilities.

Despite these experiences being similar for youth with hearing and visual impairments, their experiences with friends and jobs differ.

- Youth with hearing impairments are significantly less likely than youth with disabilities as a whole to get together with friends frequently (32 percent versus 52 percent), a difference not observed for youth with visual impairments.

- In contrast, multivariate analyses show that, irrespective of other differences in disability, functioning, and demographics, youth with visual impairments are 21 percentage points less likely to be employed currently than youth with learning disabilities; there is no difference in the probability of employment between youth with learning disabilities and those with hearing impairments.

- More than 80 percent of youth with hearing impairments who are age-eligible have driving privileges, compared with fewer than 20 percent of youth with visual impairments.

Demographic Differences across Outcome Domains

Youth with disabilities differ in many respects other than the nature of their disability, including such characteristics as age, gender, household income, and race/ethnicity. However, these differences are not associated with strong or consistent differences across outcome domains, although there are some exceptions.

Age

Age does not have an independent relationship with the likelihood that youth with disabilities see friends often or enroll in a vocational, business, or technical school, nor are there age differences in the likelihood that youth participate in volunteer or organized community group activities. Similarly, age is not associated with the likelihood of parenting or of being involved with the criminal justice system. However, some differences are evident.

- Age is significantly associated with a 23-percentage-point higher likelihood of employment and with a 12-percentage-point higher likelihood of two- or four-year college enrollment, independent of the influences of disability, functioning, and other demographic differences between youth.

- Nineteen-year-olds have experienced the largest drop over time in the proportion living with parents (from 94–67 percent) and the largest increase in having a checking account (from 8–43 percent) or personal credit card (from 8–24 percent).

- The only significant increases in earning a driver's license or learner's permit have occurred among 18- and 19-year-olds, who are more likely than younger peers to have earned those privileges (64 percent and 78 percent, respectively versus 38 percent among 15- through 17-year-olds).

Gender

The experiences of boys and girls with disabilities up to two years after high school are similar in many, although not all respects. Similarities across genders include their school-leaving status; the likelihood of being engaged in school, work, or preparation for work since leaving high school; current employment rates; and most aspects of independence, including residential arrangements, having driving privileges, using personal financial management tools, and having had or fathered a child. Significant differences are apparent regarding other experiences, however.

- Girls with disabilities are six percentage points more likely to have been enrolled in a two- or four-year college since high school than are boys, controlling for other differences between them.

- An increase over time in seeing friends frequently has occurred only among girls with disabilities (from 24–54 percent). This differential change has eliminated the difference between genders that existed in Wave–1, when boys were found to engage more frequently than girls in this behavior (38 percent versus 24 percent).

- The significant increases in the likelihood of being stopped and questioned by police other than for a traffic violation and of spending a night in jail that is evident among youth with disabilities as a whole occurs solely among boys. A 16-percentage-point increase brings to 55 percent the rate of being stopped by police among boys, and the 21 percent of boys who had spent a night in jail is a 12-percentage-point increase over the rate in 2001. The increases result in boys being significantly more likely than girls ever to have stayed overnight in jail up to two years after high school (21 percent versus 8 percent).

- Girls with disabilities are significantly less likely than boys to be single; about one-fourth are engaged, married, or in a marriage-like relationship. Girls who are living independently are significantly more likely than boys to be supporting themselves on less than $5,000 per year (82 percent versus 59 percent).

Household Income

Youth with disabilities who come from households with different income levels have some similar early post-school experiences. Their leisure-time use and social lives have not changed differentially, nor have many aspects of their independence, including their residential arrangements or parenting status. Income level also is unrelated to the likelihood of currently being employed or ever having been arrested, irrespective of other differences between youth. Also, having a better-educated head of household outweighs income in helping explain the variation in the likelihood that youth with disabilities will enroll in two- or four-year colleges up to two years after leaving high school.

However, youth with disabilities from wealthier households are more likely to be engaged in school, work, or preparation for work; whereas 93 percent of youth with disabilities from families with incomes of more than $50,000 a year are engaged in such activities after high school, 70 percent of youth from families with household incomes of $25,000 or less a year are thus engaged. Similarly, youth with disabilities from wealthier households are more likely than peers from low-income households to have earned driving privileges (79 percent versus 52 percent) and to have a personal checking account (45 percent versus 16 percent) or a credit card (26 percent versus 11 percent).

Race/Ethnicity

There are no differences across racial/ethnic groups in the likelihood of being engaged in school, work, or preparation for work shortly after high school; enrolling in college or a vocational, business, or technical school; living independently; having active friendships; having had or fathered a child; or ever having been arrested. However, independent of other differences between them, African American youth with disabilities have a 16-percentage-point lower likelihood of current employment than White youth. Also, White youth with disabilities are more likely than African American youth to have driving privileges (78 percent versus 40 percent) and a personal checking account (40 percent versus 22 percent).

Chapter 3

Perceptions, Expectations, and Outcomes of Youth with Disabilities

The National Longitudinal Transition Study-2 (NLTS2), funded by the National Center for Special Education Research at the Institute of Education Sciences, U.S. Department of Education, was initiated in 2001 to provide a national picture of the characteristics and experiences of youth with disabilities, including their self-representations of themselves, their schooling, their personal relationships, and their hopes for the future. This report presents findings drawn from the first time data were collected directly from youth on these topics; they were ages 15 through 19 at the time (2003).

The large majority of information reported in this chapter comes from responses of youth with disabilities either to a telephone interview or to a self-administered mail survey, which contained a subset of key items from the telephone interview. This report includes only data from youth who responded for themselves. Data from the two sources were combined for the analyses presented in this report. A few additional items are from in-person interviews with youth conducted in conjunction with a direct assessment of their academic skills. When similar data are available, comparisons are made between

Text in this chapter is excerpted from the executive summary of "Perceptions and Expectations of Youth with Disabilities. A Special Topic Report from the National Longitudinal Transition Study-2 (NLTS2)," by M. Wagner, L. Newman, R. Cameto, P. Levine, and C. Marder. National Center for Special Education Research, U.S. Department of Education, NCSER 2007–3006, August 2007. The full report is available online at http://www.nlts2.org/reports/2007_08/nlts2_report_2007_08_execsum.pdf.

youth with disabilities and the same-age youth in the general population.

Youth with Disabilities' Descriptions of Themselves and Their Lives

Adolescents' self-descriptions have been found to be related to multiple social and academic outcomes. To ascertain their self-perceptions, youth with disabilities were asked questions about their views of themselves, perceptions of their disability, and feelings about their lives in general.

- Between 59 and 83 percent of youth with disabilities say that each of five positive attributes are "very much" like them—being nice, being proud of themselves, being able to handle challenges, feeling useful and important, and feeling that life is full of interesting things to do. Fifty-eight percent report that they enjoyed life in the previous week "most or all of the time."

- Similarly, about 60 percent report that in the previous week they "rarely or never" felt depressed, lonely, or disliked by others.

- Approximately three in five give themselves high marks on a broad measure of self-realization that assesses how youth perceive their strengths, limitations, and confidence in their abilities and interactions with others.

- In contrast, almost one in ten youth with disabilities do not consider themselves to be useful or important "at all," and 12 percent say they "rarely or never" feel hopeful about the future.

- Fewer than one-third of those who had received special education services when they were ages 13–16 consider themselves to have a disability or special need by the time they are 15–19 years old.

Self-Evaluations of Strengths and Competencies

To document the self-representations of the competencies of youth with disabilities, youth were asked to report in telephone interviews how well they perform in six specific domains: athletics, computer use, mechanical tasks, creative arts, performing arts, and self-advocacy. In addition, two sub-scales from the *Arc's Self-Determination Scale* related to the broad concepts of personal autonomy and psychological empowerment were administered during in-person interviews with youth.

- More than half of youth with disabilities report they are at least "pretty good" in the areas of performing arts, creative arts, mechanical tasks, computer use, and physical or athletic performance.

- A comparison of parents' and youth's perceptions indicates that, overall, parents tend to hold higher opinions of their children's strengths than youth hold of themselves.

- More than half of youth with disabilities report being able to tell peers their feelings when peers upset them, and almost two-thirds say they can get adults to listen to them and get information they need.

- Among out-of-school youth who acknowledge that they have a disability or special need, approximately one-third report often providing professionals with feedback on those services.

- Half of youth with disabilities score in the high range on the measures of personal autonomy, and more than eight in ten have high scores related to psychological empowerment.

- Receiving instruction in transition planning and youth's level of participation in the transition planning process are not associated with higher personal autonomy or psychological empowerment scores.

Views of Secondary School

Research has demonstrated that the way youth feel about school can be related to their behavior and performance in school, outside of school, and in the years after leaving school. However, little research has addressed the perceptions youth with disabilities hold of their experiences in secondary school. NLTS2 addresses this gap in the knowledge base by reporting the perceptions of youth with disabilities regarding academic challenges, interpersonal challenges, school safety, services and supports received at school, affiliation with school, and enjoyment of school.

- On virtually all measures, positive views of school predominate, and strongly negative views are held by a minority of youth with disabilities.

- The majority of youth with disabilities report not finding school particularly hard, and most report having no more than occasional problems completing homework, paying attention, or getting along with teachers or other students.

- Most find school at least "pretty safe," and most report feeling at least "pretty much" a part of their school.

- Almost half agree "a lot" that they receive the services and supports they need to succeed at school, and the majority report enjoying school at least "pretty much."

- The most negative views (for example, having daily problems at school, finding school "very hard," or not liking or feeling part of school "at all") are held by 1–11 percent of youth with disabilities across measures, with one exception—three in ten youth with disabilities report they do not become involved at school, even when they have the chance.

Personal Relationships

Personal relationships can be "protective factors" against a variety of adolescent risk behaviors. NLTS2 provides the first opportunity to examine the views reported by youth with disabilities regarding their relationships with their families and friends and with other adults, and the extent to which, despite these relationships, youth report being lonely.

- For the most part, youth with disabilities report having strong, positive relationships with their parents. Parents also are the people youth with disabilities are most likely to turn to for support.

- About half of youth with disabilities report they feel very cared about by friends, and three-fourths say they can find a friend when they need one and can make friends easily. Friends are an important source of support for four in ten youth with disabilities.

- Despite these overall positive findings, a small minority of youth with disabilities report quite negative views of their personal relationships. For example, three percent report they feel their parents care about them very little or not at all, and more than twice that percentage say they are paid attention to by their family a little.

Expectations for the Future

NLTS2 has documented the perspectives of 15- through 19-year-olds regarding their future adult roles and their academic, occupational, and independence expectations.

- Most youth expect they will graduate from high school with a regular diploma. They are less confident they will attend a postsecondary school.

- The majority of youth with disabilities expect they will get a paid job, but they are less certain that these jobs will pay enough for them to be financially self-sufficient.

- Most youth think they "definitely" or "probably" will live independently in the future. Among youth who think they will not be able to live independently without supervision, half do not expect to be able to live away from home even with supervision.

- Expectations are related, in that youth who hold high expectations in one domain tend to hold high expectations in other domains.

- Youth tend to hold higher expectations for themselves than their parents hold for them. Despite this difference, parents' and youth's expectations are related to each other in that youth who hold higher expectations for their own futures also tend to have parents who hold higher expectations for them.

Disability Category Differences

Disability category differences are apparent on many of the self-representations examined in this report. Some of the perceptions or views youth report are consistent with the fundamental nature of their disabilities.

- Youth in the other health impairment category, to which youth with attention deficit/hyperactivity disorder as a primary disability typically are assigned, are more likely than those in several other disability categories to report having daily trouble paying attention in school.

- Those with orthopedic impairments are less likely to report having strong athletic or mechanical skills than computer skills.

- Youth with autism, which typically affects the ability to establish relationships with others and engage in daily activities, are less likely than those in most other categories to be involved in activities at school; they also are among the least likely to report they make friends easily or feel cared about by friends "a lot."

- Youth with emotional and/or behavioral challenges often can have relationships in which conflict is common. Consistent with

37

this, reports of infrequently having trouble getting along with others at school and of being cared about by other adults "a lot" are less common among youth with emotional disturbances than among youth in many other categories.

- Youth with disabilities such as deaf-blindness, visual impairments, or orthopedic impairments are much more likely to report having a disability than youth with learning disabilities or speech/language impairment.

More positive perceptions and expectations are apparent for some categories of youth with disabilities and more negative ones for others. Youth with visual impairments and those with mental retardation illustrate these differences.

- Youth with visual impairments are more likely than those in several other categories to report a strong sense of being able to handle things that come their way and to report rarely or never feeling depressed. They report little trouble getting along with others at school and a strong sense of affiliation with and level of involvement there. They tend to have high self-advocacy skills, confidence in their ability to find a friend, and a strong sense of being cared about by their friends.

- In contrast, compared with youth in several other categories, those with mental retardation are less likely to report there is an adult at school who knows and cares about them. They also are less likely than most categories of youth to be active participants in organized activities at school. Reports of feeling not very or not at all useful, not able to deal well with challenges, and rarely or never enjoying life are more common among youth with mental retardation than among those in most other categories. In addition, reports of feeling hopeful about the future most or all of the time are less common among these youth.

Despite these differences, there are some dimensions on which youth express similar views, regardless of their disability category. For example, there are no statistically significant differences across categories in the percentages of youth who report enjoying life most or all of the time and identifying strongly with a statement that their lives are full of interesting things to do.

Demographic Differences

Differences among youth with disabilities who are distinguished by gender, age, household income, or race/ethnicity are not common.

- There are no differences between demographic groups in their scores on measures of personal autonomy or psychological empowerment or their feelings of competence in expressing their feelings, getting adults to listen to them, or finding information they need.

- Different demographic groups share common views of being cared about by parents, friends, and other adults, and being paid attention to by their families.

However, some differences are apparent.

- Girls are more likely than boys to report being very sensitive to others' feelings, whereas boys are more likely to report being good athletes and having strong mechanical abilities.

- Adolescent girls with disabilities are more likely than boys to say they frequently turn to friends and to siblings for support, as are White youth relative to African American youth with disabilities.

- Youth from middle-income households more frequently turn to friends for support than do those from lower-income households.

- Employed older youth are less likely than younger peers to report turning frequently to their bosses or supervisors for support.

- Older youth are less likely than younger students to participate in activities at school.

Comparisons with the General Population

The picture of youth with disabilities presented in this report is similar to that of youth in the general population on several dimensions.

- Youth with disabilities and those in the general population are about equally likely to report being cared about by parents and actively turning to them and to siblings or a boyfriend or girlfriend for support.

- The two groups also report similar levels of feeling safe at school and are about equally likely to expect to receive a regular high school diploma.

However, in several respects, youth with disabilities express somewhat more negative views, experiences, or expectations than their general-population peers.

- Youth with disabilities are more likely than youth in the general population to report having daily trouble paying attention, completing their homework, and getting along with teachers and students.

- They also are more likely to have little or no sense of affiliation with school and to report strong disagreement that they enjoy school.

- However, youth with disabilities also are more likely to strongly agree that they enjoy school.

- They are less likely than youth in general to expect to attend or complete postsecondary school.

- Regarding their relationships in general, youth with disabilities are more likely than others to report pervasive feelings of loneliness and of being disliked by others, although a minority of youth with disabilities do so.

- Nonetheless, compared with youth in the general population, those with disabilities are more likely to say they receive "a lot" of attention from their families and to report enjoying life and feeling hopeful about the future most or all of the time.

Cautions in Interpreting Findings

Readers should remember the following issues when interpreting the findings in this report:

- The analyses presented in this report are descriptive; none of the findings should be interpreted as implying causal relationship, nor should differences between disability categories be interpreted as reflecting disability differences alone, because of the confounding of disability and other demographic factors.

- The report addresses the "self-representations" of youth with disabilities—for example, how they describe themselves to others. The extent of discrepancy between the perceptions youth report holding and their "true" views is unknown. "Self-representations" as measured by NLTS2 should not be interpreted as objective assessments of abilities.

Looking Ahead

This report provides the first national picture of the self-representations and expectations of youth with disabilities, how they differ across disability categories and demographic groups, and how they compare with those of youth in the general population. NLTS2 will continue to solicit the views of youth as they age, which will provide information to examine, for instance, how later achievements mesh with expectations and how views might evolve over time.

Chapter 4

Signs of Learning Disabilities

Learning Disabilities Checklist

Most people have problems with learning and behavior from time to time. During the school years, parents and educators should be on the alert for consistent (and persistent) patterns of difficulty that children and adolescents may experience over time as they may signal an underlying learning disability (LD). While variations in the course of development are to be expected, unevenness or lags in the mastery of skills and behaviors, even with children as young as 4 or 5, should not be ignored. And because LD can co-occur with other disorders, it's important to keep careful and complete records of observations and impressions so they can be shared among parent, educators and related service providers when making important decisions about needed services and supports.

Keep in mind that LD is a term that describes a heterogeneous (mixed bag) group of disorders that impact listening, speaking, reading, writing, reasoning, math, and social skills. And remember: learning disabilities do not go away. A learning disability is not something that can be outgrown or that is "cured" by medication, therapy, or expert tutoring. So, early recognition of warning signs, well-targeted screening and assessment, effective intervention, and ongoing monitoring of progress are critical to helping individuals with LD to succeed in school, in the workplace, and in life.

The following Learning Disabilities Checklist is designed as a helpful guide and not as a tool to pinpoint specific learning disabilities. The more characteristics you check, the more likely that the individual described is at risk for (or shows signs of) learning disabilities. When filling out this form, think about the person's behavior over at least the past six months. And when you're done, don't wait to seek assistance from school personnel or other professionals.

For More Information

National Center for Learning Disabilities
381 Park Ave. S., Suite 1401
New York, NY 10016-8806
Toll-Free: 888-575-7373
Phone: 212-545-7510
Fax: 212-545-9665
Websites: http://www.ncld.org; or, http://www.GetReadytoRead.org

Table 4.1. Learning Disabilities Checklist

Domains and Behaviors

* Indicates a characteristic is more likely to apply at that stage of life.
Check all that apply.

	Preschool–Kindergarten	Grades 1–4	Grades 5–8	High School and Adult
Gross and Fine Motor Skills				
Appears awkward and clumsy, dropping, spilling, or knocking things over	*	*		
Has limited success with games and activities that demand eye-hand coordination (e.g., piano lessons, basketball, baseball)	*	*	*	
Has trouble with buttons, hooks, snaps, zippers, and trouble learning to tie shoes	*	*		
Creates art work that is immature for age	*	*		
Demonstrates poor ability to color or write "within the lines"	*	*		
Grasps pencil awkwardly, resulting in poor handwriting	*	*	*	*
Experiences difficulty using small objects or items that demand precision (e.g., Legos®, puzzle pieces, tweezers, scissors)	*	*		
Dislikes and avoids writing and drawing tasks	*	*	*	
Language				
Demonstrates early delays in learning to speak	*			

table continues on next pages

45

Table 4.1. Learning Disabilities Checklist, continued

Domains and Behaviors

* Indicates a characteristic is more likely to apply at that stage of life.
Check all that apply.

	Preschool–Kindergarten	Grades 1–4	Grades 5–8	High School and Adult
Language, continued				
Has difficulty modulating voice (e.g., too soft, too loud)	*	*	*	*
Has trouble naming people or objects	*	*		
Has difficulty staying on topic	*	*		
Inserts invented words into conversation	*	*	*	
Has difficulty re-telling what has just been said	*	*	*	
Uses vague, imprecise language and has a limited vocabulary	*	*	*	*
Demonstrates slow and halting speech, using lots of fillers (e.g., uh, um, and, you know, so)	*	*	*	*
Uses poor grammar or misuses words in conversation		*	*	*
Mispronounces words frequently	*	*	*	
Confuses words with others that sound similar		*	*	*
Inserts malapropisms (slips of the tongue) into conversation (e.g., a rolling stone gathers no moths; he was a man of great statue)		*	*	*
Has difficulty rhyming	*	*		

Table 4.1. Learning Disabilities Checklist, continued

Domains and Behaviors

* Indicates a characteristic is more likely to apply at that stage of life. Check all that apply.

	Preschool– Kindergarten	Grades 1–4	Grades 5–8	High School and Adult
Language, continued				
Has limited interest in books or stories	*	*	*	
Has difficulty understanding instructions or directions	*	*	*	*
Has trouble understanding idioms, proverbs, colloquialisms, humor, and/or puns (note: take into account regional and cultural factors)		*	*	*
Has difficulty with pragmatic skills (e.g., understands the relationship between speaker and listener, stays on topic, gauges the listeners degree of knowledge, makes inferences based on a speaker's verbal and non-verbal cues)		*	*	*
Reading				
Confuses similar-looking letters and numbers	*	*		
Has difficulty recognizing and remembering sight words		*		
Frequently loses place while reading		*	*	*

47

Table 4.1. Learning Disabilities Checklist, continued

Domains and Behaviors

* Indicates a characteristic is more likely to apply at that stage of life. Check all that apply.

	Preschool– Kindergarten	Grades 1–4	Grades 5–8	High School and Adult
Reading, continued				
Confuses similar-looking words (e.g., beard/bread)		*	*	*
Reverses letter order in words (e.g., saw/was)		*	*	
Demonstrates poor memory for printed words	*	*	*	*
Has weak comprehension of ideas and themes			*	*
Has significant trouble learning to read		*	*	*
Has trouble naming letters	*	*		
Has problems associating letter and sounds, understanding the difference between sounds in words or blending sounds into words	*	*		
Guesses at unfamiliar words rather than using word analysis skills		*	*	*
Reads slowly		*	*	*
Substitutes or leaves out words while reading		*	*	*
Has poor retention of new vocabulary	*	*	*	
Dislikes and avoids reading or reads reluctantly	*	*	*	*
Written Language				
Dislikes and avoids writing and copying	*	*	*	*

Table 4.1. Learning Disabilities Checklist, continued

Domains and Behaviors

* Indicates a characteristic is more likely to apply at that stage of life. Check all that apply.

Written Language, continued

	Preschool–Kindergarten	Grades 1–4	Grades 5–8	High School and Adult
Demonstrates delays in learning to copy and write	*	*		
Writing is messy and incomplete, with many cross outs and erasures		*	*	*
Has difficulty remembering shapes of letters and numerals	*	*		
Frequently reverses letters, numbers, and symbols	*	*		
Uses uneven spacing between letters and words, and has trouble staying "on the line"		*	*	*
Copies inaccurately (e.g., confuses similar-looking letters and numbers)		*	*	*
Spells poorly and inconsistently (e.g., the same word appears differently other places in the same document)		*	*	*
Has difficulty proofreading and self-correcting work		*	*	*
Has difficulty preparing outlines and organizing written assignments			*	*
Fails to develop ideas in writing so written work is incomplete and too brief			*	*

Table 4.1. Learning Disabilities Checklist, continued

Domains and Behaviors

* Indicates a characteristic is more likely to apply at that stage of life.
Check all that apply.

	Preschool–Kindergarten	Grades 1–4	Grades 5–8	High School and Adult
Written Language, continued				
Expresses written ideas in a disorganized way			*	*
Math				
Has difficulty with simple counting and one-to-one correspondence between number symbols and items/objects	*	*		
Difficulty mastering number knowledge (e.g., recognition of quantities without counting)		*	*	*
Has difficulty with learning and memorizing basic addition and subtraction facts		*	*	*
Has difficulty learning strategic counting principles (e.g., by 2, 5, 10, 100)		*	*	*
Poorly aligns numbers resulting in computation errors			*	*
Has difficulty estimating (e.g., quantity, value)		*	*	*
Has difficulty with comparisons (e.g., less than, greater than)		*	*	*
Has trouble telling time		*	*	*
Has trouble conceptualizing the passage of time		*	*	*

Table 4.1. Learning Disabilities Checklist, continued

Domains and Behaviors

* Indicates a characteristic is more likely to apply at that stage of life. Check all that apply.

	Preschool–Kindergarten	Grades 1–4	Grades 5–8	High School and Adult
Math, continued				
Has difficulty counting rapidly or making calculations		*	*	*
Has trouble learning multiplication tables, formulas, and rules			*	*
Has trouble interpreting graphs and charts			*	*
Social/Emotional				
Does not pick up on other people's mood/feelings (e.g., may say the wrong thing at the wrong time)		*	*	*
May not detect or respond appropriately to teasing		*	*	*
Has difficulty "joining in" and maintaining positive social status in a peer group	*	*	*	*
Has trouble knowing how to share/express feelings			*	
Has trouble "getting to the point" (e.g., gets bogged down in details in conversation)			*	*
Has difficulty with self-control when frustrated	*	*		
Has difficulty dealing with group pressure, embarrassment, and unexpected challenges		*	*	*

Table 4.1. Learning Disabilities Checklist, continued

Domains and Behaviors

* Indicates a characteristic is more likely to apply at that stage of life.
Check all that apply.

	Preschool–Kindergarten	Grades 1–4	Grades 5–8	High School and Adult
Social/Emotional, continued				
Has trouble setting realistic social goals			*	*
Has trouble evaluating personal social strengths and challenges			*	*
Is doubtful of own abilities and is prone to attribute successes to luck or outside influences rather than hard work			*	*
Attention				
Fails to pay close attention to details or makes careless mistakes in schoolwork, work, or other activities			*	*
Has difficulty sustaining attention in work tasks or play activities	*	*	*	*
Does not follow through on instructions and fails to finish schoolwork, chores, or duties in the workplace		*	*	*
Has difficulty organizing tasks and activities		*	*	*
Avoids, dislikes, or is reluctant to engage in tasks that require sustained mental effort such as homework and organizing work tasks		*	*	*

Table 4.1. Learning Disabilities Checklist, continued

Domains and Behaviors

* Indicates a characteristic is more likely to apply at that stage of life.
Check all that apply.

	Preschool–Kindergarten	Grades 1–4	Grades 5–8	High School and Adult
Attention, continued				
Loses things consistently that are necessary for tasks/activities (e.g., toys, school assignments, pencils, books, or tools)		*	*	*
Is easily distracted by outside influences		*	*	*
Is forgetful in daily/routine activities		*	*	*
Other				
Confuses left and right		*	*	*
Has a poor sense of direction; slow to learn the way around a new place; easily lost or confused in unfamiliar surroundings			*	*
Finds it hard to judge speed and distance (e.g., hard to play certain games, drive a car)			*	*
Trouble reading charts and maps			*	*
Is disorganized and poor at planning			*	*
Often loses things		*	*	*
Is slow to learn new games and master puzzles		*	*	*
Has difficulty listening and taking notes at the same time			*	*

Table 4.1. Learning Disabilities Checklist, continued

Domains and Behaviors

* Indicates a characteristic is more likely to apply at that stage of life.
Check all that apply.

	Preschool–Kindergarten	Grades 1–4	Grades 5–8	High School and Adult
Other, continued				
Performs inconsistently on tasks from one day to the next		*	*	*
Has difficulty generalizing (applying) skills from one situation to another		*	*	*

54

Chapter 5

Specific Learning Disability Defined

In education, the term learning disability is used to describe specific kinds of problems that an individual has with understanding or using spoken or written language. A student with a specific learning disability may have difficulty listening, thinking, speaking, reading, writing, spelling, or doing math problems. You may have heard of dyslexia. This is a learning disability that affects reading. Specific learning disability refers to several disorders, such as dyslexia, which affect reading or language.

Learning disabilities are not visible (like those of individuals who have physical disabilities), so they often are unrecognized. They can't be fixed or cured. But special instruction, accommodations, support services, and aids can help students lessen the effects of the learning disability by using acquired methods and strategies to compensate for the difficulties one has in learning.

Most states and many schools use the Individuals with Disabilities Education Improvement Act (IDEA 2004) (Public Law 108–446) description of specific learning disability to define learning disability when determining special education eligibility and services. The IDEA 2004 definition states:

(A) General—The term means a disorder in one or more of the basic psychological processes involved in understanding or in using language, spoken or written, that may manifest itself in

National Research Center on Learning Disabilities (2007). Who is the student with a specific learning disability? [Brochure]. Lawrence, KS.

an imperfect ability to listen, think, speak, read, write, spell, or do mathematical calculations.

(B)   Disorders included—This term includes such conditions as perceptual disabilities, brain injury, minimal brain dysfunction, dyslexia, and developmental aphasia.

(C)   Disorders not included—The term does not include learning problems that are primarily the result of visual, hearing, or motor disabilities, of mental retardation, of emotional disturbances, or of any environmental, cultural, or economic disadvantage.

This is the "official" definition of a learning disability, but interpretations of this official definition can vary among schools and even among staff members within one school. The definition of specific learning disabilities is important in that it affects who is eligible for special education services, what those services will be, and who will pay for them.

Students with specific learning disabilities may have below-average to average to above-average intelligence. However, they have problems obtaining knowledge and showing their knowledge and understanding in specific skill areas, which causes them to struggle in school and do poorly compared to their peers. Having a learning disability doesn't mean a student can't learn. It just means these students may have to learn in different ways from their peers and with specific instructional aids and by using different strategies.

Schools often base learning disability determination on the difference between a student's IQ and level of achievement in specific skill areas—for example, math calculation or word recognition. Recent research and practice now encourage schools to take a broader look at the student when determining whether the student has a specific learning disability. What is the student's attention span, thinking process, memory capabilities, or comprehension? Is English the student's primary language? Does the student make progress when provided proven instructional practices? Does the student perform the same socially and behaviorally as academically? These are but a sampling of questions that might be considered when distinguishing the student with a specific learning disability from a student who has other difficulties preventing academic success.

Because of all the considerations, the process for identifying a student with specific learning disabilities remains difficult, regardless of the method used. It is crucial to design instruction formatively with continuing collection of assessment data to determine whether the instruction is helping the student learn. With such assessment feedback, the teacher can revise the instructional program as needed to ensure strong learning outcomes.

Chapter 6

Ten Things I Wish I Had Known about Learning Disabilities: One Mother's Experience

Jane Ross, founder and Executive Director of Smart Kids with Learning Disabilities, shares the lessons that she learned the hard way.

1. Trust yourself. Although his teachers said my son was fine, I knew in my heart that something was wrong: He skipped words while reading, spelled words differently each time he wrote them, and couldn't subtract to save his soul.

2. Trust your child. I knew my child was smart. But like many children with learning disabilities, he has strengths that aren't necessarily valued in the classroom—visual, spatial, and musical abilities, good interpersonal skills, and a terrific sense of humor—while struggling with the basics of reading, writing, and arithmetic.

3. Get your child tested. Even if school administrators discourage you ("He'll be out of the classroom for hours; you can't change your mind; you don't want him to be stigmatized."), testing is critical if you suspect something is wrong. Neither you nor the school can help your child if you don't know what the problem is.

---

4. Stay calm. Don't be flummoxed by the roller-coaster-like ups and downs of your child's standardized test scores. The highs and lows reflect the uneven profile of his strengths and weaknesses; take note particularly of his strengths.

5. Become an expert. At the end of the assessment process, the professionals must provide a full explanation of what is wrong—one that makes sense to you. An accurate diagnosis helps you arm yourself with information about your child's learning issues; your knowledge is the key to getting the right help.

6. Prepare for action. Once you know what he needs in order to succeed in school, gear up to ensure he gets it. You are your child's best and most effective advocate: How well he does depends, ultimately, on you.

7. Nurture his interests. Music—something my child loved—was a life preserver. The best predictor of a child's success is not grades or aptitude scores; it's the energy and commitment he gives to activities he cares about. Help him pursue his passions, whether building with Legos®, cooking, sports, music, art, dance, or collecting bugs.

8. Give them credit. Kids with learning disabilities are neither lazy nor unmotivated: They can't do better simply by trying harder. They need specific help or interventions—accommodations and some changes in the usual classroom routines—to succeed.

9. Get real. One misconception it's time to lay to rest is that reading and doing well in school equate with intelligence. Children with learning disabilities may struggle in school, but are no less intelligent than other children: They are simply wired differently.

10. Buoy them with praise. Kids with learning disabilities are generally creative and resourceful. Many innovative thinkers—scientists, inventors, performers, and entrepreneurs—have learning disabilities. With your love and support and their own hard work, there is nothing these kids cannot achieve.

Post Script: The lessons listed here were learned during years of parenting and were first published in 2000. Jane's son Ben—through her advocacy and his own hard work—learned how to marshal and build on his significant strengths. In 2004, he earned early acceptance to college.

Part Two

The Brain and Learning Disabilities

Chapter 7

Brain Basics

The brain is the most complex part of the human body. This three-pound organ is the seat of intelligence, interpreter of the senses, initiator of body movement, and controller of behavior. Lying in its bony shell and washed by protective fluid, the brain is the source of all the qualities that define our humanity. The brain is the crown jewel of the human body.

For centuries, scientists and philosophers have been fascinated by the brain, but until recently they viewed the brain as nearly incomprehensible. Now, however, the brain is beginning to relinquish its secrets. Scientists have learned more about the brain in the last ten years than in all previous centuries because of the accelerating pace of research in neurological and behavioral science and the development of new research techniques.

This chapter is a basic introduction to the human brain. It may help you understand how the healthy brain works, how to keep it healthy, and what happens when the brain is diseased or dysfunctional.

The Architecture of the Brain

The brain is like a committee of experts. All the parts of the brain work together, but each part has its own special properties. The brain

This chapter includes text from "Brain Basics: Know Your Brain," National Institute of Neurological Disorders and Stroke (NINDS), NIH Publication No. 01–3440a, updated May 1, 2007.

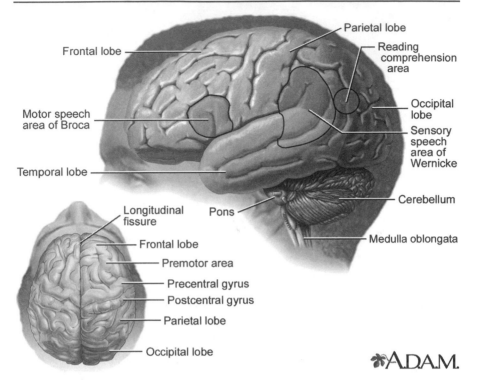

Figure 7.1. Brain (Source: "Brain: Image," © 2008 A.D.A.M., Inc. Reprinted with permission.)

can be divided into three basic units: the forebrain, the midbrain, and the hindbrain.

The hindbrain includes the upper part of the spinal cord, the brain stem, and a wrinkled ball of tissue called the cerebellum. The hindbrain controls the body's vital functions such as respiration and heart rate. The cerebellum coordinates movement and is involved in learned rote movements. When you play the piano or hit a tennis ball you are activating the cerebellum. The uppermost part of the brainstem is the midbrain, which controls some reflex actions and is part of the circuit involved in the control of eye movements and other voluntary movements. The forebrain is the largest and most highly developed part of the human brain: it consists primarily of the cerebrum and the structures hidden beneath it.

When people see pictures of the brain, it is usually the cerebrum that they notice. The cerebrum sits at the topmost part of the brain and is the source of intellectual activities. It holds your memories, allows you to plan, enables you to imagine and think. It allows you to recognize friends, read books, and play games.

The cerebrum is split into two halves (hemispheres) by a deep fissure. Despite the split, the two cerebral hemispheres communicate with each other through a thick tract of nerve fibers that lies at the base of this fissure. Although the two hemispheres seem to be mirror images of each other, they are different. For instance, the ability to form words seems to lie primarily in the left hemisphere, while the right hemisphere seems to control many abstract reasoning skills.

For some as-yet-unknown reason, nearly all of the signals from the brain to the body and vice-versa cross over on their way to and from the brain. This means that the right cerebral hemisphere primarily controls the left side of the body and the left hemisphere primarily controls the right side. When one side of the brain is damaged, the opposite side of the body is affected. For example, a stroke in the right hemisphere of the brain can leave the left arm and leg paralyzed.

The Geography of Thought

Each cerebral hemisphere can be divided into sections, or lobes, each of which specializes in different functions. To understand each lobe and its specialty we will take a tour of the cerebral hemispheres, starting with the two frontal lobes, which lie directly behind the forehead. When you plan a schedule, imagine the future, or use reasoned arguments, these two lobes do much of the work. One of the ways the frontal lobes seem to do these things is by acting as short-term storage sites, allowing one idea to be kept in mind while other ideas are considered. In the rearmost portion of each frontal lobe is a motor area which helps control voluntary movement. A nearby place on the left frontal lobe called the Broca area allows thoughts to be transformed into words.

When you enjoy a good meal—the taste, aroma, and texture of the food—two sections behind the frontal lobes called the parietal lobes are at work. The forward parts of these lobes, just behind the motor areas, are the primary sensory areas. These areas receive information about temperature, taste, touch, and movement from the rest of the body. Reading and arithmetic are also functions in the repertoire of each parietal lobe.

As you look at the words and pictures on this page, two areas at the back of the brain are at work. These lobes, called the occipital lobes, process images from the eyes and link that information with images stored in memory. Damage to the occipital lobes can cause blindness.

The last lobes on our tour of the cerebral hemispheres are the temporal lobes, which lie in front of the visual areas and nest under the parietal and frontal lobes. Whether you appreciate symphonies or rock music, your brain responds through the activity of these lobes. At the top of each temporal lobe is an area responsible for receiving information from the ears. The underside of each temporal lobe plays a crucial role in forming and retrieving memories, including those associated with music. Other parts of this lobe seem to integrate memories and sensations of taste, sound, sight, and touch.

The Cerebral Cortex

Coating the surface of the cerebrum and the cerebellum is a vital layer of tissue the thickness of a stack of two or three dimes. It is called the cortex, from the Latin word for bark. Most of the actual information processing in the brain takes place in the cerebral cortex. When people talk about "gray matter" in the brain they are talking about this thin rind. The cortex is gray because nerves in this area lack the insulation that makes most other parts of the brain appear to be white. The folds in the brain add to its surface area and therefore increase the amount of gray matter and the quantity of information that can be processed.

The Inner Brain

Deep within the brain, hidden from view, lie structures that are the gatekeepers between the spinal cord and the cerebral hemispheres. These structures not only determine our emotional state, they also modify our perceptions and responses depending on that state, and allow us to initiate movements that you make without thinking about them. Like the lobes in the cerebral hemispheres, these structures—the hypothalamus, thalamus, and hippocampus—come in pairs: each is duplicated in the opposite half of the brain.

The hypothalamus, about the size of a pearl, directs a multitude of important functions. It wakes you up in the morning, and gets the adrenaline flowing during a test or job interview. The hypothalamus is also an important emotional center, controlling the molecules that make you feel exhilarated, angry, or unhappy. Near the hypothalamus lies the thalamus, a major clearinghouse for information going to and from the spinal cord and the cerebrum.

An arching tract of nerve cells leads from the hypothalamus and the thalamus to the hippocampus. This tiny nub acts as a memory indexer—sending memories out to the appropriate part of the cerebral hemisphere for long-term storage and retrieving them when necessary. The basal ganglia are clusters of nerve cells surrounding the thalamus. They are responsible for initiating and integrating movements.

Making Connections

The brain and the rest of the nervous system are composed of many different types of cells, but the primary functional unit is a cell called the neuron. All sensations, movements, thoughts, memories, and feelings are the result of signals that pass through neurons. Neurons consist of three parts. The cell body contains the nucleus, where most of the molecules that the neuron needs to survive and function are manufactured. Dendrites extend out from the cell body like the branches of a tree and receive messages from other nerve cells. Signals then pass from the dendrites through the cell body and may travel away from the cell body down an axon to another neuron, a muscle cell, or cells in some other organ. The neuron is usually surrounded by many support cells. Some types of cells wrap around the axon to form an insulating sheath. This sheath can include a fatty molecule called myelin, which provides insulation for the axon and helps nerve signals travel faster and farther. Axons may be very short, such as those that carry signals from one cell in the cortex to another cell less than a hair's width away. Or axons may be very long, such as those that carry messages from the brain all the way down the spinal cord.

Scientists have learned a great deal about neurons by studying the synapse—the place where a signal passes from the neuron to another cell. When the signal reaches the end of the axon it stimulates tiny sacs. These sacs release chemicals known as neurotransmitters into the synapse. The neurotransmitters cross the synapse and attach to receptors on the neighboring cell. These receptors can change the properties of the receiving cell. If the receiving cell is also a neuron, the signal can continue the transmission to the next cell.

Some Key Neurotransmitters at Work

Acetylcholine is called an excitatory neurotransmitter because it generally makes cells more excitable. It governs muscle contractions and causes glands to secrete hormones. Alzheimer disease, which initially affects memory formation, is associated with a shortage of acetylcholine.

GABA (gamma-aminobutyric acid) is called an inhibitory neurotransmitter because it tends to make cells less excitable. It helps control muscle activity and is an important part of the visual system. Drugs that increase GABA levels in the brain are used to treat epileptic seizures and tremors in patients with Huntington disease.

Serotonin is an inhibitory neurotransmitter that constricts blood vessels and brings on sleep. It is also involved in temperature regulation. Dopamine is an inhibitory neurotransmitter involved in mood and the control of complex movements. The loss of dopamine activity in some portions of the brain leads to the muscular rigidity of Parkinson disease. Many medications used to treat behavioral disorders work by modifying the action of dopamine in the brain.

Chapter 8

How the Brain Learns

How the Brain Learns throughout Life

Neuroscientists have well established that the brain has a highly robust and well-developed capacity to change in response to environmental demands, a process called plasticity. This involves creating and strengthening some neuronal connections and weakening or eliminating others. The degree of modification depends on the type of learning that takes place, with long-term learning leading to more profound modification. It also depends on the period of learning, with infants experiencing extraordinary growth of new synapses. But a profound message is that plasticity is a core feature of the brain throughout life.

There are optimal or "sensitive periods" during which particular types of learning are most effective, despite this lifetime plasticity. For sensory stimuli such as speech sounds, and for certain emotional and cognitive experiences such as language exposure, there are relatively tight and early sensitive periods. Other skills, such as vocabulary acquisition, do not pass through tight sensitive periods and can be learned equally well at any time over the lifespan.

Excerpted from "Executive Summary, Understanding the Brain: The Birth of a Learning Science," © 2007 Organisation for Economic Co-operation and Development. Reprinted with permission. For additional information about this publication, visit www.oecd.org/bookshop?926029125. Note: Omnigraphics has modified the original text of this document by changing the spelling from British to American spelling norms.

Neuroimaging of adolescents now shows us that the adolescent brain is far from mature, and undergoes extensive structural changes well past puberty. Adolescence is an extremely important period in terms of emotional development partly due to a surge of hormones in the brain; the still underdeveloped prefrontal cortex among teenagers may be one explanation for their unstable behavior. We have captured this combination of emotional immaturity and high cognitive potential in the phrase "high horsepower, poor steering."

In older adults, fluency or experience with a task can reduce brain activity levels—in one sense this is greater processing efficiency. But the brain also declines the more we stop using it and with age. Studies have shown that learning can be an effective way to counteract the reduced functioning of the brain: the more there are opportunities for older and elderly people to continue learning (whether through adult education, work, or social activities), the higher the chances of deferring the onset or delaying the acceleration of neurodegenerative diseases.

The Importance of Environment

Findings from brain research indicate how nurturing is crucial to the learning process, and are beginning to provide indication of appropriate learning environments. Many of the environmental factors conducive to improved brain functioning are everyday matters—the quality of social environment and interactions, nutrition, physical exercise, and sleep—which may seem too obvious and so easily overlooked in their impact on education. By conditioning our minds and bodies correctly, it is possible to take advantage of the brain's potential for plasticity and to facilitate the learning process. This calls for holistic approaches which recognize the close interdependence of physical and intellectual well-being and the close interplay of the emotional and cognitive.

In the center of the brain is the set of structures known as the limbic system, historically called the "emotional brain." Evidence is now accumulating that our emotions do re-sculpt neural tissue. In situations of excessive stress or intense fear, social judgment and cognitive performance suffer through compromise to the neural processes of emotional regulation. Some stress is essential to meet challenges and can lead to better cognition and learning, but beyond a certain level, it has the opposite effect. Concerning positive emotions, one of the most powerful triggers that motivate people to learn is the illumination that comes with the grasp of new concepts—the brain responds very well to this. A primary goal of early education should be to ensure that children have this experience of "enlightenment" as early as possible and become aware of just how pleasurable learning can be.

Managing one's emotions is one of the key skills of being an effective learner; self-regulation is one of the most important behavioral and emotional skills that children and older people need in their social environments. Emotions direct (or disrupt) psychological processes, such as the ability to focus attention, solve problems, and support relationships. Neuroscience, drawing on cognitive psychology and child development research, starts to identify critical brain regions whose activity and development are directly related to self-control.

Language, Literacy, and the Brain

The brain is biologically primed to acquire language right from the very start of life; the process of language acquisition needs the catalyst of experience. There is an inverse relationship between age and the effectiveness of learning many aspects of language—in general, the younger the age of exposure, the more successful the learning—and neuroscience has started to identify how the brain processes language differently among young children compared with more mature people. This understanding is relevant to education policies especially regarding foreign language instruction which often does not begin until adolescence. Adolescents and adults, of course, can also learn a language anew, but it presents greater difficulties.

The dual importance in the brain of sounds (phonetics) and of the direct processing of meaning (semantics) can inform the classic debate in teaching reading between the development of specific phonetic skills, sometimes referred to as "syllabic instruction," and "whole language" text immersion. Understanding how both processes are at work argues for a balanced approach to literacy instruction that may target more phonetics or more "whole language" learning, depending on the morphology of the language concerned.

Much of the brain circuitry involved in reading is shared across languages but there are some differences, where specific aspects of a language call on distinct functions, such as different decoding or word recognition strategies. Within alphabetical languages, the main difference discussed in this report is the importance of the "depth" of a language's orthography: a "deep" language (which maps sounds onto letters with a wide range of variability) such as English or French contrasts with "shallow," much more "consistent" languages such as Finnish or Turkish. In these cases, particular brain structures get brought into play to support aspects of reading which are distinctive to these particular languages.

Dyslexia is widespread and occurs across cultural and socio-economic boundaries. Atypical cortical features which have been localized in the left hemisphere in regions to the rear of the brain are commonly associated with dyslexia, which results in impairment in processing the sound elements of language. While the linguistic consequences of these difficulties are relatively minor (for example, confusing words which sound alike), the impairment can be much more significant for literacy as mapping phonetic sounds to orthographic symbols is the crux of reading in alphabetic languages. Neuroscience is opening new avenues of identification and intervention.

Numeracy and the Brain

Numeracy, like literacy, is created in the brain through the synergy of biology and experience. Just as certain brain structures are designed through evolution for language, there are analogous structures for the quantitative sense. And, also as with language, genetically defined brain structures alone cannot support mathematics as they need to be coordinated with those supplementary neural circuits not specifically destined for this task but shaped by experience to do so. Hence, the important role of education—whether in schools, at home, or in play; and hence, the valuable role for neuroscience in helping address this educational challenge.

Although the neuroscience research on numeracy is still in its infancy, the field has already made significant progress in the past decade. It shows that even very simple numerical operations are distributed in different parts of the brain and require the coordination of multiple structures. The mere representation of numbers involves a complex circuit that brings together sense of magnitude, and visual and verbal representations. Calculation calls on other complex distributed networks, varying according to the operation in question: subtraction is critically dependent on the inferior parietal circuit, while addition and multiplication engage yet others. Research on advanced mathematics is currently sparse, but it seems that it calls on at least partially distinct circuitry.

Understanding the underlying developmental pathways to mathematics from a brain perspective can help shape the design of teaching strategies. Different instructional methods lead to the creation of neural pathways that vary in effectiveness: drill learning, for instance, develops neural pathways that are less effective than those developed through strategy learning. Support is growing from neuroscience for teaching strategies which involve learning in rich detail rather than the identification of correct or incorrect responses. This is broadly consistent with formative assessment.

Though the neural underpinnings of dyscalculia—the numerical equivalent of dyslexia—are still under-researched, the discovery of biological characteristics associated with specific mathematics impairments suggests that mathematics is far from a purely cultural construction: it requires the full functioning and integrity of specific brain structures. It is likely that the deficient neural circuitry underlying dyscalculia can be addressed through targeted intervention because of the "plasticity"—the flexibility—of the neural circuitries involved in mathematics.

Dispelling "Neuromyths"

Over the past few years, there has been a growing number of misconceptions circulating about the brain—"neuromyths." They are relevant to education as many have been developed as ideas about, or approaches to, how we learn. These misconceptions often have their origins in some element of sound science, which makes identifying and refuting them the more difficult. As they are incomplete, extrapolated beyond the evidence, or plain false, they need to be dispelled in order to prevent education running into a series of dead ends.

They are grouped as follows:

- "There is no time to lose as everything important about the brain is decided by the age of three."

- "There are critical periods when certain matters must be taught and learned."

- "But I read somewhere that we only use 10% of our brain anyway."

- "I'm a left-brain, she's a right-brain person."

- "Let's face it—men and boys just have different brains from women and girls."

- "A young child's brain can only manage to learn one language at a time."

- "Improve your memory."

- "Learn while you sleep."

Chapter 9

Neuropsychological Evaluation

Neuropsychological Evaluation Frequently Asked Questions (FAQ)

What is a neuropsychological evaluation?

A neuropsychological evaluation is a comprehensive assessment of cognitive and behavioral functions using a set of standardized tests and procedures. Various mental functions are systematically tested, including, but not limited to:

- Intelligence
- Problem solving and conceptualization
- Planning and organization
- Attention, memory, and learning
- Language
- Academic skills
- Perceptual and motor abilities
- Emotions, behavior, and personality

This chapter includes: "Neuropsychological Evaluation FAQ," and "Evaluation of Developmental Learning Disabilities and Attentional Disorders FAQ," © 2008 Ernest J. Bordini, Ph.D. and Neuropsychology Central. All rights reserved. Reprinted with permission.

Who is qualified to conduct a neuropsychological evaluation?

A neuropsychological evaluation can only be done by a licensed psychologist who has had specialized training and experience in the field, which include:

- pre-doctoral training in psychology and neuropsychology which includes an organized graduate course of study in neuropsychology;

- formal postdoctoral training focusing on brain-behavior relationships and neuropsychological assessment;

- professional board (American Board of Clinical Neuropsychology [ABCN], American Board of Professional Neuropsychology [ABPN]) recognition in the specialized techniques of neuropsychological assessment and interpretation require the listed training as well as peer-reviewed competence and examination.

When is neuropsychological evaluation needed?

A neuropsychological evaluation is recommended for any case in which brain-based impairment in cognitive function or behavior is suspected. Typical referrals are made to diagnose or rule out the following conditions, and to describe their impact on a person's cognitive functioning:

- Traumatic brain injury
- Strokes
- Developmental learning disabilities
- Attention deficit disorders
- Psychiatric or neuropsychiatric disorders
- Seizure disorders
- Medical illness or treatments
- Effects of toxic chemicals or chronic substance abuse
- Dementing conditions (for example, Alzheimer disease)

A neuropsychological evaluation is particularly useful for tracking progress in rehabilitation after brain injury or other neurological disease. Neuropsychological evaluation can assist greatly in planning educational and vocational programs. It can also be invaluable for disability determination or for forensic (legal) purposes.

Are all neuropsychological evaluations the same?

No. A neuropsychological evaluation is not a fixed series of tests which anyone can give. Specialized training allows the neuropsychologist to select, administer, and interpret the particular battery, tests, and procedures which will yield the most comprehensive understanding of an individual's strengths and weaknesses. While each neuropsychological examination is tailored to the needs of the individual client, some neuropsychologists, particularly in forensic settings rely on established batteries of tests supplemented by tests which explain or examine additional areas of function in more detail.

What is an exam like?

Generally, a neuropsychological evaluation involves a wide variety of tasks, most of which are done sitting at a table or at bedside in a hospital. There are no invasive procedures, no pain, no needles, or electrodes. The evaluation often takes six to eight hours of face-to-face contact, but can vary widely depending on what information is being sought. The evaluation can be scheduled in a single appointment or in a series of appointments.

How are the test results used?

That depends on the reason for the evaluation. Neuropsychological evaluations may:

- confirm or clarify a diagnosis;
- provide a profile of strengths and weaknesses to guide rehabilitation, educational, vocational, or other services;
- document changes in functioning since prior examinations, including effects of treatment;
- clarify what compensatory strategies would help;
- result in referrals to other specialists, such as educational therapists, cognitive rehabilitation professionals, neurologists, psychiatrists, psychologists, social workers, nurses, special education teachers, or vocational counselors.

Evaluation of Developmental Learning Disabilities and Attentional Disorders FAQ

Why choose a neuropsychologist to assess learning disability (LD)?

Neuropsychologists are specially trained to understand and evaluate the relationships between brain functioning, behavior, psychological functioning, and results of structured tests. These comprehensive evaluations include assessment of executive mental functions, such as planning, organizing, prioritizing, and monitoring one's performance. This assessment contributes to the diagnosis of subtle disabilities, and clarifies the nature of any cognitive problems underlying LD.

At what age should a neuropsychological evaluation be done?

Any age at which a problem is suspected, from preschool to adulthood.

What about attention deficit hyperactivity disorders (ADD, AD/HD) and neuropsychology?

Neuropsychological evaluation is an objective method for diagnosing attentional disorders, because it specifically measures attention and related cognitive skill deficits usually implicated in AD/HD syndromes. The evaluation usually involves an integration of medical and educational history, behavioral data, and test results. As such, it can be used to determine if there is a true neuropsychological basis for behavioral and attention difficulties. A neuropsychological evaluation also provides an opportunity to detect other problems often associated with AD/HD, such as learning disabilities.

What are some reasons for referring students to a neuropsychologist?

- To confirm a diagnosis of learning disability or attention deficit disorder.
- To understand the neuropsychological reasons for a student's learning difficulty.
- To determine if academic difficulties are due to cognitive or motivational deficits.

- To explain the declining achievement of a previously successful student.

- To assess the effectiveness of treatments.

- To obtain recommendations for how to accommodate the learning disability of attention deficit disorder.

- To identify any neurological or psychiatric factors associated with attention and learning problems.

How can neuropsychological evaluation help with work or college?

Many colleges have support programs for LD adults, and are aware of their obligation to make appropriate provisions for LD adults. Students who are properly diagnosed by qualified professionals can be eligible for accommodations such as extended time for testing and alternative examination formats. A neuropsychological examination can offer specific recommendations to employers, vocational counselors, educators, or consultants, which can help the individual adapt to the work or school setting.

For More Information

Clinical Psychology Associates of North Central Florida, P.A.
2121 N.W. 40th Terrace, Suite B
Gainesville, FL 32605
Phone: 352-336-2888
Fax: 352-371-1730
Websites: http://cpancf.com; and, http://www.ldassessment.com
E-mail: info@cpancf.com

Clinical Psychology Associates of North Central Florida, P.A. (http://cpancf.com) has more information on learning disability resources and the neuropsychological assessment of learning disability on its http://ldassessment.com website and their articles and archives page, http://www.cpancf.com/Articles_Tips_Archives.asp.

Chapter 10

Executive Function Impacts Learning

What Is Executive Function?

"Executive function" is a term used to describe a set of mental processes that helps us connect past experience with present action. We use executive function when we perform such activities as planning, organizing, strategizing, and paying attention to and remembering details.

People with executive function problems have difficulty with planning, organizing, and managing time and space. They also show weakness with "working memory" (or "seeing in your mind's eye"), which is an important tool in guiding one's actions.

As with other manifestations of learning disabilities (LD), disorders in executive function can run in families. Problems can be seen at any age but tend to be increasingly apparent as children move through the early elementary grades; the demands of completing schoolwork independently can often trigger signs that there are difficulties in this area.

How Does Executive Function Affect Learning?

In school, at home, or in the workplace, we're called on all day, every day, to self-regulate behavior. Normally, features of executive function are seen in our ability to:

- make plans;
- keep track of time;
- keep track of more than one thing at once;
- meaningfully include past knowledge in discussions;
- engage in group dynamics;
- evaluate ideas;
- reflect on our work;
- change our minds and make mid-course and corrections while thinking, reading, and writing;
- finish work on time;
- ask for help;
- wait to speak until we're called on; or
- seek more information when we need it.

These skills allow us to finish our work on time, ask for help when needed, wait to speak until we're called on and seek more information. Problems with executive function may be manifested when a person:

- has difficulty planning a project;
- has trouble comprehending how much time a project will take to complete;
- struggles to tell a story (verbally or in writing), having trouble communicating details in an organized, sequential manner;
- has difficulty with the mental strategies involved in memorization and retrieving information from memory;
- has trouble initiating activities or tasks, or generating ideas independently; or
- has difficulty retaining information while doing something with it, for example, remembering a phone number while dialing.

How Are Problems with Executive Function Identified?

There is no single test or even battery of tests that identifies all of the different features of executive function. Educators, psychologists, speech-language pathologists, and others have used measures including the *Wisconsin Card Sorting Test* (Berg, 1948), the *Category Test* (Reitan,

1979), the *Trail Making Test* (Reitan, 1979), and the *Progressive Figures and Color Form Tests* (Reitan and Wolfson, 1985) to name a few.

Careful observation and trial-teaching are invaluable in identifying, and better understanding, weaknesses in this area.

What Are Some Strategies to Help?

There are many effective strategies one can use when faced with the challenge of problems with executive function. Here are some methods to try:

General Strategies

- Take step-by-step approaches to work; rely on visual organizational aids.
- Use tools like time organizers, computers, or watches with alarms.
- Prepare visual schedules and review them several times a day.
- Ask for written directions with oral instructions whenever possible.
- Plan and structure transition times and shifts in activities.

Managing Time

- Create checklists and "to do" lists, estimating how long tasks will take.
- Break long assignments into chunks and assign time frames for completing each chunk.
- Use visual calendars at to keep track of long term assignments, due dates, chores, and activities.
- Use management software such as the Franklin Day Planner, Palm Pilot, or Lotus Organizer.
- Be sure to write the due date on top of each assignment.

Managing Space and Materials

- Organize work space.
- Minimize clutter.

- Consider having separate work areas with complete sets of supplies for different activities.

- Schedule a weekly time to clean and organize the work space.

Managing Work

- Make a checklist for getting through assignments. For example, a student's checklist could include such items as: get out pencil and paper; put name on paper; put due date on paper; read directions; and so forth.

- Meet with a teacher or supervisor on a regular basis to review work; troubleshoot problems.

The Bottom Line

The brain continues to mature and develop connections well into adulthood, and a person's executive function abilities are shaped by both physical changes in the brain and by life experiences, in the classroom and in the world at large. Early attention to developing efficient skills in this area can be very helpful, and as a rule, direct instruction, frequent reassurance, and explicit feedback are strongly recommended.

Chapter 11

Reading Instruction Changes the Brain

What the Research Shows

Psychological science can help more kids learn to read. Scientists are using new brain imaging technology to study what happens in the brain when children read. By comparing images of children who are known to have reading difficulties with those of children who are strong readers, researchers are learning more about how to help children overcome reading problems. Furthermore, using new before and after images that show what happens to children's brains after they get systematic, research-based reading instruction, the images show that the right teaching methods can actually normalize brain function and thereby improve a child's reading skills.

Reading problems, the most common of which is called dyslexia, affect nearly one out of every five children, boys and girls equally, and can continue into adulthood. In the first stage of scientific reading research, experts hypothesized that many reading problems, especially in figuring out the different sounds made by different letters (decoding), were caused by a problem in the brain and had more to do with sound than sight. Special imaging studies of the brain proved the hypothesis correct, joining other psychological studies in confirming that dyslexia—although it can make a child feel dumb and be a problem in school—does not reflect visual problems or lower intelligence.

In the next stage of research, psychologists are testing whether certain kinds of reading instruction can actually change the brain. A 2005 study of 32 children—17 who were at low risk for reading problems and 16 who were at high risk—confirmed that systematic instruction in reading can give children who might otherwise be at risk the ability to read as well as other children who are successful readers.

In that study, researchers including Panagiatos Simos, Ph.D., Andrew Papanicolaou, Ph.D., and Jack Fletcher, Ph.D., of the University of Texas Health Science Center at Houston, compared the brain activity patterns of kindergartners with either good or poor pre-reading skills and followed them into first grade. Using magnetic source imaging (MSI), the researchers showed how different parts of the brain get active when people undertake certain tasks, such as reading. MSI can track events at the level of millionths of a second—the speed of a working brain.

The images showed that children who became skilled readers by the end of first grade had, as early as kindergarten, effective brain-activation patterns for reading. Children who had a bumpier start with reading skills showed different patterns. However, 13 of the 16 children with reading difficulties responded to systematic reading instruction. After a year of teachers directly teaching them the "alphabetic principle" (how letters work together to make words), comprehension (the meaning of words), and fluency (accurately reading words aloud), the students with previous reading difficulties became average readers. What's more, the MSI images showed that their brains started to bring critical areas—areas that they hadn't used before—into the reading process during the course of first grade. This study followed another MSI study from Papanicolaou's lab that revealed that these areas of the brain did not function correctly in children who showed early signs of reading problems.

As a result, by the end of first grade, the brains of those children who began the grade with good reading skills, and the brains of those who'd been at risk for reading problems but got high-quality instruction, functioned in very similar ways. The brains of the few children who didn't respond to instruction worked a lot like those of older children with significant reading problems.

Benita Blachman, Ph.D., of Syracuse University, and her colleagues reported in 2004 that children in second and third grades with poor word-reading skills who got eight months of instruction in letter sounds and spelling while reading text (an experimental group), instead of regular remedial-reading programs (a control group), showed significantly greater gains in reading real words, non-words, and passages, in reading rate and in spelling. When re-tested a year later, they had mostly held those gains.

A 2004 study of the same students by Sally Shaywitz, M.D., and Bennett Shaywitz, M.D., of Yale University gave more evidence that reading problems come from the abnormal processing of sounds. Previous studies by these researchers showed that when kids without reading problems tried to distinguish between similar spoken syllables, speech areas in the left brain worked much harder than matching areas in the right brain (whose function is still unknown). But when children with reading problems made the same attempt, those parts of the right brain actually worked harder, going into overdrive after a brief delay. In that study of Blachman's students, the researchers also found that when students with dyslexia learned to read through the intervention, these critical left-hemisphere areas became active. That finding is helping psychologists and their medical colleagues to identify a cen tral marker of the problem that makes it so hard for people with dyslexia to process similar but different sounds, whether spoken or written. This skill, called phonological processing, is fundamental to reading.

What the Research Means

Reading research has made significant progress over the past 30 years, accelerating in the last few years as researchers who do intervention collaborate with brain-imaging researchers. Many studies over the last three decades have confirmed that reading has more to do with mentally "hearing" letter sounds and words than with seeing them, thus making it clear that children with reading problems are not lazy or unintelligent. Instead, they have specific brain-based differences in how they process information.

By using brain images to study reading, psychologists and their colleagues in medicine and education have found a biological explanation for the 2004 finding that research-based teaching can significantly improve how students with dyslexia read and spell. And in another 2004 study, they found evidence that effective instruction normalizes brain function.

The 2005 study showed that children who might otherwise have trouble learning to read can be identified and taught before their reading problems are apparent. When taught, their brains will change in as little as a year. This news is encouraging: Most kids who are at risk for reading problems can still learn to read.

How the Research Can Be Used

Research has underscored the importance of quality instruction in reading basics: phonological awareness, the alphabetic principle, orthography (the rules of spelling and writing), and comprehension. When children get started with the basics, they become engaged and read quickly enough to make reading effortless and fun. Children as young as beginning kindergarten—if not earlier—should be screened to determine their level of risk for reading difficulties, and research-based reading programs should be incorporated in the elementary-school curriculum. A child who is at risk may need more intense instruction, but the earlier the better.

Sources and Further Reading

Blachman , B. A. (1994). What we have learned from longitudinal studies of phonological processing and reading, and some... *Journal of Learning Disabilities, 27(5)*, p287.

Blachman , B. A., Fletcher, J. M., Schatschneider, C., Francis, D. J., Clonan, S. M., Shaywitz, B. A., Shaywitz, S. E. (2004). Effects of intensive reading remediation for second and third graders and a 1-year follow-up. *Journal of Educational Psychology, 96(3)*, 444–461.

Breier, J. I., Simos, P.G., Fletcher, J. M., Castillo, E. M., Zhang, W., and Papanicolaou, A.C. (2003). Abnormal activation of temporoparietal language areas during phonetic analysis in children with dyslexia. *Neuropsychology, 17(4)*, 610–621.

Foorman, B., Fletcher, J. and Francis, D. (1997). A scientific approach to reading instruction. Learning Disabilities Online. Available: http://www.ldonline.org/ld_indepth/reading/cars.html.

Shaywitz, B. A., Shaywitz, S. E., Blachman, B. A., Pugh, K. R., Fulbright, R. K., Skudlarski, P., et al. (2004). Development of left occipito-temporal systems for skilled reading in children after a phonologically based intervention. *Biological Psychiatry*, 55, 926–933.

Shaywitz, S. E. (1996, November). Dyslexia. *Scientific American*, 77–83.

Shaywitz, S. E. (2003). *Overcoming Dyslexia: A new and complete science-based program for reading problems at any level*. New York: Alfred A. Knopf.

Simos, P. G., Fletcher, J. M., Sarkari, S., Billingsley, R. L., Castillo, E. M., Pataraia, E., Francis, D. J., Denton, C., Papanicolaou, A. C. (2005). Early development of neurophysiological processes involved in normal reading and reading disability: A magnetic source imaging study. *Neuropsychology, 19(6)*.

Chapter 12

Brain Imaging and Research Findings about Learning Disabilities

Chapter Contents

Section 12.1

Diffuse Optical Imaging: An Advance in Brain Imaging

"Advance in Brain Imaging," *NIH Research Matters*,
National Institutes of Health (NIH), July 16, 2007.

Brain imaging is becoming an increasingly important tool in many research areas, including sleep, addiction, and other behaviors, and in diseases such as autism, Alzheimer disease, and Parkinson disease. Its expanding use is driving the development of new, more flexible tools. Researchers have now developed a high-performance, portable system that offers unique advantages over current brain imaging systems.

The large scanners currently in use make brain imaging difficult in many situations—for example, with patients in intensive care units, research subjects performing complex tasks, or for infants and young children who need sedation. Diffuse optical imaging (DOI) is a mobile system that uses a small, flexible imaging cap. In contrast to positron emission tomography (PET), which uses ionizing radiation, DOI uses safe, infrared light for imaging. DOI detects blood dynamics in a manner similar to functional magnetic resonance imaging (fMRI), which primarily measures levels of one form of hemoglobin, the molecule that carries oxygen in our blood. DOI can measure levels of hemoglobin both when it is carrying oxygen and when it isn't, enabling researchers to form a more complete picture of blood activity in the brain. Despite these advantages, however, DOI has been limited by its low resolution, lack of ability to measure area volumes, and the complexity of the equipment.

A research team led by Dr. Joseph Culver of the Washington University School of Medicine set out to develop a more advanced optical imaging system with improved image quality. Their work was supported in part by NIH's National Institute of Neurological Disorders and Stroke (NINDS) and National Institute of Biomedical Imaging and Bioengineering (NIBIB). In the online edition of *Proceedings of the National Academy of Sciences* on July 6, 2007, they reported the development of a high-performance, high-density diffuse optical tomography (DOT) system.

The researchers demonstrated their system by functionally mapping the adult human visual cortex. This brain region is ideal for testing new brain imaging techniques because its structure and function have already been comprehensively mapped using other methods. The results from the high-density DOT system were consistent with previous fMRI and PET mappings of the visual cortex.

The study demonstrated that high-density DOT can be a practical and powerful tool for functional brain mapping. The system is also scalable, which will allow for mapping larger brain regions. The researchers anticipate that this advance will open the path for a wide range of new studies of both developing and diseased brains.

—by Harrison Wein, Ph.D.

Section 12.2

Imaging Study Reveals Brain Function of Poor Readers Can Improve

NIH News, National Institutes of Health (NIH), April 19, 2004.

A brain imaging study has shown that, after they overcome their reading disability, the brains of formerly poor readers begin to function like the brains of good readers, showing increased activity in a part of the brain that recognizes words. The study appeared in the May 1, 2004 issue of *Biological Psychiatry* and was funded by the National Institute of Child Health and Human Development (NICHD), one of the National Institutes of Health.

"These images show that effective reading instruction not only improves reading ability, but actually changes the brain's functioning so that it can perform reading tasks more efficiently," said Duane Alexander, M.D., Director of the NICHD.

The research team was led by Bennett Shaywitz, M.D., and Sally Shaywitz, M.D., of Yale University, in New Haven, Connecticut. Other authors of the study were from Syracuse University, in Syracuse, New York; Vanderbilt University, in Nashville, Tennessee; and the NICHD.

According to Dr. Sally Shaywitz, the results show that "teaching matters and good teaching can change the brain in a way that has the potential to benefit struggling readers."

Along with testing the children's reading ability, the researchers used functional magnetic resonance imaging (fMRI), a sophisticated brain imaging technology, to observe the children's brain functioning as they read.

In all, 77 children between the ages of six and about nine and a half took part in the study. Of these, 49 had difficulty reading, and 29 children were good readers. Of the 49 poor readers, 12 received the standard instruction in reading that was available through their school systems. The remaining 37 were enrolled in an intensive reading program based on instruction in phonemic awareness and phonics.

In the study, the 37 poor readers in the intensive reading program outpaced the 12 poor readers in the standard instruction groups, making strong gains in three measures of reading skill: accuracy, fluency, and comprehension. These gains were still apparent when the children were tested again a year later. Moreover, fMRI scans showed that the brains of the 37 formerly poor readers began functioning like the brains of good readers. Specifically, the poor readers showed increased activity in an area of the brain that recognizes words instantly without first having to decipher them.

The intensive reading program the 37 children took had strong components in phonemic awareness and phonics. Phonemic awareness refers to the ability to identify the individual sounds that make up spoken words. The word "bag," for example, is made up of three such elemental units of speech, which can be represented as bbb, aaa, and ggg. The brain strings together the 40 phonemes making up the English language to produce hundreds and thousands of words. In speech, this process is unconscious and automatic.

Beginning in the 1970s, NICHD-funded researchers learned that developing a conscious awareness of the smaller sounds in words was essential to mastering the next step in learning to read, phonics. Phonics refers to the ability to match spoken phonemes to the individual letters of the alphabet that represent them. Once children master phonics, the NICHD-funded studies showed, they could make sense of words they haven't seen before, without first having to memorize them.

Further NICHD-supported research found that instruction in phonemic awareness was an essential part of a comprehensive program in reading instruction that could help most poor readers overcome their disability.

In the 1990s, the Shaywitzes had used fMRI to learn that reading ability resides in the brain's left half, or hemisphere. Within the hemisphere, three brain regions work together to control reading. In the left front of the brain, one area recognizes phonemes. Further back, another brain area "maps" phonemes to the letters that represent them. Still another brain area serves as a kind of long-term storage system. Once a word is learned, this brain region recognizes it automatically, without first having to decipher it phonetically.

Poor readers, the researchers had learned in the earlier studies, have difficulty accessing this automatic recognition center. Instead, they rely almost exclusively on the phoneme center and the mapping center. Each time poor readers see a word, they must puzzle over it, as if they were seeing it for the first time.

In the current study, the researchers discovered that as the 37 poor readers progressed through their instruction program their brains began to function more like the brains of good readers. Specifically, the brains of these children showed increased activation in the automatic recognition center.

Section 12.3

Separate Genes Influence Speed and Accuracy in Decoding Written Words

"Separate Genes Influence Speed, Accuracy in Decoding Written Words in Dyslexia," by Joel Schwartz, © 2005 University of Washington Office of News and Information. Reprinted with permission.

Researchers trying to tease out the genetic basis of dyslexia have discovered a location on chromosome 2 that may contain one or more genes that contribute to the reading disorder and make it difficult for people to rapidly pronounce pseudo words.

The team from the University of Washington, headed by medical geneticists Dr. Wendy Raskind and Ellen Wijsman and developmental psychologist Virginia Berninger, cautioned that the new findings do not mean that scientists have found "the gene" responsible for dyslexia.

"Just as with heart disease, no single gene will provide the answer to what causes dyslexia," said Raskind. "When you look at something that is inherited, there could be multiple genes, perhaps as many as a hundred, that contribute to it. And when you look at any character-istic of a person, you must consider the environmental background. There are other factors besides genes that could modify a behavior."

The study, published in the March 2005 issue of the journal *Molecular Psychiatry*, is noteworthy for two reasons. First, it points to a new location containing genes that contribute to dyslexia. Second, the gene or genes at that location are involved in speed of decoding—changing written words into spoken words without clues to their meaning—a basic and persistent component of dyslexia.

Building on previous findings by the UW team on familial patterns of accuracy and rates of decoding, the research also provides the first evidence identifying separate genetic influences on these abilities. "In other published and in-press research, we have shown that accuracy of decoding may be a bridge to reading at one stage of learning to read and rate of decoding may be a bridge at a later stage. Effective in-structional techniques for each bridge are not necessarily the same and typically require more than teaching as usual," said Berninger, who heads the UW's Learning Disabilities Center.

The UW researchers used pseudo words, or what Berninger calls "jibberwacky," which are similar to the nonsense syllables in Lewis Carroll's poem "Jabberwocky." Examples of these pseudo words are "chimwoggle," "meb" and "crong." The "jibberwacky" was used to test 108 first- through ninth-grade children diagnosed with dyslexia and their families—parents, grandparents, siblings at least 6.5 years old, aunts, and uncles. In all, 874 people were involved in the study.

Raskind and Wijsman said they used three different analytic approaches to search for genetic influences affecting how fast and accurately people could pronounce non-words. For accuracy alone, they found five different potential contributing locations on four different chromosomes. When they examined influences on speed and accuracy, they found three other locations on different chromosomes. However, the signal from chromosome 2 was the most robust, particularly when the researchers only looked at speed and not accuracy in decoding. They said evidence points to a possible combination of genes on chromosomes 2, 10, and 11 affecting speed.

The researchers focused on how dyslexics translate written words into spoken words without meaning cues because of a large body of evidence pointing to it as a hallmark deficit in dyslexia. The UW group also has published a finding that this deficit is detectable in children and adults.

Dyslexia is a complex learning disorder that affects 5–10 percent of school-age children in the United States. It typically is characterized by early difficulties in learning to name letters and associate sounds with letters. Later on, children with dyslexia have difficulty pronouncing real words and pseudo words when they are not in a sentence or do not have meaning cues. Such children can have problems with fluent reading and spelling as well.

The results of the new study provide further evidence that dyslexia has biological roots and is a learning disorder that requires specialized instruction. Earlier UW research has shown that there are chemical differences in brain function and how the brains of dyslexic and non-dyslexic children use oxygen during sound processing tasks.

That research also showed that dyslexics can be successfully treated. A set of specialized instructional approaches developed at the UW not only helped dyslexic children improve their reading skills, but also showed that their brains change in response to instruction designed for this genetic influence on learning to decode quickly. These approaches show children the regularity of decoding written English words and how to apply this regularity quickly, efficiently, and strategically. "It was not phonics as usual," said Berninger, "but could be implemented in schools so that parents do not have to seek costly treatment outside the schools."

The National Institute of Child Health and Development supported the research. Co-authors of the UW study are Robert Igo, Nicola Chapman and Mark Matsushita, medical genetics research scientists; Dr. Zoran Brkanac, acting assistant professor of psychiatry and behavioral sciences; Jennifer Thompson, former clinical coordinator; Ted Holzman, computer research consultant; and Mary Brown, undergraduate student.

Section 12.4

Medication Boosts Brain Activity in Children with Attention and Reading Disorders

National Institute of Biomedical Imaging and Bioengineering (NIBIB),
August 11, 2005.

Using a sensitive new functional magnetic resonance imaging (fMRI) technique, scientists have identified a brain region that under-functions in adolescents with attention deficit/hyperactivity disorder (AD/HD) or a reading disorder. In addition, the researchers found, a standard treatment using the drug methylphenidate causes that brain region to become more strongly activated.

AD/HD affects three to five percent of American school-aged children, with symptoms that include an inability to restrain impulsive behavior or to pay attention for long periods of time. These symptoms, often lasting into adulthood, are associated with lower achievement levels in school and at work. The signaling pathways in the brain that are involved in AD/HD have come under intensive study in recent years. But most of this research has focused on impulsivity. Inattention has been more difficult to study, partly because the neural circuitry of attention extends throughout different brain regions.

"A number of distributed systems are responsible for attention," says Dr. John Gore, director of the Institute for Imaging Science at

Vanderbilt University. Collaborator Dr. Keith Shafritz, of the Center for Brain Imaging and Analysis at Duke University, adds, "We wanted to find out what role each particular brain region plays in attentional circuitry." AD/HD offers a chance to look closely at the attention-related regions one by one.

Tracing a picture of how the brain functions when people focus or shift their attention requires a technique for detecting subtle shifts in activity patterns. With the help of a grant from the National Institute of Biomedical Imaging and Bioengineering, Drs. Gore and Shafritz developed a specialized and sensitive method of analyzing fMRI scans of the brain.

Although the use of fMRI to examine AD/HD is not new, this recent research is innovative in several respects. It is the first double-blind, placebo-controlled study to look at the effects of methylphenidate on brain activity. "This is a more stringent type of study," says Dr. Shafritz. "We didn't know and the children didn't know whether they were taking the real medication or a placebo, so their subjective opinions could not influence the results." This was also the first neuroimaging study to compare the brain activity of AD/HD subjects to that of people with another, similar disorder—in this case a reading disorder. Also, says Dr. Gore, "This is one of very few fMRI studies to look at a psychoactive drug to see what areas it affects during a particular mental task." More commonly, studies look at how a drug affects the outcome of a particular task, rather than how the results are produced.

The main goal of the study was to discover which brain regions function abnormally both in individuals with AD/HD and in individuals with a reading disorder. The two disorders often occur together. The study population comprised four groups: fifteen adolescents with AD/HD alone, eight with reading disorder alone, four with both reading disorder and AD/HD, and a control group of fourteen who had neither disorder. Except for those in the control group, each person underwent two brain scans while performing two attention-related tasks—one after receiving a dose of methylphenidate and one after receiving a placebo.

In the unmedicated portion of the experiment, the subjects with AD/HD or reading disorder had significantly less activity than the control subjects in a part of the brain known as the striatum. After they received methylphenidate, however, their activity in this brain area rose to match that of the control group, but their performance on the attention tasks did not improve. "This is a surprising finding," says Dr. Shafritz. "We had expected that an increase in activation would equal an increase in performance, but we found no correlation."

These results leave the scientists with scant answers but plenty of room for more investigation. One new question is why AD/HD and reading disorder, which affect children in two different ways, yield fMRI scans that show similar brain dysfunctions and a similar response to medication. Another topic to explore is the primary effect of methylphenidate. Does it moderate impulsivity and hyperactivity more than it bolsters attention? With Duke psychologist Dr. Jeff Epstein, Dr. Shafritz is now developing a study to look at potential differences in brain response to different drug treatments for AD/HD. He expects that study to open yet more questions. Besides support from NIBIB, the scientists received funding from the National Institute of Mental Health and the National Institute of Child Health and Human Development.

Reference

Shafritz KM, et al., The effects of methylphenidate on neural systems of attention in attention deficit hyperactivity disorder. *American Journal of Psychiatry* 161:1990–1997, 2004.

Chapter 13

Brain Matures Late in Attention Deficit/Hyperactivity Disorder (AD/HD), But Follows Normal Pattern

In youth with attention deficit/hyperactivity disorder (AD/HD), the brain matures in a normal pattern but is delayed three years in some regions, on average, compared to youth without the disorder, an imaging study by researchers at the National Institutes of Health's (NIH) National Institute of Mental Health (NIMH) has revealed. The delay in AD/HD was most prominent in regions at the front of the brain's outer mantle (cortex), important for the ability to control thinking, attention, and planning. Otherwise, both groups showed a similar back-to-front wave of brain maturation with different areas peaking in thickness at different times.

"Finding a normal pattern of cortex maturation, albeit delayed, in children with AD/HD should be reassuring to families and could help to explain why many youth eventually seem to grow out of the disorder," explained Philip Shaw, M.D., NIMH Child Psychiatry Branch, who led research team.

Previous brain imaging studies failed to detect the developmental lag because they focused on the size of the relatively large lobes of the brain. The sharp differences emerged only after a new image analysis technique allowed the researchers to pinpoint the thickening and thinning of thousands of cortex sites in hundreds of children and teens, with and without the disorder.

"If you're just looking at the lobes, you have only four measures instead of 40,000," explained Shaw. "You don't pick up the focal, regional

National Institute of Mental Health (NIMH), November 12, 2007.

changes where this delay is most marked." Among 223 youth with AD/HD, half of 40,000 cortex sites attained peak thickness at an average age of 10.5, compared to age 7.5 in a matched group of youth without the disorder.

Shaw, Judith Rapoport, M.D., of the NIMH Child Psychiatry Branch, Alan Evans, M.D., of McGill University, and colleagues reported on their magnetic resonance imaging (MRI) study during the week of November 12, 2007, in the online edition of the *Proceedings of the National Academy of Sciences.*

The researchers scanned most of the 446 participants—ranging from preschoolers to young adults—at least twice at about three-year intervals. They focused on the age when cortex thickening during childhood gives way to thinning following puberty, as unused neural connections are pruned for optimal efficiency during the teen years.

In both AD/HD and control groups, sensory processing and motor control areas at the back and top of the brain peaked in thickness earlier in childhood, while the frontal cortex areas responsible for higher-order executive control functions peaked later, during the teen years. These frontal areas support the ability to suppress inappropriate actions and thoughts, focus attention, remember things from moment to moment, work for reward, and control movement—all functions that are often disturbed in people with AD/HD.

Circuitry in the frontal and temporal (at the side of the brain) areas that integrate information from the sensory areas with the higher-order functions showed the greatest maturational delay in youth with AD/HD. For example, one of the last areas to mature, the middle of the prefrontal cortex, lagged five years in those with the disorder.

The motor cortex emerged as the only area that matured faster than normal in the youth with AD/HD, in contrast to the late-maturing frontal cortex areas that direct it. This mismatch might account for the restlessness and fidgety symptoms common among those with the disorder, the researchers suggested.

They also noted that the delayed pattern of maturation observed in AD/HD is the opposite of that seen in other developmental brain disorders like autism, in which the volume of brain structures peak at a much earlier-than-normal age.

The findings support the theory that AD/HD results from a delay in cortex maturation. In future studies, the researchers hope to find genetic underpinnings of the delay and ways of boosting processes of recovery from the disorder.

"Brain imaging is still not ready for use as a diagnostic tool in AD/HD," noted Shaw. "Although the delay in cortex development was marked, it could only be detected when a very large number of children with the disorder were included. It is not yet possible to detect such delay from the brain scans of just one individual. The diagnosis of AD/HD remains clinical, based on taking a history from the child, the family, and teachers."

Also participating in the research were: Kristen Eskstrand, Wendy Sharp, Jonathan Blumenthal, Dede Greenstein, Liv Clasen, and Jay Giedd, M.D., NIMH.

Part Three

Specific Learning Disabilities

Chapter 14

Auditory Processing Disorder

Auditory processing disorder (APD), also known as central auditory processing disorder (CAPD), is a complex problem affecting about 5% of school-aged children. These kids can't process the information they hear in the same way as others because their ears and brain don't fully coordinate. Something adversely affects the way the brain recognizes and interprets sounds, most notably the sounds composing speech.

Kids with APD often do not recognize subtle differences between sounds in words, even when the sounds are loud and clear enough to be heard. These kinds of problems typically occur in background noise, which is a natural listening environment. So kids with APD have the basic difficulty of understanding any speech signal presented under less than optimal conditions.

Detecting APD

Kids with APD are thought to hear normally because they can usually detect pure tones that are delivered one by one in a very quiet environment (such as a sound-treated room). Those who can normally detect sounds and recognize speech in ideal listening conditions are not considered to have hearing difficulties.

"Auditory Processing Disorder," November 2007, reprinted with permission from www.kidshealth.org. Copyright © 2007 The Nemours Foundation. This information was provided by KidsHealth, one of the largest resources online for medically reviewed health information written for parents, kids, and teens. For more articles like this one, visit www.KidsHealth.org, or www.TeensHealth.org.

However, the ability to detect the presence of sounds is only one part of the processing that occurs in the auditory system. So, most kids with APD do not have a loss of hearing sensitivity, but have a hearing problem in the sense that they do not process auditory information normally.

If the auditory deficits aren't identified and managed early, many of these kids will have speech and language delays and academic problems.

Symptoms of APD can range from mild to severe and can take many different forms. If you think your child might have a problem with how he or she processes sounds, consider these questions:

- Is your child easily distracted or unusually bothered by loud or sudden noises?

- Are noisy environments upsetting to your child?

- Does your child's behavior and performance improve in quieter settings?

- Does your child have difficulty following directions, whether simple or complicated?

- Does your child have reading, spelling, writing, or other speech-language difficulties?

- Is abstract information difficult for your child to comprehend?

- Are verbal (word) math problems difficult for your child?

- Is your child disorganized and forgetful?

- Are conversations hard for your child to follow?

APD is an often misunderstood problem because many of the behaviors noted above can also appear in other conditions like learning disabilities, attention deficit hyperactivity disorder (AD/HD), and even depression. Although APD is often confused with AD/HD, it is possible to have both. It is also possible to have APD and specific language impairment or learning disabilities.

Causes

The many possible causes of APD include head trauma, lead poisoning, and chronic ear infections. Sometimes the cause is unknown. Because there are many different possibilities—even combinations of causes—each child must be assessed individually.

Diagnosis

Audiologists (hearing specialists) can determine if a child has APD. Although speech-language pathologists can get an idea by interacting with the child, only audiologists can perform auditory processing testing and determine if there really is a problem.

However, some of the skills a child needs to be evaluated for auditory processing disorder don't develop until age eight or nine. Younger kids' brains just haven't matured enough to accept and process a lot of information. Therefore, many children diagnosed with APD can develop better skills with time.

Once diagnosed, kids with APD usually work with a speech therapist. The audiologist will also recommend that they return for yearly follow-up evaluations.

Problem Areas for Kids with CAPD

The five main problem areas that can affect both home and school activities in kids with APD are:

1. **Auditory Figure-Ground Problems:** This is when the child can't pay attention when there's noise in the background. Noisy, low-structured classrooms could be very frustrating.

2. **Auditory Memory Problems:** This is when the child has difficulty remembering information such as directions, lists, or study materials. It can be immediate (for example, "I can't remember it now") and/or delayed (for example, "I can't remember it when I need it for later").

3. **Auditory Discrimination Problems:** This is when the child has difficulty hearing the difference between sounds or words that are similar (coat/boat or ch/sh). This problem can affect following directions, reading, spelling, and writing skills, among others.

4. **Auditory Attention Problems:** This is when the child can't maintain focus for listening long enough to complete a task or requirement (such as listening to a lecture in school). Although health, motivation, and attitude might also affect attention, among other factors, a child with CAPD cannot (not will not) maintain attention.

5. **Auditory Cohesion Problems:** This is when higher-level listening tasks are difficult. Auditory cohesion skills—drawing inferences from conversations, understanding riddles, or comprehending verbal math problems—require heightened auditory processing and language levels. They develop best when all the other skills (levels 1 through 4) are intact.

How Can I Help My Child?

Strategies applied at home and school can alleviate some of the problem behaviors associated with APD. Because it's common for kids with CAPD to have difficulty following directions, for example, these tactics might help:

- Since most kids with APD have difficulty hearing amid noise, it's very important to reduce the background noise at home and at school.

- Have your child look at you when you're speaking.

- Use simple, expressive sentences.

- Speak at a slightly slower rate and at a mildly increased volume.

- Ask your child to repeat the directions back to you and to keep repeating them aloud (to you or to himself or herself) until the directions are completed.

- For directions that are to be completed at a later time, writing notes, wearing a watch, and maintaining a household routine also help. General organization and scheduling also can be beneficial.

It's especially important to teach your child to notice noisy environments, for example, and move to quieter places when listening is necessary.

Other strategies that might help:

- Provide your child with a quiet study place (not the kitchen table).

- Maintain a peaceful, organized lifestyle.

- Encourage good eating and sleeping habits.

- Assign regular and realistic chores, including keeping a neat room and desk.

- Build your child's self-esteem.

Be sure to keep in regular contact with school officials about your child's progress. Kids with APD aren't typically put in special education programs. Instead, teachers can make it easier for kids by altering seating plans so the child can sit in the front of the room or with the back to the window, or providing additional aids for study, like an assignment pad or a tape recorder.

One of the most important things that both parents and teachers can do is to acknowledge that CAPD is real. Symptoms and behaviors are not within the child's control. What is within the child's control is recognizing the problems associated with APD and applying the strategies recommended both at home and school.

A positive, realistic attitude and healthy self-esteem in a child with APD can work wonders. And kids with APD can go on to be just as successful as other classmates. Although some children do, however, grow up to be adults with APD, with coping strategies and by using techniques taught to them in speech therapy, they can be very successful adults.

Chapter 15

Communication Disorders

Chapter Contents

Section 15.1

The Impact of Language Difficulties

"Language Abilities and the Impact of Language Difficulties," by Matthew Cruger, Ph.D. Reprinted with permission from the New York University Child Study Center, http://www.aboutoutkids.org, © 2005. All rights reserved.

When does language start?

Think of your child when he or she was an infant and recall the way that he or she cooed, warbled, and gurgled, even before saying a first word. Your child was practicing for later communication but neither the brain nor the vocal apparatus were developed enough for the use of words to communicate his or her needs. As children grow, however, they come to recognize that sets of particular sounds, when organized in a certain way, have meaning. Children also gradually learn that words go together in many different ways and that they can communicate their ideas to other people. These language abilities develop automatically for most children because they regularly listen to and talk with members of their families.

Indeed, studies have shown that talking to young children is important, and that families differ in how much they talk to their infants. Even before children turn 12–15 months old (a milestone around which most children will utter their first words), parents may have exposed them to thousands of new words and millions of words may have been spoken in their presence. Studies of how families communicate before the age of 18 months show that children whose parents talked to them a lot had stronger skills when they began school than children whose parents had spoken to them less. For the average child, the best foundation for academic success is increased exposure to language.

What are the basic building blocks of language?

By the age of four or five, children typically have the ability to name many objects, understand straightforward communications, follow two and three step instructions, and listen to and comprehend short stories. These skills are called receptive language abilities because they involve the understanding of information spoken by others. Most children at that age also have the capacity to repeat information told to them and to express their ideas according to specific rules, called syntax, which is equivalent to the rules of grammar. These are called expressive language skills. As children develop, they demonstrate greater abilities to listen to and understand lengthier communications, they can remember and retain more verbal information, and they also add skills involved in understanding figurative communications and pragmatic language rules, like turn taking in dialogues and the methods of practical and social language use.

How much learning is based on these language skills?

Many aspects of school instruction involve language skills. For example, a teacher may deliver a brief lecture as a form of teaching, and classroom discussions often serve as an opportunity to learn new information. Children are also expected to remember what was said to them for later use. Children with receptive or expressive language difficulties will likely struggle in school because they cannot easily learn in these conditions. These children cannot always keep up with the pace of verbal instruction, they may not consistently understand the content of ideas being discussed, and they may not have strong skills for communicating what they do or do not know. As a result, they may become withdrawn in school or appear inattentive because they lose their focus when they do not understand what is being discussed. For these children, language skills need to be evaluated and, when necessary, speech and language therapy should be instituted. As language skills improve, they feel more productive in the classroom.

How do language abilities influence a child's performance in reading, math, and writing?

Some language skills play a significant role in academic development. Young children should be able to rhyme, to understand that letters stand for specific sounds, and to detect individual speech sounds called phonemes in words. They can then recognize and manipulate speech sounds. This skill, which is the foundation of learning to read, has been labeled phonological awareness or phonological decoding. As an example, when a child learns to read he must sound out each letter before he recognizes the word. Children with difficulties in phonological awareness will not consistently recognize the sounds associated with each letter and will struggle to learn to read fluently. Research studies have shown that these problems in phonological decoding are evident in almost all cases of developmental dyslexia or reading disorder. Difficulties manipulating speech sounds for the purposes of reading and writing are called language-based, but they are not the same difficulties as seen in children with receptive and expressive language difficulties; as dyslexic children often understand other people's oral communication and verbally express their ideas with ease.

What can be done to help children with language-based learning difficulties?

If you suspect your child has a learning disability, a psychoeducational evaluation is recommended in order to identify the cause and severity of his or her difficulties. The Committee for Special Education through the Board of Education in your school district can complete these assessments, or a local psychologist may be able to evaluate your child for the presence of these problems. These difficulties do not resolve by themselves as your child grows older, so if a disorder is diagnosed, specialized interventions are necessary. Early intervention is crucial so that the child does not fall further and further behind her peers.

What is the emotional impact of language difficulties or learning disorders?

Children who are diagnosed with a language-based learning disability or a language disorder can feel demoralized and defeated by their struggles. Many children with these difficulties become aware that they are not performing as well as other children and they may withdraw or avoid academic challenges. Helping these children overcome these weaknesses is imperative so that they can experience more success when approaching academic challenges.

Section 15.2

Speech and Language Impairments

Text in this section is excerpted from "Speech and Language Impairments," National Dissemination Center for Children with Disabilities (NICHCY), Fact Sheet 11, January 2004; and "Statistics on Voice, Speech, and Language," National Institute on Deafness and Other Communication Disorders (NIDCD), April 1, 2008.

Defining Speech and Language Impairments

Speech and language disorders refer to problems in communication and related areas such as oral motor function. These delays and disorders range from simple sound substitutions to the inability to understand or use language or use the oral-motor mechanism for functional speech and feeding. Some causes of speech and language disorders include hearing loss, neurological disorders, brain injury, mental retardation, drug abuse, physical impairments such as cleft lip or palate, and vocal abuse or misuse. Frequently, however, the cause is unknown.

Characteristics

A child's communication is considered delayed when the child is noticeably behind his or her peers in the acquisition of speech or language skills. Sometimes a child will have greater receptive (understanding) than expressive (speaking) language skills, but this is not always the case.

Speech disorders refer to difficulties producing speech sounds or problems with voice quality. They might be characterized by an interruption in the flow or rhythm of speech, such as stuttering, which is called disfluency. Speech disorders may be problems with the way sounds are formed, called articulation or phonological disorders, or they may be difficulties with the pitch, volume, or quality of the voice. There may be a combination of several problems. People with speech disorders have trouble using some speech sounds, which can also be a symptom of a delay. They may say "see" when they mean "ski" or they may have trouble using other sounds like "l" or "r." Listeners may have trouble understanding what someone with a speech disorder is trying to say. People with voice disorders may have trouble with the way their voices sound.

A language disorder is an impairment in the ability to understand or use words in context, both verbally and nonverbally. Some characteristics of language disorders include improper use of words and their meanings, inability to express ideas, inappropriate grammatical patterns, reduced vocabulary, and inability to follow directions. One or a combination of these characteristics may occur in children who are affected by language learning disabilities or developmental language delay. Children may hear or see a word but not be able to understand its meaning. They may have trouble getting others to understand what they are trying to communicate.

Educational Implications

Because all communication disorders carry the potential to isolate individuals from their social and educational surroundings, it is essential to find appropriate timely intervention. While many speech and language patterns can be called "baby talk" and are part of a young child's normal development, they can become problems if they are not outgrown as expected. In this way an initial delay in speech and language or an initial speech pattern can become a disorder which can cause difficulties in learning. Because of the way the brain develops, it is easier to learn language and communication skills before the age of five. When children have muscular disorders, hearing problems, or developmental delays, their acquisition of speech, language, and related skills is often affected.

Speech-language pathologists assist children who have communication disorders in various ways. They provide individual therapy for the child; consult with the child's teacher about the most effective ways to facilitate the child's communication in the class setting; and work closely with the family to develop goals and techniques for effective therapy in class and at home. The speech-language pathologist may assist vocational teachers and counselors in establishing communication goals related to the work experiences of students and suggest strategies that are effective for the important transition from school to employment and adult life.

Technology can help children whose physical conditions make communication difficult. The use of electronic communication systems allow nonspeaking people and people with severe physical disabilities to engage in the give and take of shared thought.

Vocabulary and concept growth continues during the years children are in school. Reading and writing are taught and, as students get older, the understanding and use of language becomes more complex. Communication skills are at the heart of the education experience. Speech or language therapy may continue throughout a student's school years either in the form of direct therapy or on a consultant basis.

Statistics on Voice, Speech, and Language

The functions, skills, and abilities of voice, speech, and language are related. Some dictionaries and textbooks use the terms almost interchangeably. But, for scientists and medical professionals, it is important to distinguish among them.

Head trauma can have an adverse effect on all three. Males who are between 15 and 24 years of age tend to be more vulnerable because of their high-risk lifestyles. Young children and individuals over 75 years of age are also more susceptible to head injury. Falls around the home are the leading cause of injury for infants, toddlers, and elderly people. Violent shaking of an infant or toddler is another significant cause. The leading causes for adolescents and adults are automobile and motorcycle accidents, but injuries that occur during violent crimes are also a major source. Approximately 200,000 Americans die each year from their injuries. An additional half million or more are hospitalized. About ten percent of the surviving individuals have mild to moderate problems that threaten their ability to live independently. Another 200,000 have serious problems that may require institutionalization or some other form of close supervision.

Speech

- The prevalence of speech sound disorder in young children is 8–9 percent. By the first grade, roughly five percent of children have noticeable speech disorders; the majority of these speech disorders have no known cause.

- Usually by six months of age an infant babbles or produces repetitive syllables such as "ba, ba, ba" or "da, da, da." Babbling soon turns into a type of nonsense speech called jargon that often has the tone and cadence of human speech but does not contain real words. By the end of their first year, most children have mastered the ability to say a few simple words. By 18 months of age, most children can say 8–10 words, and by age two, they are putting words together in crude sentences such as "more milk."

At ages three, four, and five a child's vocabulary rapidly increases, and he or she begins to master the rules of language.

- It is estimated that more than three million Americans stutter. Stuttering affects individuals of all ages but occurs most frequently in young children between the ages of 2–6 who are developing language. Boys are three times more likely to stutter than girls. Most children, however, outgrow their stuttering, and it is estimated that fewer than one percent of adults stutter.

- Autism is one of the most common developmental disabilities, affecting individuals of all races and ethnic and socioeconomic backgrounds. Current estimates suggest that approximately 400,000 individuals in the United States have autism. Autism is three to four times more likely to affect boys than girls and occurs in individuals of all levels of intelligence. Approximately 75 percent are of low intelligence while ten percent may demonstrate high intelligence in specific areas such as math.

Humans express thoughts, feelings, and ideas orally to one another through a series of complex movements that alter and mold the basic tone created by voice into specific, decodable sounds. Speech is produced by precisely coordinated muscle actions in the head, neck, chest, and abdomen. Speech development is a gradual process that requires years of practice. During this process, a child learns how to regulate these muscles to produce understandable speech.

However, by the first grade, roughly five percent of children have noticeable speech disorders; the majority of these speech disorders have no known cause. One category of speech disorder is fluency disorder, or stuttering, which is characterized by a disruption in the flow of speech. It includes repetitions of speech sounds, hesitations before and during speaking, and the prolonged emphasis of speech sounds. More than 15 million individuals in the world stutter, and most began stuttering at a very early age. The majority of speech sound disorders in the preschool years occur in children who are developing normally in all other areas. Speech disorders also may occur in children who have developmental disabilities.

Children with specific speech sound disorder, which has also been termed articulation disorder or phonological disorder, have clinically significant difficulties producing the speech sounds of their language expected for their age. The extent of these patterns of errors will affect the intelligibility of their speech to some degree and in some cases rendering the speech unintelligible to those unfamiliar with the child.

These estimates have focused on children in the early school years and the prevalence estimates range from two percent among the oldest children who were eight years old, to 24.6 percent among the youngest who were five years old. Much of this variability can be attributed to different diagnostic standards. The median prevalence estimate across these studies falls in the range of 8–9 percent. These studies all showed a greater rate of impairment in boys than girls with male to female ratios ranging from 1.5 to 2.4. Speech sound disorders have been shown to occur with specific language impairments (SLI), particularly among children referred for clinical services. Risk factors for speech sound disorders consist of family histories of speech sound disorder.

Language

- Between 6–8 million people in the United States have some form of language impairment.

- Research suggests that the first six months are the most crucial to a child's development of language skills. For a person to become fully competent in any language, exposure must begin as early as possible, preferably before school age.

- Anyone can acquire aphasia (a loss of the ability to use or understand language), but most people who have aphasia are in their middle to late years. Men and women are equally affected. It is estimated that approximately 80,000 individuals acquire aphasia each year. About one million persons in the United States currently have aphasia.

- More than 160 cases of Landau-Kleffner syndrome (LKS)—a childhood disorder involving loss of the ability to understand and use spoken language—have been reported from 1957 through 1990. Approximately 80 percent of children with LKS have one or more epileptic seizures that usually occur at night. Most children outgrow the seizures, and electrical brain activity on the EEG usually returns to normal by age 15.

Language is the expression of human communication through which knowledge, belief, and behavior can be experienced, explained, and shared. This sharing is based on systematic, conventionally used signs, sounds, gestures, or marks that convey understood meanings within a group or community. Recent research identifies "windows of opportunity" for acquiring language—written, spoken, or signed—that exist within the first few years of life.

121

Between 6–8 million individuals in the United States have some form of language impairment. Disorders of language affect children and adults differently. For children who do not use language normally from birth, or who acquire impaired language during childhood, language may not be fully developed or acquired. Many children who are deaf in the United States use a natural sign language known as American Sign Language (ASL). ASL shares an underlying organization with spoken language and has its own syntax and grammar. Many adults acquire disorders of language because of stroke, head injury, dementia, or brain tumors. Language disorders also are found in adults who have failed to develop normal language skills because of mental retardation, autism, hearing impairment, or other congenital or acquired disorders of brain development.

Primary or specific language impairments (SLI) are diagnosed in children who have clinically significant impairments in their development of spoken language in the absence of sensory or neurodevelopmental disorders. Spoken language in this case includes the ability to understand words, sentences, and connected speech, as well as the ability to express messages using appropriate vocabulary, grammar, and discourse. Standards for the diagnosis of SLI vary; and therefore, prevalence estimates across studies vary accordingly. Variation in prevalence also appears to be affected by a pattern of recovery for many children during the early preschool years. Much greater stability over age is seen in children during the school years.

The typical range of prevalence estimates of SLI during the preschool and early school years was between 2% and 8% with an overall median prevalence of 5.95%. Most studies reported a greater prevalence of SLI in boys than girls. The male to female sex ratios varied from .98:1 to 2.30:1. Risk factors for SLI have been found to concentrate on family factors. Limited parental education, and parental history of speech, language, or learning problems have been found to be associated with elevated rates of SLI. In contrast, breast feeding has been shown to serve as a protective factor even in the context of parental education. Reading impairments have been widely shown to be strongly associated with SLI.

Section 15.3

Apraxia of Speech

National Institute on Deafness and Other Communication
Disorders (NIDCD), updated January 10, 2008.

What is apraxia of speech?

Apraxia of speech, also known as verbal apraxia or dyspraxia, is a speech disorder in which a person has trouble saying what he or she wants to say correctly and consistently. It is not due to weakness or paralysis of the speech muscles (the muscles of the face, tongue, and lips). The severity of apraxia of speech can range from mild to severe.

What are the types and causes of apraxia?

There are two main types of speech apraxia: acquired apraxia of speech and developmental apraxia of speech. Acquired apraxia of speech can affect a person at any age, although it most typically occurs in adults. It is caused by damage to the parts of the brain that are involved in speaking, and involves the loss or impairment of existing speech abilities. The disorder may result from a stroke, head injury, tumor, or other illness affecting the brain. Acquired apraxia of speech may occur together with muscle weakness affecting speech production (dysarthria) or language difficulties caused by damage to the nervous system (aphasia).

Developmental apraxia of speech (DAS) occurs in children and is present from birth. It appears to affect more boys than girls. This speech disorder goes by several other names, including developmental verbal apraxia, developmental verbal dyspraxia, articulatory apraxia, and childhood apraxia of speech. DAS is different from what is known as a developmental delay of speech, in which a child follows the "typical" path of speech development but does so more slowly than normal.

The cause or causes of DAS are not yet known. Some scientists believe that DAS is a disorder related to a child's overall language development. Others believe it is a neurological disorder that affects the brain's ability to send the proper signals to move the muscles involved in speech. However, brain imaging and other studies have not found evidence of specific brain lesions or differences in brain structure in children with DAS. Children with DAS often have family members who have a history of communication disorders or learning disabilities. This observation and recent research findings suggest that genetic factors may play a role in the disorder.

What are the symptoms?

People with either form of apraxia of speech may have a number of different speech characteristics, or symptoms. One of the most notable symptoms is difficulty putting sounds and syllables together in the correct order to form words. Longer or more complex words are usually harder to say than shorter or simpler words. People with apraxia of speech also tend to make inconsistent mistakes when speaking. For example, they may say a difficult word correctly but then have trouble repeating it, or they may be able to say a particular sound one day and have trouble with the same sound the next day. People with apraxia of speech often appear to be groping for the right sound or word, and may try saying a word several times before they say it correctly. Another common characteristic of apraxia of speech is the incorrect use of "prosody"—that is, the varying rhythms, stresses, and inflections of speech that are used to help express meaning.

Children with developmental apraxia of speech generally can understand language much better than they are able to use language to express themselves. Some children with the disorder may also have other problems. These can include other speech problems, such as dysarthria; language problems such as poor vocabulary, incorrect grammar, and difficulty in clearly organizing spoken information; problems with reading, writing, spelling, or math; coordination or "motor-skill" problems; and chewing and swallowing difficulties.

The severity of both acquired and developmental apraxia of speech varies from person to person. Apraxia can be so mild that a person has trouble with very few speech sounds or only has occasional problems pronouncing words with many syllables. In the most severe cases, a person may not be able to communicate effectively with speech, and may need the help of alternative or additional communication methods.

How is it diagnosed?

Professionals known as speech-language pathologists play a key role in diagnosing and treating apraxia of speech. There is no single factor or test that can be used to diagnose apraxia. In addition, speech-language experts do not agree about which specific symptoms are part of developmental apraxia. The person making the diagnosis generally looks for the presence of some, or many, of a group of symptoms, including those described previously. Ruling out other contributing factors, such as muscle weakness or language-comprehension problems, can also help with the diagnosis.

To diagnose developmental apraxia of speech, parents and professionals may need to observe a child's speech over a period of time. In formal testing for both acquired and developmental apraxia, the speech-language pathologist may ask the person to perform speech tasks such as repeating a particular word several times or repeating a list of words of increasing length (for example, love, loving, lovingly). For acquired apraxia of speech, a speech-language pathologist may also examine a person's ability to converse, read, write, and perform non-speech movements. Brain-imaging tests such as magnetic resonance imaging (MRI) may also be used to help distinguish acquired apraxia of speech from other communication disorders in people who have experienced brain damage.

How is it treated?

In some cases, people with acquired apraxia of speech recover some or all of their speech abilities on their own. This is called spontaneous recovery. Children with developmental apraxia of speech will not outgrow the problem on their own. Speech-language therapy is often helpful for these children and for people with acquired apraxia who do not spontaneously recover all of their speech abilities.

Speech-language pathologists use different approaches to treat apraxia of speech, and no single approach has been proven to be the most effective. Therapy is tailored to the individual and is designed to treat other speech or language problems that may occur together with apraxia. Each person responds differently to therapy, and some people will make more progress than others. People with apraxia of speech usually need frequent and intensive one-on-one therapy. Support and encouragement from family members and friends are also important.

In severe cases, people with acquired or developmental apraxia of speech may need to use other ways to express themselves. These might include formal or informal sign language, a language notebook with pictures or written words that the person can show to other people, or an electronic communication device such as a portable computer that writes and produces speech.

What research is being done?

Researchers are searching for the causes of developmental apraxia of speech, including the possible role of abnormalities in the brain or other parts of the nervous system. They are also looking for genetic factors that may play a role in DAS. Other research on DAS is aimed at identifying more specific criteria and new techniques that can be used to diagnose the disorder and distinguish it from other communication disorders. Research on acquired apraxia of speech includes studies to pinpoint the specific areas of the brain that are involved in the disorder. In addition, researchers are studying the effectiveness of various treatment approaches for acquired and developmental apraxia of speech.

Chapter 16

Dyscalculia: Math Learning Disability

What Is Dyscalculia?

Dyscalculia is a term referring to a wide range of lifelong learning disabilities involving math. There is no single form of math disability, and difficulties vary from person to person and affect people differently in school and throughout life.

What Are the Effects of Dyscalculia?

Since disabilities involving math can be so different, the effects they have on a person's development can be just as different. For instance, a person who has trouble processing language will face different challenges in math than a person who has difficulty with visual-spatial relationships. Another person with trouble remembering facts and keeping a sequence of steps in order will have yet a different set of math-related challenges to overcome.

Early Childhood

Building a solid foundation in math involves many different skills. Young children with learning disabilities can have difficulty learning the meaning of numbers (number sense), trouble with tasks like sorting objects by shape, size or color; recognizing groups and patterns;

---

and comparing and contrasting using concepts like smaller or bigger or taller or shorter. Learning to count, recognizing numbers, and matching numbers with amounts can also be difficult for these children.

School-Age Children

As math learning continues, school-age children with language processing disabilities may have difficulty solving basic math problems using addition, subtraction, multiplication, and division. They struggle to remember and retain basic math facts (for example, times tables), and have trouble figuring out how to apply their knowledge and skills to solve math problems.

Difficulties may also arise because of weakness in visual-spatial skills, where a person may understand the needed math facts, but have difficulty putting them down on paper in an organized way. Visual-spatial difficulties can also make understanding what is written on a board, or in a textbook, challenging.

Teenagers and Adults

If basic math facts are not mastered, many teenagers and adults with dyscalculia may have difficulty moving on to more advanced math applications. Language processing disabilities can make it hard for a person to get a grasp of the vocabulary of math. Without the proper vocabulary and a clear understanding of what the words represent, it is difficult to build on math knowledge.

Success in more advanced math procedures requires that a person be able to follow multi-step procedures. For individuals with learning disabilities, it may be hard to visualize patterns, different parts of a math problem, or identify critical information needed to solve equations and more complex problems.

What Are the Warning Signs?

Since math disabilities are varied, the signs that a person may have a difficulty in this area can be just as varied. However, having difficulty learning math skills does not necessarily mean a person has a learning disability. All students learn at different paces, and particularly among young people, it takes time and practice for formal math procedures to make practical sense.

If a person has trouble in any of the following areas, additional help may be beneficial.

- Good at speaking, reading, and writing, but slow to develop counting and math problem-solving skills

- Good memory for printed words, but difficulty reading numbers, or recalling numbers in sequence

- Good with general math concepts, but frustrated when specific computation and organization skills need to be used

- Trouble with the concept of time—chronically late, difficulty remembering schedules, trouble with approximating how long something will take

- Poor sense of direction, easily disoriented and easily confused by changes in routine

- Poor long-term memory of concepts—can do math functions one day, but is unable to repeat them the next day

- Poor mental math ability—trouble estimating grocery costs or counting days until vacation

- Difficulty playing strategy games like chess, bridge, or role-playing video games

- Difficulty keeping score when playing board and card games

How Is Dyscalculia Identified?

When a teacher or trained professional evaluates a student for learning disabilities in math, the student is interviewed about a full range of math-related skills and behaviors. Pencil and paper math tests are often used, but an evaluation needs to accomplish more. It is meant to reveal how a person understands and uses numbers and math concepts to solve advanced-level, as well as everyday, problems. The evaluation compares a person's expected and actual levels of skill and understanding while noting the person's specific strengths and weaknesses. Following are some of the areas that may be addressed:

- Ability with basic math skills like counting, adding, subtracting, multiplying, and dividing

- Ability to predict appropriate procedures based on understanding patterns—knowing when to add, subtract, multiply, divide, or do more advanced computations

- Ability to organize objects in a logical way

- Ability to measure, telling time, using money

- Ability to estimate number quantities

- Ability to self-check work and find alternate ways to solve problems

Treating Dyscalculia

Helping a student identify his or her strengths and weaknesses is the first step to getting help. Following identification, parents, teachers, and other educators can work together to establish strategies that will help the student learn math more effectively. Help outside the classroom lets a student and tutor focus specifically on the difficulties that student is having, taking pressure off from moving to new topics too quickly. Repeated reinforcement and specific practice of straightforward ideas can make understanding easier. Other strategies for inside and outside the classroom include the following:

- Use of graph paper for students who have difficulty organizing ideas on paper.

- Work on finding different ways to approach math facts; for example, instead of just memorizing the multiplication tables, explain that 8 x 2 = 16, so if 16 is doubled, 8 x 4 must = 32.

- Practice estimating as a way to begin solving math problems.

- Introduce new skills beginning with concrete examples and later moving to more abstract applications.

- For language difficulties, explain ideas and problems clearly and encourage students to ask questions as they work.

- Provide a place to work with few distractions and have pencils, erasers, and other tools on hand as needed.

Help students become aware of their strengths and weaknesses. Understanding how a person learns best is a big step in achieving academic success and confidence.

Chapter 17

Dysgraphia: Writing Learning Disability

The word dysgraphia simply means difficulty expressing thoughts in writing. In other words, it just means writing difficulty. And generally it is used to refer to extremely poor handwriting and may even be identified to as a disorder of written expression. As with dyslexia, confusion often arises when we start dealing with the term dysgraphia as it relates to special education services.

Each state has its own criteria (based upon the federal definition of LD) which determine if a student has a learning disability as it is defined by special education rules. When a student's writing difficulties are severe enough to meet this criteria, special education services are indicated. On the other hand, dysgraphia has no clearly defined criteria. A student with any degree of handwriting difficulty may be considered dysgraphic by some educational specialists. This frequently occurs when a student receives an educational evaluation outside of the public school system.

So, being labeled as dysgraphic may or may not indicate the need for special education services. It should be noted that most students with learning disabilities experience difficulty with handwriting and probably could be considered dysgraphic. However, the term is seldom used within public schools because of the lack of any strict or measurable criteria.

"Dysgraphia," © 2006–2007 LDinfo Publishing. Reprinted with permission. For additional information from LDinfo, including learning disability terms and definitions, special education rules, and other support for parents and teachers, visit www.ldinfo.com.

Underlying Causes of Dysgraphia

Sequencing Problems

As with dyslexia, written language difficulty is often believed to be the result of underlying visual or perceptual processing weakness. However, research on brain functioning has not found much evidence to support the notion of a visual basis for dysgraphia. In fact, what usually appears to be a perceptual problem (reversing letters or numbers, writing words backwards, writing letters out of order, and very sloppy handwriting) usually seems to be directly related to sequential or rational information processing. In other words, when students experience difficulty sequencing and organizing detailed information, they often have difficulty with the sequence of letters and words as they write. As a result, the student either needs to slow way down in order to write correctly or experiences rather extreme difficulty with the mechanics of writing (for example, spelling or punctuation). Usually, they have difficulty even when they do slow down. And by slowing down or getting stuck with the details of writing, they often lose the great thoughts that they are trying to write about. Sometimes the creative writing skills of such a student are surprisingly strong when the mechanics of writing don't get in the way. This is because their conceptual processing skills are often quite strong enabling them to express deeper meaning in spite of difficulty with the details.

Attention Deficit/Hyperactivity Disorder (AD/HD)

Students with an attention deficit disorder (especially with hyperactivity) often experience rather significant difficulty with writing in general and handwriting in particular. This is because AD/HD students also have difficulty organizing and sequencing detailed information. In addition, AD/HD students are often processing information at a very rapid rate and simply don't have the fine-motor coordination needed to keep up with their thoughts.

Auditory Processing Weakness

Other students experience writing difficulty because of a general auditory or language processing weakness. Because of their difficulty learning and understanding language in general, they obviously have difficulty with language expression. And written language is the most difficult form of language expression. A generalized auditory processing weakness is frequently referred to as a verbal or language-based learning disability and typically affects the areas of reading and writing. Math may be a relative strength.

Visual Processing Weakness

Although most writing disabled or dysgraphic students do not have visual or perceptual processing problems, some students with a visual processing weakness will experience difficulty with writing speed and clarity simply because they aren't able to fully process the visual information as they are placing it on the page. Again, this is probably the least likely cause of a written language problem. A visual processing weakness is sometimes referred to as a nonverbal learning disability and typically affects the areas of spelling and math much more than reading.

Writing Strategies for Dysgraphic Students

1. Outline your thoughts. It is very important to get the main ideas down on paper without having to struggle with the details of spelling or punctuation. Try writing just one key word or phrase for each paragraph, and then go back later to fill in the details.

2. Draw a picture of a thought for each paragraph.

3. Dictate your ideas into a tape recorder then listen and write them down later.

4. Really practice keyboarding skills. It may be difficult at first, but after you have learned the pattern of the keys, typing will be faster and clearer than handwriting.

5. Use a computer to organize information and check spelling. Even if your keyboarding skills aren't great, a computer can sure help with the details.

6. Continue practicing handwriting. As frustrating as it may be, there will be times throughout your life that you will need to be able to write things down and maybe even share your handwriting with others. It will continue to improve as long as you keep working at it.

7. Talk to yourself as you write. This may provide valuable auditory feedback.

If spelling lists are a problem, try the following:

8. Look at each word, then close your eyes and visualize how it looks, letter by letter. Stay with one word until you can clearly visualize it.

9. Spell each word out loud while looking at it, then look away and spell it out loud again several times before writing it down.

10. Try spelling with scrabble tiles so that you can keep re-arranging the letters until they look right.

11. Break the spelling list down into manageable sections of only three to five words. Then take a break after mastering each section.

Chapter 18

Dyslexia

Chapter Contents

Section 18.1

Understanding Dyslexia

Sarah hates reading aloud in class. She's never been a good reader, and even when she recognizes the words on the page, she seems to have trouble saying them correctly. School has never been her favorite place anyway because her teachers always complain about her writing and her spelling. She often gets discouraged, thinking that she's not as smart as other students.

Fortunately, Sarah has discovered she has talents that others don't. She's great at dreaming up costume and scenery ideas in drama club, and she's one of the best artists in her school. Sometimes she wonders how she can do so well in some areas of her life and so poorly in others.

What Sarah, her parents, and her teachers don't realize is that Sarah has dyslexia.

What Is Dyslexia?

Dyslexia (pronounced: dis-lek-see-ah) is a type of learning disability. A person with a learning disability has trouble processing words or numbers. There are several kinds of learning disabilities; dyslexia is the term used when people have difficulty learning to read, even though they are smart enough and are motivated to learn. The word dyslexia comes from two Greek words: *dys*, which means abnormal or impaired, and *lexis*, which refers to language or words.

Dyslexia is not a disease. It's a condition that you are born with, and it often runs in families. People with dyslexia are not stupid or lazy. Most have average or above-average intelligence, and they work very hard to overcome their learning problems.

What Causes Dyslexia?

Research has shown that dyslexia happens because of the way the brain processes information. Pictures of the brain, taken with modern imaging tools, have shown that when people with dyslexia read, they use different parts of the brain than people without dyslexia. These pictures also show that the brains of people with dyslexia don't work efficiently during reading. So that's why reading seems like such slow, hard work.

Most people think that dyslexia causes people to reverse letters and numbers and see words backwards. But reversals occur as a normal part of development, and are not seen only in people with dyslexia. The main problem in dyslexia is trouble recognizing phonemes (pronounced: fo-neems), which are the basic sounds of speech (the "b" sound in "bat" is a phoneme, for example). Therefore, it's a struggle to make the connection between the sound and the letter symbol for that sound, and to blend sounds into words.

This makes it hard to recognize short, familiar words or to sound out longer words. It takes a lot of time for a person with dyslexia to sound out a word. The meaning of the word is often lost, and reading comprehension is poor. It is not surprising that people with dyslexia have trouble spelling. They may also have trouble expressing themselves in writing and even speaking. Dyslexia is a language processing disorder, so it can affect all forms of language, either spoken or written.

Some people have milder forms of dyslexia, so they may have less trouble in these other areas of spoken and written language. Some people work around their dyslexia, but it takes a lot of effort and extra work. Dyslexia isn't something that goes away on its own or that a person outgrows. Fortunately, with proper help, most people with dyslexia learn to read. They often find different ways to learn and use those strategies all their lives.

What Is It Like to Have Dyslexia?

If you have dyslexia, you might have trouble reading even simple words you've seen many times. You probably will read slowly and feel that you have to work extra-hard when reading. You might mix up the letters in a word, for example, reading the word "now" as "won" or "left" as "felt." Words may blend together and spaces are lost. Phrases might appear like this:

> Thew ord sare n otsp aced cor rect ly.
> We spell wrds xatle as tha snd to us.
> Sometimesalthelettersarepushedtogether

You might have trouble remembering what you've read. You may remember more easily when the same information is read to you or heard on tape. Word problems in math may be especially hard, even if you've mastered the basics of arithmetic. If you're doing a presentation in front of the class, you might have trouble finding the right words or names for various objects. Spelling and writing usually are very hard for people with dyslexia.

How Is Dyslexia Diagnosed?

People with dyslexia frequently find ways to work around their disability, so no one will know they're having trouble. This may save some embarrassment, but getting help could make school and reading easier. Most people are diagnosed as children, but it's not unusual for people to be diagnosed as teens or even adults.

In preschool and elementary school children, some signs of dyslexia include difficulty with:

- Learning to talk;
- Pronouncing longer words;
- Rhyming;
- Learning the alphabet, days of the weeks, colors, shapes, and numbers;
- Learning to read and write his or her name;
- Learning the connection between letters and sounds;
- Decoding simple words;
- Using "b" and "d" accurately;
- Reading and spelling words with the correct letter sequence— for example, "top" versus "pot;"
- Hand fine-motor coordination.

In older children, teenagers, and adults, these same signs of dyslexia may still be present. In addition, they probably will:

- Read and spell far below grade level;
- Avoid reading and writing;
- Work slowly on reading and writing assignments and tests;
- Struggle with learning a foreign language.

A teen's parents or teachers might suspect dyslexia if they notice these problems:

- Poor reading skills, despite having normal intelligence
- Poor spelling and writing skills
- Difficulty finishing assignments and tests within time limits
- Difficulty remembering the right names for things
- Difficulty memorizing written lists and phone numbers
- Difficulty with directions (telling right from left or up from down) or reading maps

If someone has one of these problems, it doesn't mean he or she has dyslexia, but someone who shows several of these signs should be tested for the condition.

A physical exam should be done to rule out any medical problems, including hearing and vision tests. Then a school psychologist or learning specialist should give several standardized tests to measure language, reading, spelling, and writing abilities. Sometimes a test of thinking ability (intelligence quotient [IQ] test) is given. Some people with dyslexia have trouble in other school skills, like handwriting and math, or they may have trouble paying attention or remembering things. If this is the case, more testing will be done.

Dealing with Dyslexia

Although dealing with dyslexia can be tough, help is available. Under federal law, someone diagnosed with a learning disability like dyslexia is entitled to extra help from the public school system. A child or teen with dyslexia usually needs to work with a specially trained teacher, tutor, or reading specialist to learn how to read and spell better. The best type of help teaches awareness of speech sounds in words and letter-sound correspondences (called phonics). The teacher or tutor should use special learning and practice activities for dyslexia.

A student with dyslexia may get more time to complete assignments or tests, permission to tape class lectures, or copies of lecture notes. Using a computer with spelling checkers can be helpful for written assignments. For older students in challenging classes, services are available that provide any book on tape, even textbooks. Computer software is also available that "reads" printed material aloud. Ask your parent, teacher, or learning disability services coordinator how to get these services if you need them.

Treatment with eye exercises or glasses with tinted lenses will not help a person with dyslexia. It's not an eye problem, it's a language processing problem, so teaching language processing skills is the most important part of treatment.

Emotional support for people with dyslexia is very important. They often get frustrated because no matter how hard they try, they can't seem to keep up with other students. They often feel that they are stupid or worthless, and may cover up their difficulties by acting up in class or by becoming the class clown. They may try to get other students to do their work for them. They may pretend that they don't care about their grades or that they think school is dumb.

Family and friends can help people with dyslexia by understanding that they aren't stupid or lazy, and that they are trying as hard as they can. It's important to recognize and appreciate each person's strengths, whether they're in sports, drama, art, creative problem solving, or something else.

People with dyslexia shouldn't feel limited in their academic or career choices. Most colleges make special accommodations for students with dyslexia, offering them trained tutors, learning aids, computer software, reading assignments on tape, and special arrangements for exams. People with dyslexia can become doctors, politicians, corporate executives, actors, artists, teachers, or whatever else they choose.

Section 18.2

What Is Having Dyslexia Like?

Peter works so hard at reading, but it just never gets easier. He knows he's smart so why can't he read like the other kids? Peter has a problem called dyslexia.

Dyslexia (say: dis-lek-see-uh) is a learning problem some kids have. Dyslexia makes it tough to read and spell. The problem is inside the brain, but it doesn't mean the person is dumb. Plenty of smart and talented people struggle with dyslexia.

But dyslexia doesn't have to keep a kid down. With some help and a lot of hard work, a kid who has dyslexia can learn to read and spell.

How Does Reading Happen?

To understand dyslexia, it helps to understand reading. Reading is a real workout for your brain. You need to do the following steps—and all at once:

1. Understand the way speech sounds make up words.

2. Focus on printed marks (letters and words).

3. Connect speech sounds to letters.

4. Blend letter sounds smoothly into words.

5. Control eye movements across the page.

6. Build images and ideas.

7. Compare new ideas with what is already known.

8. Store the ideas in memory.

Phew! Kids who have dyslexia struggle with the beginning steps, so that makes doing the rest of the steps even harder. It's no surprise, then, that trying to read and dealing with dyslexia makes a kid's brain really tired, really fast.

How Kids Become Readers

Most kids start learning to read by learning how speech sounds make up words. Then they connect those sounds to alphabet letters. For example, they learn that the letter "b" makes a "buh" sound.

Then kids learn to blend those sounds into words. They learn that "b" and "at" makes "bat." Eventually, most kids don't have to sound words out and can instantly recognize words they've seen many times before.

But it's tougher for kids who have dyslexia. They may struggle to remember simple words they have seen many times and to sound out longer words. Why is it so hard?

Dyslexia means that a person's brain has trouble processing letters and sounds. That makes it tough to break words into separate speech sounds, like b-a-t for bat. When it's hard to do that, it's really hard to connect speech sounds to different letters, like "buh" for b, and blend them into words.

So a kid who has dyslexia will read slowly and might make a lot of mistakes. Sometimes he or she will mix up letters in a word, such as reading the word "was" as "saw." Words may blend together wrong and look like this:

> Thew ord sare n otsp aced cor rect ly.
> We spell wrds xatle az tha snd to us.
> Sometimesallthelettersarepushedtogether

What's It Like to Have Dyslexia?

Even before kindergarten, a kid who has dyslexia usually has trouble with letters and sounds. Later, a teacher might say that the kid is smart, but doesn't seem to be getting the hang of reading. Other times, it's a parent who notices the kid is struggling. The best thing to do is to go to a specialist who can help figure out what's wrong.

A specialist in learning disabilities knows a lot about learning problems that kids have and what to do about them. During a visit with a specialist, a kid might take some tests. But the idea isn't to get a good grade; it's to spot problems. Discovering a learning disability is the first step toward getting help that will make it easier for the kid to learn.

Making Reading Easier

Most kids with dyslexia can learn to read with the right kind of teaching. They might learn new ways for remembering sounds. For example, "p" and "b" are called brother sounds because they're both "lip poppers." You have to press your lips together to make the sound.

Thinking about the way the mouth needs to move to make sounds can help kids read more easily. Learning specialists know lots of special activities like this to teach reading to kids who have dyslexia.

Kids with dyslexia also might use flash cards or tape classroom lessons and homework assignments instead of taking notes about them. They may need parents and tutors to help them stay caught up.

Extra time for tests is really important, so kids with dyslexia have enough time to finish and show their teacher how much they have learned. Computers help a lot, too. You can get programs that "read" books out loud from the computer or even download recorded books to an iPod®.

How Do Kids with Dyslexia Feel?

Kids who have dyslexia might get frustrated, angry, or sad because reading and spelling are so hard. They may not like being in a different reading group than their friends or having to see a special reading tutor.

But getting this help is so important and will help them go on to do great things in life. Some of the most creative and successful people have dyslexia, but it didn't stop them from chasing their dreams.

Section 18.3

Decoding Dyslexia

Excerpted from "DCDC2: Demystifying and Decoding Dyslexia," by Michelle D. Jones-London, Ph.D., National Institute of Neurological Disorders and Stroke (NINDS), January 31, 2007.

A recent study shows that variations in a gene called DCDC2 may disrupt the normal formation of brain circuits that are necessary for fluent reading, leading to dyslexia. After further research, genetic screening for these variations could identify affected children early in their lives and possibly prevent the misdiagnosis of other learning disabilities that resemble dyslexia.

"We have good statistical data that variations of the DCDC2 gene are strongly associated with reading disability, also known as dyslexia. These results reconfirm that dyslexia is strongly genetic and is not a consequence of just environmental factors," says lead investigator Jeffrey Gruen, M.D., Associate Professor of Pediatrics at Yale University School of Medicine in New Haven, Connecticut. This study was funded in part by the National Institute of Neurological Disorders and Stroke (NINDS) and appeared in the November 22, 2005, issue of *Proceedings of the National Academy of Sciences*.[1]

Dyslexia is a common disorder that causes people to have difficulties with accurate or fluent word recognition and hinders the development of reading skills. The brain-based learning disability specifically impairs a person's ability to read. These affected individuals typically read at levels significantly lower than expected despite having normal intelligence. "Unfortunately, people assume that if you read poorly that correlates with having a low intelligence quotient (IQ). This study confirms that dyslexic children can be typically smart and can have strong IQs. The reading disability is not a global effect on entire brain function," says Dr. Gruen.

The researchers examined variations in a gene, doublecortin domain containing 2 (DCDC2), and found that specific variations including a large deletion may be inherited in up to 20 percent of people affected with dyslexia. The study demonstrates that DCDC2 is involved in neuronal migration (the movement of neurons to their target regions during early brain development). The researchers tested the hypothesis that down-regulation of DCDC2 affects brain or neuronal circuits using embryonic rats. Brain sections of these rats showed an abnormal migration pattern of neurons, in which the neurons failed to reach their target destination.

In humans, the DCDC2 gene is strongly expressed in the same brain regions (cortex, hypothalamus, amygdala, and hippocampus) of normal and dyslexic readers, suggesting that changes in the gene's function, rather than a deletion of the entire gene, cause the disorder. The gene in people with dyslexia is altered but still somewhat functional, which may explain why dyslexia is frequently associated with subtle changes and not extreme learning disability.

Previous clinical studies have shown that up to 50 percent of children of dyslexic parents have dyslexia themselves. These and other studies of heritability led researchers to hunt for genes that influence the disorder. In recent years, two other genes have also been linked to dyslexia, EKN1 and KIAA0319. KIAA0319 is also involved in neuronal migration.

The DCDC2 gene and its strong relationship to dyslexia have already been replicated in an independent study in Germany.[2] "This is powerful because those researchers studied subjects who speak a different language and used different reading tests, yet they still found this same gene involvement. This illustrates a strong role for human genetics in the expression of the disorder," says Dr. Gruen.

Although the disorder varies from person to person, common characteristics among people with dyslexia include difficulty with phonological processing (the manipulation of sounds) and rapid visual-verbal responding. Researchers estimate that 10–17 percent of the population in the U.S. has dyslexia. Dyslexia is also equally prevalent in non-English-speaking countries. It is a common misconception that dyslexia is simply a person who sees words backwards. Only 30 percent of dyslexics have trouble with reversing letters and numbers.

"Traditionally, many people are under the impression that dyslexia is an issue with visualizing letters differently. However, we now know that dyslexics just learn to read differently—most learn to read by sight memorization not phonetically," says Dr. Gruen. Anatomically, dyslexics have normal brains; however, the brain areas activated in reading may be different. Several studies using fMRI, an imaging technique that studies activity in the brain, have shown that dyslexics display different patterns of brain activity than other people when they read.

"Some kids just learn differently. Not all children learn to read with our current one-size fits all methods," says Dr. Gruen. "The earlier we can identify children at risk, the earlier we can start intervention when studies have shown that remediation works best. Even with the future capabilities of genetic testing for dyslexia, the biggest problem is still the lack of infrastructure for early intervention in schools."

Dr. Gruen cautions that although we can now draw a path from the disease to the gene, the reverse is not necessarily proven yet. That is, predicting the outcome for a person who has the gene and determining if the person will have the disorder is still not possible. The next steps of the research will examine other variations including deletions or changes in this particular gene family. The investigators will also examine brain imaging in children and adults given reading tasks and then see how that relates to DCDC2 variations. Ultimately, identifying dyslexia genes may provide opportunities for early identification of the disorder and help to distinguish dyslexia from other learning disabilities.

References

1. Meng H, Smith S, Hager K, Held M, Liu J, Olson R, Pennington B, DeFries J, Gelernter J, O'Reilly-Pol T, Somlo S, Skudlarski P, Shaywitz S, Shaywitz B, Marchione K, Wang Y, Murugan P, LoTurco J, Grier P, Gruen J. "DCDC2 is associated with reading disability and modulates neuronal development in the brain." *Proceedings of the National Academy of Sciences*, November 22, 2005, Vol. 102, pp. 17053–17058.

2. Schumacher J, Anthoni H, Dahdouh F, Konig I, Hillmer A, Kluck N, Manthey M, Plume E, Warnke A, Remschmidt H, Hulsmann J, Cichon S, Lindgren C, Propping P, Zuccheli M, Ziegler A, Peyrard-Janvid M, Schulte-Korne G, Nothen M, Kere J. "Strong genetic evidence of DCDC2 as a susceptibility gene for dyslexia." *The American Journal of Human Genetics*, January 2006, Vol. 78, pp. 52–62.

Chapter 19

Nonverbal Learning Disorders

What is nonverbal learning disability (NLD or NVLD)?

Kids with nonverbal learning disability are very verbal, and may not have academic problems until they get into the upper grades in school. Often their biggest problem is with social skills.

NLD is very like Asperger syndrome. It may be that the diagnoses of Asperger syndrome (AS) and NLD simply "provide different perspectives on a heterogeneous, yet overlapping, group of individuals sharing at least some common aspects.[1]" AS and NLD are generally thought to describe pretty much the same kind of disorder, but to differ in severity—with AS describing more severe symptoms.

What are the signs of nonverbal learning disability?

- Great vocabulary and verbal expression
- Excellent memory skills
- Attention to detail, but misses the big picture
- Trouble understanding reading
- Difficulty with math, especially word problems
- Poor abstract reasoning

"Non-verbal Learning Disability (NLD or NVLD)." Used with permission of the University of Michigan Health System, July 2008. Written by Kyla Boyse, R.N. http://www.med.umich.edu/1lib/yourchild/nld.htm.

- Physically awkward; poor coordination
- Messy and laborious handwriting
- Concrete thinking; taking things very literally
- Trouble with nonverbal communication, like body language, facial expression, and tone of voice
- Poor social skills; difficulty making and keeping friends
- Fear of new situations
- Trouble adjusting to changes
- May be very naïve and lack common sense
- Anxiety, depression, low self-esteem
- May withdraw, becoming agoraphobic (abnormal fear of open spaces)

What are some parenting tips for kids with NLD?

- Keep the environment predictable and familiar.
- Provide structure and routine.
- Prepare your child for changes, giving logical explanations.
- Pay attention to sensory input from the environment, like noise, temperature, smells, or many people being around.
- Help your child learn coping skills for dealing with anxiety and sensory difficulties.
- Be logical, organized, clear, concise, and concrete. Avoid jargon, double meanings, sarcasm, nicknames, and teasing.
- State your expectations clearly.
- Be very specific about cause and effect relationships.
- Work with your child's school to modify homework assignments, testing (time and content), grading, art, and physical education.
- Have your child use the computer at school and at home for schoolwork.
- Help your child learn organizational and time management skills.
- Make use of your child's verbal skills to help with social interactions and nonverbal experiences, for example, giving a verbal explanation of visual material.

- Teach your child about nonverbal communication (facial expressions, gestures). Help them learn how to tell from others' reactions whether they are communicating well.

- Learn about social competence and how to teach it.

- Help your child out in group activities.

- Get your child into the therapies they need, such as: occupational or physical therapy, psychological, or speech and language (to address social issues) therapy.

How can parents help kids with poor social skills?

According to Mel Levine, in a book chapter titled "Unpopular Children"[2] there are many ways parents can help kids with social skills problems. Here are some ways parents can help their kids:

- Steer your child toward a playmate they have something in common with and set up a play date. This is a way to get some social skills experience in a small, controlled, less-threatening way.

- See if you can find a small-group social skills training program in your school system, medical system, or community. This kind of program will probably not be available in smaller communities.

- Encourage your child to develop interests that will build their self-esteem and help them relate to other kids. For example, if your child is interested in Pokémon®, pursuing this interest may open social doors for them with schoolmates.

- Talk to your child in private after you have gone with them to a group activity. You can discuss with them how they could improve the way they interact with other kids. For example, you might point out that other kids don't feel comfortable when your child stands so close to them. Help them practice the social skills you explain to them through role-playing.

- Bullying is unacceptable. Your child's school must make every effort to prevent it. If talking to your child's teachers and principal does not put an end to the victimization, ask your child's doctor to write a letter to the school, and pursue the issue up to higher channels in the school district if necessary.

- These kids need as few handicaps as possible, so make sure your child is getting the counseling, therapies, and medication they need to treat any other problems or medical conditions they might have.

- Reassure your child that you value them for who they are. It's a little tricky to help your child improve social skills, and at the same time nurture their confidence to hold onto their unique individuality.

Literature Cited

1. Klin, A, Volkmar, FR. *Asperger's syndrome: guidelines for assessment and diagnosis.* Yale Child Study Center, Developmental Disabilities Clinic. Available from: URL: http://info.med.yale.edu/childstdy/autism/asdiagnosis.html.

2. Levine, MD. Unpopular Children. In: Parker, S, Zuckerman, B, editors. *Behavioral and developmental pediatrics: a handbook for primary care.* Boston: Little, Brown and Company; 1995. p. 327.

Chapter 20

Visual Processing Disorders

Visual Processing Disorders: In Detail

There are lots of ways the brain processes visual information. Weaknesses in a particular kind of visual processing can often be seen in specific difficulties with practical, everyday tasks.

Following is an explanation of each of the types of visual processing. Each category also includes:

- Possible difficulties that can occur if there is a weakness in that area;

- Possible strategies that may help overcome the difficulties.

Be aware that weakness can occur in one or more category at the same time.

It is also important to note that many people without any kind of visual processing disorder experience problems with learning and behavior from time to time. However, if a person consistently displays difficulties with these tasks over time, testing for visual processing disorders by trained professionals should be considered.

Visual Discrimination

The skill: Using the sense of sight to notice and compare the features of different items to distinguish one item from another.

Difficulties observed:

- Seeing the difference between two similar letters, shapes, or objects
- Noticing the similarities and differences between certain colors, shapes, and patterns

Types of helpful strategies:

- Clearly space words or problems on a page.
- Anticipate confusions and point out examples of correct responses.

Visual Figure-Ground Discrimination

The skill: Discriminating a shape or printed character from its background.

Difficulties observed:

- Finding a specific bit of information on a printed page full of words and numbers
- Seeing an image within a competing background

Types of helpful strategies:

- Practice with "find the item" challenges, such as "Where's Waldo?"
- Use an index card or marker when reading to blot out distraction of other words.
- Highlight useful information while reading.

Visual Sequencing

The skill: The ability to see and distinguish the order of symbols, words, or images.

Difficulties observed:

- Using a separate answer sheet

- Staying in the right place while reading a paragraph; for example, skipping lines, reading the same line over and over

- Reversing or misreading letters, numbers and words

- Understanding math equations

Types of helpful strategies:

- Combine reading with oral presentation.

- Color code written instruction.

Visual Motor Processing

The skill: Using feedback from the eyes to coordinate the movement of other parts of the body.

Difficulties observed:

- Writing within lines or margins of a piece of paper

- Copying from a board or book

- Moving around without bumping into things

- Participating in sports that require well-timed and precise movements in space

Types of helpful strategies:

- Allow use of a computer.

- Allow use of a tape recorder for lectures.

- Substitute oral reports for written ones.

- Provide a "note buddy" to check that topic notes are clear and well-organized.

Visual Memory

The skill: There are two kinds of visual memory.

- Long-term visual memory is the ability to recall something seen some time ago.

- Short-term visual memory is the ability to remember something seen very recently.

Difficulties observed:

- Remembering the spelling of familiar words with irregular spelling
- Reading comprehension
- Using a calculator or keyboard with speed and accuracy
- Remembering phone numbers

Types of helpful strategies:

- Provide handouts that are clearly written.
- Provide oral instruction to reinforce written directions.

Visual Closure

The skill: The ability to know what an object is when only parts of it are visible.

Difficulties observed:

- Recognizing a picture of a familiar object from a partial image; for example, a truck without its wheels
- Identifying a word with a letter missing
- Recognizing a face when one feature (such as the nose) is missing

Types of helpful strategies:

- Practice with jigsaw puzzles and rebus-type games.

Spatial Relationships

The skill: The ability to understand how objects are positioned in space in relation to oneself. This involves the understanding of distance (near or far), as well as the relationship of objects and characters described on paper or in a spoken narrative.

Difficulties observed:

- Getting from one place to another
- Spacing letters and words on paper
- Judging time
- Reading maps

Types of helpful strategies:

- Practice estimating distance with ball games and using a tape measure.

- Create maps and travel logs.

- Practice social skills that focus on judging appropriate physical proximity to others.

Visual Processing Disorders: By Age Group

Basics you should know about visual processing disorders.

- Visual processing disorders are also known as visual perceptual processing disorders.

- They affect how the brain perceives and processes what the eye sees.

- These disorders can occur without impaired vision of any kind.

- Like all learning disabilities, visual processing disorders can be a lifelong challenge.

- People with visual processing disorders have problems with the way they interpret information, but what others will notice in people with these disorders is the behavior that happens after the difficulties occur.

- There are several types of visual processing disorders, each affecting different aspects of visual information processing.

Visual Processing Disorders at Different Ages

Many people experience problems with learning and behavior occasionally, but if a person consistently displays difficulties with these tasks over time, testing for visual processing disorders by trained professionals should be considered.

Early Childhood

Common difficulties:

- Misunderstanding or confusing written symbols (example: +, x, /, &)

- Easily distracted, especially by competing visual information

- Writing within margins or on lines or aligning numbers in math problems

- Judging distances (for example: bumping into things, placing objects too close to an edge)

- Fluidity of movement (for example: getting out of the way of a moving ball, knocking things over)

- Differentiating colors or similarly shaped letters and numbers (for example: b, d; p, q; 6, 9; 2, 5)

Accommodation and modification strategies:

- Use books, worksheets, and other materials with enlarged print.

- Read written directions aloud. Varying teaching methods (written and spoken words; images and sounds) can help promote understanding.

- Be aware of the weakness but don't overemphasize it. While helping a child work on the weakness is important; it is just as important to build other skills and function in any setting.

- Break assignments and chores into clear, concise steps. Often multiple steps can be difficult to visualize and complete.

- Give examples and point out the important details of visual information (the part of a picture that contains information for a particular question).

- Provide information about a task before starting to focus attention on the activity.

School-Age Children

Common difficulties:

- Organizing and solving math problems
- Finding and retaining important information in reading assignments or tests
- Writing coherent, well-organized essays
- Copying from board or books
- Sewing or other types of fine motor activities
- Writing neatly and quickly
- Reading with speed and precision

Accommodation and modification strategies:

- Allow student to write answers on the same sheet of paper as the questions, or offer opportunities for student to explain answers orally.

- Provide paper for writing and math work that has darker or raised lines to make the boundaries more distinct.

- Organize assignments to be completed in smaller steps instead of one large finished product.

- Use a ruler as a reading guide (to keep focus on one line at a time) and a highlighter (to immediately emphasize important information).

- Provide a tape recorder to supplement note-taking.

- Have a proof-reading buddy for notes and essays.

Teenagers and Adults

Common difficulties:

- Accurately identifying information from pictures, charts, graphs, or maps

- Organizing information from different sources into one cohesive document

- Finding specific information on a printed page (for example: getting a number out of the phone book)

- Remembering directions to a location

Accommodation and modification strategies:

- Color code important information.

- Have a proof-reading buddy for all written materials.

- Use a tape recorder when getting important information.

- Before writing letters or essays, create an outline to simplify and organize ideas.

Part Four

Other Health Conditions That Impede Learning

Chapter 21

Attention Deficit/Hyperactivity Disorder (AD/HD)

Chapter Contents

Section 21.1

AD/HD in Children

Excerpted from "Attention Deficit Hyperactivity Disorder,"
National Institute of Mental Health (NIMH), 2007.

Attention deficit/hyperactivity disorder (AD/HD) is a condition that becomes apparent in some children in the preschool and early school years. It is hard for these children to control their behavior or pay attention. It is estimated that between 3–5 percent of children have AD/HD, or approximately two million children in the United States. This means that in a classroom of 25 to 30 children, it is likely that at least one will have AD/HD.

A child with AD/HD faces a difficult but not insurmountable task ahead. In order to achieve his or her full potential, he or she should receive help, guidance, and understanding from parents, guidance counselors, and the public education system. This chapter offers information on AD/HD and its management, including research on medications and behavioral interventions, as well as helpful resources on educational options.

Symptoms

The principal characteristics of AD/HD are inattention, hyperactivity, and impulsivity. These symptoms appear early in a child's life. Because many normal children may have these symptoms, but at a low level, or the symptoms may be caused by another disorder, it is important that the child receive a thorough examination and appropriate diagnosis by a well-qualified professional.

Symptoms of AD/HD will appear over the course of many months, often with the symptoms of impulsiveness and hyperactivity preceding those of inattention, which may not emerge for a year or more. Different symptoms may appear in different settings, depending on the demands the situation may pose for the child's self-control. A child who can't sit still or is otherwise disruptive will be noticeable in school, but the inattentive daydreamer may be overlooked. The impulsive child who acts before thinking may be considered just a discipline problem, while the child who is passive or sluggish may be viewed as merely unmotivated. Yet both may have different types of AD/HD. All children are sometimes restless, sometimes act without thinking, and sometimes daydream the time away. When the child's hyperactivity, distractibility, poor concentration, or impulsivity begin to affect performance in school, social relationships with other children, or behavior at home, AD/HD may be suspected. But because the symptoms vary so much across settings, AD/HD is not easy to diagnose. This is especially true when inattentiveness is the primary symptom.

According to the most recent version of the *Diagnostic and Statistical Manual of Mental Disorders (DSM-IV-TR)*, there are three patterns of behavior that indicate AD/HD. People with AD/HD may show several signs of being consistently inattentive. They may have a pattern of being hyperactive and impulsive far more than others of their age. Or they may show all three types of behavior. This means that there are three subtypes of AD/HD recognized by professionals. These are the predominantly hyperactive-impulsive type (that does not show significant inattention); the predominantly inattentive type (that does not show significant hyperactive-impulsive behavior) sometimes called attention deficit disorder (ADD)—an outdated term for this entire disorder; and the combined type (that displays both inattentive and hyperactive-impulsive symptoms).

Hyperactivity-Impulsivity

Hyperactive children always seem to be on the go or constantly in motion. They dash around touching or playing with whatever is in sight, or talk incessantly. Sitting still at dinner or during a school lesson or story can be a difficult task. They squirm and fidget in their seats or roam around the room. Or they may wiggle their feet, touch everything, or noisily tap their pencil. Hyperactive teenagers or adults may feel internally restless. They often report needing to stay busy and may try to do several things at once.

Impulsive children seem unable to curb their immediate reactions or think before they act. They will often blurt out inappropriate comments, display their emotions without restraint, and act without regard for the later consequences of their conduct. Their impulsivity may make it hard for them to wait for things they want or to take their turn in games. They may grab a toy from another child or hit when they're upset. Even as teenagers or adults, they may impulsively choose to do things that have an immediate but small payoff rather than engage in activities that may take more effort yet provide much greater but delayed rewards.

Some signs of hyperactivity-impulsivity are:

- feeling restless, often fidgeting with hands or feet, or squirming while seated;

- running, climbing, or leaving a seat in situations where sitting or quiet behavior is expected;

- blurting out answers before hearing the whole question; and,

- having difficulty waiting in line or taking turns.

Inattention

Children who are inattentive have a hard time keeping their minds on any one thing and may get bored with a task after only a few minutes. If they are doing something they really enjoy, they have no trouble paying attention. But focusing deliberate, conscious attention to organizing and completing a task or learning something new is difficult.

Homework is particularly hard for these children. They will forget to write down an assignment, or leave it at school. They will forget to bring a book home, or bring the wrong one. The homework, if finally finished, is full of errors and erasures. Homework is often accompanied by frustration for both parent and child.

The *DSM-IV-TR* lists these signs of inattention:

- Often becoming easily distracted by irrelevant sights and sounds

- Often failing to pay attention to details and making careless mistakes

- Rarely following instructions carefully and completely losing or forgetting things like toys, or pencils, books, and tools needed for a task

- Often skipping from one uncompleted activity to another

Children diagnosed with the predominantly inattentive type of AD/HD are seldom impulsive or hyperactive, yet they have significant problems paying attention. They appear to be daydreaming, easily confused, slow moving, and lethargic. They may have difficulty processing information as quickly and accurately as other children. When the teacher gives oral or even written instructions, this child has a hard time understanding what he or she is supposed to do and makes frequent mistakes. Yet the child may sit quietly, unobtrusively, and even appear to be working, but is not fully attending to or understanding the task and the instructions.

These children do not show significant problems with impulsivity and overactivity in the classroom, on the school ground, or at home. They may get along better with other children than the more impulsive and hyperactive types of AD/HD, and they may not have the same sorts of social problems so common with the combined type of AD/HD. So, their problems with inattention are often overlooked. But they need help just as much as children with other types of AD/HD, who cause more obvious problems in the classroom.

Is It Really AD/HD?

Not everyone who is overly hyperactive, inattentive, or impulsive has AD/HD. Since most people sometimes blurt out things they did not mean to say, or jump from one task to another, or become disorganized and forgetful, how can specialists tell if the problem is AD/HD?

Because everyone shows some of these behaviors at times, the diagnosis requires that such behavior be demonstrated to a degree that is inappropriate for the person's age. The diagnostic guidelines also contain specific requirements for determining when the symptoms indicate AD/HD. The behaviors must appear early in life, before age seven, and continue for at least six months. Above all, the behaviors must create a real handicap in at least two areas of a person's life such as in the schoolroom, on the playground, at home, in the community, or in social settings. So someone who shows some symptoms but whose schoolwork or friendships are not impaired by these behaviors would not be diagnosed with AD/HD. Nor would a child who seems overly active on the playground but functions well elsewhere receive an AD/HD diagnosis.

To assess whether a child has AD/HD, specialists consider several critical questions: Are these behaviors excessive, long-term, and pervasive? That is, do they occur more often than in other children the same age? Are they a continuous problem, not just a response to a temporary situation? Do the behaviors occur in several settings or only in one specific place like the playground or in the schoolroom? The person's pattern of behavior is compared against a set of criteria and characteristics of the disorder as listed in the *DSM-IV-TR*.

Diagnosis

Some parents see signs of inattention, hyperactivity, and impulsivity in their toddler long before the child enters school. The child may lose interest in playing a game or watching a television show, or may run around completely out of control. But because children mature at different rates and are very different in personality, temperament, and energy levels, it is useful to get an expert's opinion of whether the behavior is appropriate for the child's age. Parents can ask their child's pediatrician, or a child psychologist or psychiatrist, to assess whether their toddler has an attention deficit/hyperactivity disorder or is, more likely at this age, just immature or unusually exuberant.

AD/HD may be suspected by a parent or caretaker or may go unnoticed until the child runs into problems at school. Given that AD/HD tends to affect functioning most strongly in school, sometimes the teacher is the first to recognize that a child is hyperactive or inattentive and may point it out to the parents and consult with the school psychologist. Because teachers work with many children, they come to know how average children behave in learning situations that require attention and self-control. However, teachers sometimes fail to notice the needs of children who may be more inattentive and passive yet who are quiet and cooperative, such as those with the predominantly inattentive form of AD/HD.

Professionals Who Make the Diagnosis

If AD/HD is suspected, to whom can the family turn? What kinds of specialists do they need? Ideally, the diagnosis should be made by a professional in your area with training in AD/HD or in the diagnosis of mental disorders. Child psychiatrists and psychologists, developmental or behavioral pediatricians, or behavioral neurologists are those most often trained in differential diagnosis. Clinical social workers may also have such training.

What Causes AD/HD?

One of the first questions a parent will have is "Why? What went wrong?" "Did I do something to cause this?" There is little compelling evidence at this time that AD/HD can arise purely from social factors or child-rearing methods. Most substantiated causes appear to fall in the realm of neurobiology and genetics. This is not to say that environmental factors may not influence the severity of the disorder, and especially the degree of impairment and suffering the child may experience, but that such factors do not seem to give rise to the condition by themselves.

166

The parents' focus should be on looking forward and finding the best possible way to help their child. Scientists are studying causes in an effort to identify better ways to treat, and perhaps someday, to prevent AD/HD. They are finding more and more evidence that AD/HD does not stem from the home environment, but from biological causes. Knowing this can remove a huge burden of guilt from parents who might blame themselves for their child's behavior.

Over the last few decades, scientists have come up with possible theories about what causes AD/HD. Some of these theories have led to dead ends, some to exciting new avenues of investigation.

Environmental Agents

Studies have shown a possible correlation between the use of cigarettes and alcohol during pregnancy and risk for AD/HD in the offspring of that pregnancy. As a precaution, it is best during pregnancy to refrain from both cigarette and alcohol use.

Another environmental agent that may be associated with a higher risk of AD/HD is high levels of lead in the bodies of young preschool children. Since lead is no longer allowed in paint and is usually found only in older buildings, exposure to toxic levels is not as prevalent as it once was. Children who live in old buildings in which lead still exists in the plumbing or in lead paint that has been painted over may be at risk.

Brain Injury

One early theory was that attention disorders were caused by brain injury. Some children who have suffered accidents leading to brain injury may show some signs of behavior similar to that of AD/HD, but only a small percentage of children with AD/HD have been found to have suffered a traumatic brain injury.

Food Additives and Sugar

It has been suggested that attention disorders are caused by refined sugar or food additives, or that symptoms of AD/HD are exacerbated by sugar or food additives. In 1982, the National Institutes of Health held a scientific consensus conference to discuss this issue. It was found that diet restrictions helped about five percent of children with AD/HD, mostly young children who had food allergies. A more recent study on the effect of sugar on children, using sugar one day and a sugar substitute on alternate days, without parents, staff, or children knowing which substance was being used, showed no significant effects of the sugar on behavior or learning.

In another study, children whose mothers felt they were sugar-sensitive were given aspartame as a substitute for sugar. Half the mothers were told their children were given sugar, half that their children were given aspartame. The mothers who thought their children had received sugar rated them as more hyperactive than the other children and were more critical of their behavior.

Genetics

Attention disorders often run in families, so there are likely to be genetic influences. Studies indicate that 25 percent of the close relatives in the families of AD/HD children also have AD/HD, whereas the rate is about five percent in the general population. Many studies of twins now show that a strong genetic influence exists in the disorder. Researchers continue to study the genetic contribution to AD/HD and to identify the genes that cause a person to be susceptible to AD/HD.

Recent Studies on Causes of AD/HD

Some knowledge of the structure of the brain is helpful in understanding the research scientists are doing in searching for a physical basis for attention deficit/hyperactivity disorder. One part of the brain that scientists have focused on in their search is the frontal lobes of the cerebrum. The frontal lobes allow us to solve problems, plan ahead, understand the behavior of others, and restrain our impulses. The two frontal lobes, the right and the left, communicate with each other through the corpus callosum, (nerve fibers that connect the right and left frontal lobes).

The basal ganglia are the interconnected gray masses deep in the cerebral hemisphere that serve as the connection between the cerebrum and the cerebellum and, with the cerebellum, are responsible for motor coordination. The cerebellum is divided into three parts. The middle part is called the vermis.

All of these parts of the brain have been studied through the use of various methods for seeing into or imaging the brain. These methods include functional magnetic resonance imaging (fMRI) positron emission tomography (PET), and single photon emission computed tomography (SPECT). The main or central psychological deficits in those with AD/HD have been linked through these studies. By 2002 the researchers in the National Institute of Mental Health (NIMH) Child Psychiatry Branch had studied 152 boys and girls with AD/HD, matched with 139 age- and gender-matched controls without AD/HD. The children were scanned at least twice, some as many as four times over a decade. As a group, the AD/HD children showed 3-4 percent smaller brain volumes in all regions—the frontal lobes, temporal gray matter, caudate nucleus, and cerebellum.

This study also showed that the AD/HD children who were on medication had a white matter volume that did not differ from that of controls. Those never-medicated patients had an abnormally small volume of white matter. The white matter consists of fibers that establish long-distance connections between brain regions. It normally thickens as a child grows older and the brain matures.

Although this long-term study used MRI to scan the children's brains, the researchers stressed that MRI remains a research tool and cannot be used to diagnose AD/HD in any given child. This is true for other neurological methods of evaluating the brain, such as PET and SPECT.

Disorders That Sometimes Accompany AD/HD

Learning Disabilities

Many children with AD/HD—approximately 20 to 30 percent—also have a specific learning disability (LD). In preschool years, these disabilities include difficulty in understanding certain sounds or words or difficulty in expressing oneself in words. In school age children, reading or spelling disabilities, writing disorders, and arithmetic disorders may appear. A type of reading disorder, dyslexia, is quite widespread. Reading disabilities affect up to eight percent of elementary school children.

Tourette Syndrome

A very small proportion of people with AD/HD have a neurological disorder called Tourette syndrome. People with Tourette syndrome have various nervous tics and repetitive mannerisms, such as eye blinks, facial twitches, or grimacing. Others may clear their throats frequently, snort, sniff, or bark out words. These behaviors can be controlled with medication. While very few children have this syndrome, many of the cases of Tourette syndrome have associated AD/HD. In such cases, both disorders often require treatment that may include medications.

Oppositional Defiant Disorder

As many as one-third to one-half of all children with AD/HD—mostly boys—have another condition, known as oppositional defiant disorder

(ODD). These children are often defiant, stubborn, non-compliant, have outbursts of temper, or become belligerent. They argue with adults and refuse to obey.

Conduct Disorder

About 20 to 40 percent of AD/HD children may eventually develop conduct disorder (CD), a more serious pattern of antisocial behavior. These children frequently lie or steal, fight with or bully others, and are at a real risk of getting into trouble at school or with the police. They violate the basic rights of other people, are aggressive toward people or animals, destroy property, break into people's homes, commit thefts, carry or use weapons, or engage in vandalism. These children or teens are at greater risk for substance use experimentation, and later dependence and abuse. They need immediate help.

Anxiety and Depression

Some children with AD/HD often have co-occurring anxiety or depression. If the anxiety or depression is recognized and treated, the child will be better able to handle the problems that accompany AD/HD. Conversely, effective treatment of AD/HD can have a positive impact on anxiety as the child is better able to master academic tasks.

Bipolar Disorder

There are no accurate statistics on how many children with AD/HD also have bipolar disorder. Differentiating between AD/HD and bipolar disorder in childhood can be difficult. In its classic form, bipolar disorder is characterized by mood cycling between periods of intense highs and lows. But in children, bipolar disorder often seems to be a rather chronic mood dysregulation with a mixture of elation, depression, and irritability. Furthermore, there are some symptoms that can be present both in AD/HD and bipolar disorder, such as a high level of energy and a reduced need for sleep. Of the symptoms differentiating children with AD/HD from those with bipolar disorder, elated mood and grandiosity of the bipolar child are distinguishing characteristics.

Treatment of AD/HD

Every family wants to determine what treatment will be most effective for their child. This question needs to be answered by each family in consultation with their health care professional. To help families make this important decision, the National Institute of Mental Health (NIMH) has funded many studies of treatments for AD/HD and has conducted the most intensive study ever undertaken for evaluating the treatment of this disorder. This study is known as the Multimodal Treatment Study of Children with Attention Deficit Hyperactivity Disorder (MTA). The NIMH is now conducting a clinical trial for younger children ages 3 to 5.5 years (Treatment of AD/HD in Preschool-Age Children).

The Multimodal Treatment Study of Children with Attention Deficit Hyperactivity Disorder

The MTA study included 579 (95–98 at each of six treatment sites) elementary school boys and girls with AD/HD, who were randomly assigned to one of four treatment programs: (1) medication management alone; (2) behavioral treatment alone; (3) a combination of both; or (4) routine community care. In each of the study sites, three groups were treated for the first 14 months in a specified protocol and the fourth group was referred for community treatment of the parents' choosing. All of the children were reassessed regularly throughout the study period. An essential part of the program was the cooperation of the schools, including principals and teachers. Both teachers and parents rated the children on hyperactivity, impulsivity and inattention, and symptoms of anxiety and depression, as well as social skills.

The results of the study indicated that long-term combination treatments and the medication-management alone were superior to intensive behavioral treatment and routine community treatment. And in some areas—anxiety, academic performance, oppositional behaviors, parent-child relations, and social skills—the combined treatment was usually superior. Another advantage of combined treatment was that children could be successfully treated with lower doses of medicine, compared with the medication-only group.

Which Treatment Should My Child Have?

For children with AD/HD, no single treatment is the answer for every child. A child may sometimes have undesirable side effects to a medication that would make that particular treatment unacceptable. And if a child with AD/HD also has anxiety or depression, a treatment combining medication and behavioral therapy might be best. Each child's needs and personal history must be carefully considered.

When a child's schoolwork and behavior improve soon after starting medication, the child, parents, and teachers tend to applaud the drug for causing the sudden changes. Unfortunately, when people see such immediate improvement, they often think medication is all that is needed. But medications do not cure AD/HD; they only control the symptoms on the day they are taken. Although the medications help the child pay better attention and complete school work, they can't increase knowledge or improve academic skills. The medications help the child to use those skills he or she already possesses.

Behavioral therapy, emotional counseling, and practical support will help AD/HD children cope with everyday problems and feel better about themselves.

Facts to Remember about Medication for AD/HD

- Medications for AD/HD help many children focus and be more successful at school, home, and play. Avoiding negative experiences now may actually help prevent addictions and other emotional problems later.

- About 80 percent of children who need medication for AD/HD still need it as teenagers. Over 50 percent need medication as adults.

Section 21.2

AD/HD in Adults

This section includes excerpts from "Attention Deficit Hyperactivity Disorder," National Institute of Mental Health (NIMH), 2007; and, "Harvard Study Suggests Significant Prevalence of ADHD Symptoms among Adults," NIMH, April 1, 2006.

Attention deficit/hyperactivity disorder (AD/HD) is a highly publicized childhood disorder that affects approximately three percent to five percent of all children. What is much less well known is the probability that, of children who have AD/HD, many will still have it as adults. Several studies done in recent years estimate that between 30 percent and 70 percent of children with AD/HD continue to exhibit symptoms in the adult years.

The first studies on adults who were never diagnosed as children as having AD/HD, but showed symptoms as adults, were done in the late 1970s by Drs. Paul Wender, Frederick Reimherr, and David Wood. These symptomatic adults were retrospectively diagnosed with AD/HD after the researchers' interviews with their parents. The researchers developed clinical criteria for the diagnosis of adult AD/HD (the Utah Criteria), which combined past history of AD/HD with current evidence of AD/HD behaviors. Other diagnostic assessments are now available; among them are the widely used Conners Rating Scale and the Brown Attention Deficit Disorder Scale.

Typically, adults with AD/HD are unaware that they have this disorder—they often just feel that it is impossible to get organized, to stick to a job, to keep an appointment. The everyday tasks of getting up, getting dressed and ready for the day's work, getting to work on time, and being productive on the job can be major challenges for the AD/HD adult.

Diagnosing AD/HD in an Adult

Diagnosing an adult with AD/HD is not easy. Many times, when a child is diagnosed with the disorder, a parent will recognize that he or she has many of the same symptoms the child has and, for the first time, will begin to understand some of the traits that have given him or her trouble for years—distractibility, impulsivity, restlessness. Other adults will seek professional help for depression or anxiety and will find out that the root cause of some of their emotional problems is AD/HD. They may have a history of school failures or problems at work. Often they have been involved in frequent automobile accidents.

To be diagnosed with AD/HD, an adult must have childhood-onset, persistent, and current symptoms. The accuracy of the diagnosis of adult AD/HD is of utmost importance and should be made by a clinician with expertise in the area of attention dysfunction. For an accurate diagnosis, a history of the patient's childhood behavior, together with an interview with his life partner, a parent, close friend, or other close associate, will be needed. A physical examination and psychological tests should also be given. Comorbidity with other conditions may exist such as specific learning disabilities, anxiety, or affective disorders.

A correct diagnosis of AD/HD can bring a sense of relief. The individual has brought into adulthood many negative perceptions of himself that may have led to low esteem. Now he can begin to understand why he has some of his problems and can begin to face them. This may mean, not only treatment for AD/HD, but also psychotherapy that can help him cope with the anger he feels about the failure to diagnose the disorder when he was younger.

Treatment of AD/HD in an Adult

Medications: As with children, if adults take a medication for AD/HD, they often start with a stimulant medication. The stimulant medications affect the regulation of two neurotransmitters, norepinephrine and dopamine. The newest medication approved for AD/HD by the U.S. Food and Drug Administration (FDA), atomoxetine (Strattera®), has been tested in controlled studies in both children and adults and has been found to be effective.

Antidepressants are considered a second choice for treatment of adults with AD/HD. The older antidepressants, the tricyclics, are sometimes used because they, like the stimulants, affect norepinephrine and dopamine. Venlafaxine (Effexor®), a newer antidepressant, is also used for its effect on norepinephrine. Bupropion (Wellbutrin®), an antidepressant with an indirect effect on the neurotransmitter dopamine, has been useful in clinical trials on the treatment of AD/HD in both children and adults. It has the added attraction of being useful in reducing cigarette smoking.

In prescribing for an adult, special considerations are made. The adult may need less of the medication for his weight. A medication may have a longer half-life in an adult. The adult may take other medications for physical problems such as diabetes or high blood pressure. Often the adult is also taking a medication for anxiety or depression. All of these variables must be taken into account before a medication is prescribed.

Education and psychotherapy: Although medication gives needed support, the individual must succeed on his own. To help in this struggle, both psychoeducation and individual psychotherapy can be helpful. A professional coach can help the AD/HD adult learn how to organize his life by using props—a large calendar posted where it will be seen in the morning, date books, lists, reminder notes, and have a special place for keys, bills, and the paperwork of everyday life. Tasks can be organized into sections, so that completion of each part can give a sense of accomplishment. Above all, AD/HD adults should learn as much as they can about their disorder.

Psychotherapy can be a useful adjunct to medication and education. First, just remembering to keep an appointment with the therapist is a step toward keeping to a routine. Therapy can help change a long-standing poor self-image by examining the experiences that produced it. The therapist can encourage the AD/HD patient to adjust to changes brought into his life by treatment—the perceived loss of impulsivity and love of risk-taking, the new sensation of thinking before acting. As the patient begins to have small successes in his new ability to bring organization out of the complexities of his or her life, he or she can begin to appreciate the characteristics of AD/HD that are positive—boundless energy, warmth, and enthusiasm.

Harvard Study Suggests Significant Prevalence of AD/HD Symptoms among Adults

A recent National Institute of Mental Health (NIMH)-funded survey tracking the prevalence of attention deficit/hyperactivity symptoms found that an estimated 4.4 percent of adults ages 18–44 in the United States experience symptoms and some disability. The survey is known as the National Comorbidity Survey Replication (NCS-R) and is part of a series of tracking surveys supported by NIMH and conducted by researchers at Harvard Medical School to assess the state of mental health of the nation. The NCS-R is a nationally representative survey of English-speaking residents ages 18 and older.

The results of the survey raise awareness about the possibility that many children who have AD/HD continue to have related symptoms as adults. It points to the need for long-term, follow-up assessments of children diagnosed with AD/HD to determine if the disorder lingers past adolescence and into adulthood.

In the survey, those with attention deficit/hyperactivity symptoms were more likely to be white males who were divorced and unemployed or unable to work. They also tended to have more problems with alcohol and drug abuse—problems that are known to be associated with AD/HD. In addition, the study found that while many people with AD/HD problems are in treatment for other mental disorders and substance abuse, a smaller proportion receive treatment for their AD/HD symptoms.

Adult AD/HD symptoms often coexist with other mental and emotional disorders, such as depression or anxiety, and can significantly impair a person's ability to function productively. The researchers also note that because AD/HD assessments have been traditionally targeted to children, AD/HD is difficult to diagnose in adults.

Moreover, the symptoms tend to be more varied and subtler in adults than in children, suggesting that clinicians may need to consider a wider variety of possible symptoms for the condition to allow for better assessment in adults. Until biomarkers for AD/HD are identified that will allow clinicians to differentiate between AD/HD and other conditions with similar symptoms, diagnosis must depend on careful and comprehensive clinical evaluation. Treatment decisions are best left to individual patients and their doctors, taking into account the potential risks and benefits posed by the various treatment options.

Reference

Kessler RC, Adler L, Barkley R, Biederman J, Conners CK, Demler O, Faraone SV, Greenhill LL, Howes MJ, Secnik K, Spencer T, Ustun TB, Walters EE, Zaslavsky AM. The Prevalence and Correlates of Adult ADHD in the United States: Results from the National Comorbidity Survey Replication. *American Journal of Psychiatry*. 2006. 163: 724–732.

Chapter 22

Chromosome-Based Disorders Increase Risk of Learning Disabilities

Chapter Contents

Section 22.1

47,XYY Syndrome

Genetics Home Reference, U.S. National Library of Medicine, January 2006.

What is 47,XYY syndrome?

47,XYY syndrome is characterized by an extra copy of the Y chromosome in each of a male's cells. Most often this chromosomal change causes no unusual physical features or medical problems. Males with 47,XYY syndrome are sometimes taller than average and have an increased risk of learning disabilities and delayed speech and language skills. Developmental delays and behavioral problems are also possible, but the characteristics vary widely among affected boys and men. Most males with 47,XYY syndrome have normal sexual development and are able to conceive children.

How common is 47,XYY syndrome?

About one in 1,000 males is born with an extra copy of the Y chromosome in each cell. Five to ten boys with 47,XYY syndrome are born in the United States each day.

What are the genetic changes related to 47,XYY syndrome?

47,XYY syndrome, is related to the Y chromosome. People normally have 46 chromosomes in each cell. Two of the 46 chromosomes are sex chromosomes, called X and Y. Females have two X chromosomes (46,XX), and males have one X chromosome and one Y chromosome (46,XY).

47,XYY syndrome is caused by the presence of an extra copy of the Y chromosome in each of a male's cells. As a result of the extra Y chromosome, each cell has a total of 47 chromosomes instead of 46. It remains uncertain why an extra copy of the Y chromosome is associated with tall stature and learning problems in some boys and men.

Some males with 47,XYY syndrome have an extra Y chromosome in only some of their cells. These cases are called 46,XY/47,XYY mosaics.

Can 47,XYY syndrome be inherited?

47,XYY syndrome usually is not inherited, but occurs as a random event during the formation of sperm cells. An error in cell division called nondisjunction can result in sperm cells with an extra copy of the Y chromosome. If one of these atypical reproductive cells contributes to the genetic makeup of a child, the child will have an extra Y chromosome in each of the body's cells.

In some cases, the addition of an extra Y chromosome results from nondisjunction during cell division in early embryonic development. These cases are usually 46,XY/47,XYY mosaics.

What other names do people use for 47,XYY syndrome?

- XYY karyotype
- XYY syndrome
- YY syndrome

Section 22.2

Klinefelter Syndrome

National Institute of Child Health and Human Development (NICHD), May 24, 2007.

What is Klinefelter syndrome?

Klinefelter syndrome, also known as the XXY condition, is a term used to describe males who have an extra X chromosome in most of their cells. Instead of having the usual XY chromosome pattern that most males have, these men have an XXY pattern.

Klinefelter syndrome is named after Dr. Henry Klinefelter, who first described a group of symptoms found in some men with the extra X chromosome. Even though all men with Klinefelter syndrome have the extra X chromosome, not every XXY male has all of those symptoms. Because not every male with an XXY pattern has all the symptoms of Klinefelter syndrome, it is common to use the term XXY

179

male to describe these men, or XXY condition to describe the symptoms.

Scientists believe the XXY condition is one of the most common chromosome abnormalities in humans. About one of every 500 males has an extra X chromosome, but many do not have any symptoms.

What are the symptoms of the XXY condition?

Not all males with the condition have the same symptoms or to the same degree. Symptoms depend on how many XXY cells a man has, how much testosterone is in his body, and his age when the condition is diagnosed.

The XXY condition can affect three main areas of development:

Physical development: As babies, many XXY males have weak muscles and reduced strength. They may sit up, crawl, and walk later than other infants. After about age four, XXY males tend to be taller and may have less muscle control and coordination than other boys their age.

As XXY males enter puberty, they often do not make as much testosterone as other boys. This can lead to a taller, less muscular body, less facial and body hair, and broader hips than other boys. As teens, XXY males may have larger breasts, weaker bones, and a lower energy level than other boys.

By adulthood, XXY males look similar to males without the condition, although they are often taller. They are also more likely than other men to have certain health problems, such as autoimmune disorders, breast cancer, vein diseases, osteoporosis, and tooth decay. XXY males can have normal sex lives, but they usually make little or no sperm. Between 95 percent and 99 percent of XXY males are infertile because their bodies do not make a lot of sperm.

Language development: As boys, between 25 percent and 85 percent of XXY males have some kind of language problem, such as learning to talk late, trouble using language to express thoughts and needs, problems reading, and trouble processing what they hear. As adults, XXY males may have a harder time doing work that involves reading and writing, but most hold jobs and have successful careers.

Social development: As babies, XXY males tend to be quiet and undemanding. As they get older, they are usually quieter, less self-confident, less active, and more helpful and obedient than other boys.

As teens, XXY males tend to be quiet and shy. They may struggle in school and sports, meaning they may have more trouble fitting in with other kids. However, as adults, XXY males live lives similar to men without the condition; they have friends, families, and normal social relationships.

What are the treatments for the XXY condition?

The XXY chromosome pattern can not be changed. But, there are a variety of ways to treat the symptoms of the XXY condition. One of the most important factors for all types of treatment is starting it as early in life as possible.

Educational treatments: As children, many XXY males qualify for special services to help them in school. Teachers can also help by using certain methods in the classroom, such as breaking bigger tasks into small steps.

Therapeutic options: A variety of therapists, such as physical, speech, occupational, behavioral, mental health, and family therapists, can often help reduce or eliminate some of the symptoms of the XXY condition, such as poor muscle tone, speech or language problems, or low self-confidence.

Medical treatments: Testosterone replacement therapy (TRT) can greatly help XXY males get their testosterone levels into normal range. Having a more normal testosterone level can help develop bigger muscles, deepen the voice, and grow facial and body hair. TRT often starts when a boy reaches puberty. Some XXY males can also benefit from fertility treatment to help them father children.

Section 22.3

Triple X Syndrome

Genetics Home Reference, U.S. National Library of Medicine, January 2006.

What is triple X syndrome?

Triple X syndrome, also called trisomy X or 47,XXX, is characterized by the presence of one extra X chromosome in each of a female's cells. Most often, this chromosomal change causes no unusual physical features or medical problems. Females with triple X syndrome are sometimes taller than average and have an increased risk of learning disabilities and delayed speech and language skills. Developmental delays and behavioral problems are also possible, but these characteristics vary widely among affected girls and women. Most females with triple X syndrome have normal sexual development and are able to conceive children.

How common is triple X syndrome?

This condition occurs in about one in 1,000 newborn girls. Five to ten girls with triple X syndrome are born in the United States each day.

What are the genetic changes related to triple X syndrome?

Triple X syndrome is related to the X chromosome. People normally have 46 chromosomes in each cell. Two of the 46 chromosomes are sex chromosomes, called X and Y. Females have two X chromosomes (46,XX), and males have one X chromosome and one Y chromosome (46,XY).

Triple X syndrome results from an extra copy of the X chromosome in each of a female's cells. As a result of the extra X chromosome, each cell has a total of 47 chromosomes (47,XXX) instead of 46. It remains uncertain why an extra copy of the X chromosome is associated with tall stature and learning problems in some girls and women.

Some females with triple X syndrome have an extra X chromosome in only some of their cells. These cases are called 46,XX/47,XXX mosaics.

Can triple X syndrome be inherited?

Trisomy X usually is not inherited, but occurs as a random event during the formation of reproductive cells (eggs and sperm). An error in cell division called nondisjunction can result in reproductive cells with an abnormal number of chromosomes. For example, an egg or sperm cell may gain an extra copy of the X chromosome as a result of nondisjunction. If one of these atypical reproductive cells contributes to the genetic makeup of a female child, the child will have an extra X chromosome in each of the body's cells.

In some cases, trisomy X results from nondisjunction during cell division in early embryonic development. These cases are usually 46,XX/47,XXX mosaics.

What other names do people use for triple X syndrome?

- Triple X syndrome
- Trisomy X
- 47,XXX
- XXX syndrome

Section 22.4

Turner Syndrome

National Institute of Child Health and Human Development (NICHD),
February 21, 2007.

What is Turner syndrome?

Turner syndrome is a disorder caused by a partially or completely missing X chromosome. It is a condition that only affects females.

Most people have 46 chromosomes in each cell—23 from their mother and 23 from their father. The 23rd pair of chromosomes is called the sex chromosomes—X and Y—because they determine whether a person is male or female. Most females have XX in most of their cells and most males have XY in most of their cells. Females with Turner syndrome are missing all or part of one of their X chromosomes.

What are the symptoms of Turner syndrome?

People with Turner syndrome can have a wide variety of symptoms. Some people may have more severe problems, and others may have mild symptoms. Turner syndrome may affect many areas, including the following:

- **Appearance:** Features may include short neck, low hairline at the back of the neck, low-set ears, hands, and feet that are swollen or puffy at birth, and soft nails that turn upward.

- **Stature:** Children with Turner grow more slowly than other kids and without treatment tend to be very short as adults.

- **Puberty and reproduction:** Most individuals with Turner syndrome lose ovarian function in early childhood and do not start puberty at a normal age. These women usually cannot become pregnant naturally.

- **Cardiovascular:** Some individuals with Turner syndrome have structural problems with their hearts or major blood vessels. For this reason, everyone with Turner syndrome needs a thorough cardiologic evaluation at the time of diagnosis. High blood pressure also affects about 20 percent of girls and 40 percent of adults with Turner syndrome.

- **Kidney:** Some people with Turner syndrome have kidneys that appear to be structurally abnormal, but their kidney function is usually normal.

- **Osteoporosis:** Women with Turner syndrome who do not get adequate estrogen often get osteoporosis, which can cause loss of height and increased bone fractures.

- **Diabetes:** People with Turner syndrome are at higher risk for type II diabetes.

- **Thyroid:** Many people with Turner have thyroid problems, usually hypothyroidism (reduced thyroid function).

- **Cognitive:** Even though people with Turner syndrome have normal intelligence, some have problems with specific visual-spatial coordination tasks (such as mentally rotating objects in space) and may have trouble learning math (geometry and arithmetic).

What are the treatments for Turner syndrome?

Although there is no cure for Turner syndrome, there are some treatments that can help minimize the symptoms.

- Human growth hormone (hGH) given in early childhood can often increase adult height by a few inches.

- Estrogen replacement therapy (ERT) can help start up secondary sexual development that normally begins at puberty for girls without Turner (such as breast development or developing wider hips). Health care providers may prescribe ERT to girls who have not started menstruating by age 15.

- Assistive reproductive therapies, such as egg donation, may help some women with Turner get pregnant

Section 22.5

Williams Syndrome

"Williams Syndrome Information Page," National Institute of Neurological Disorders and Stroke (NINDS), February 14, 2007.

What is Williams syndrome?

Williams syndrome (WS) is a rare genetic disorder characterized by mild to moderate mental retardation or learning difficulties, a distinctive facial appearance, and a unique personality that combines over-friendliness and high levels of empathy with anxiety. The most significant medical problem associated with WS is cardiovascular disease caused by narrowed arteries. WS is also associated with elevated blood calcium levels in infancy. A random genetic mutation (deletion of a small piece of chromosome 7), rather than inheritance, most often causes the disorder. However, individuals who have WS have a 50 percent chance of passing it on if they decide to have children.

The characteristic facial features of WS include puffiness around the eyes, a short nose with a broad nasal tip, wide mouth, full cheeks, full lips, and a small chin. People with WS are also likely to have a long neck, sloping shoulders, short stature, limited mobility in their joints, and curvature of the spine. Some individuals with WS have a star-like pattern in the iris of their eyes. Infants with WS are often irritable and colicky, with feeding problems that keep them from gaining weight. Chronic abdominal pain is common in adolescents and adults. By age 30, the majority of individuals with WS have diabetes or pre-diabetes and mild to moderate sensorineural hearing loss (a form of deafness due to disturbed function of the auditory nerve). For some people, hearing loss may begin as early as late childhood.

WS also is associated with a characteristic cognitive profile of mental strengths and weaknesses composed of strengths in verbal short-term memory and language, combined with severe weakness in visuospatial construction (the skills used to copy patterns, draw, or write). Within language, the strongest skills are typically in concrete, practical vocabulary, which in many cases is in the low average to average range for the general population. Abstract or conceptual-relational vocabulary is much more limited. Most older children and adults with WS speak fluently and use good grammar. More than 50% of children with WS have attention deficit disorders (ADD or AD/HD), and about 50% have specific phobias, such as a fear of loud noises. The majority of individuals with WS worry excessively.

Is there any treatment?

There is no cure for Williams syndrome, nor is there a standard course of treatment. Because WS is an uncommon and complex disorder, multidisciplinary clinics have been established at several centers in the United States. Treatments are based on an individual's particular symptoms. People with WS require regular cardiovascular monitoring for potential medical problems, such as symptomatic narrowing of the blood vessels, high blood pressure, and heart failure.

What is the prognosis?

The prognosis for individuals with WS varies. Some degree of mental retardation is found in most people with the disorder. Some adults are able to function independently, complete academic or vocational school, and live in supervised homes or on their own; most live with a caregiver. Parents can increase the likelihood that their child will be able to live semi-independently by teaching self-help skills early. Early intervention and individualized educational programs designed with the distinct cognitive and personality profiles of WS in mind also help individuals maximize their potential. Medical complications associated with the disorder may shorten the lifespan of some individuals with WS.

What research is being done?

The National Institutes of Health (NIH), and the National Institute of Neurological Disorders and Stroke (NINDS), have funded many of the research studies exploring the genetic and neurobiological origins of WS. In the early 1990s, researchers located and identified the genetic mutation responsible for the disorder: the deletion of a small section of chromosome 7 that contains approximately 25 genes. NINDS continues to support WS researchers including, for example, groups that are attempting to link specific genes with the corresponding facial, cognitive, personality, and neurological characteristics of WS.

Chapter 23

Dyspraxia and Apraxia: Sensory Integration Disorders

Developmental Dyspraxia

Developmental dyspraxia is a disorder characterized by an impairment in the ability to plan and carry out sensory and motor tasks. Generally, individuals with the disorder appear "out of sync" with their environment. Symptoms vary and may include poor balance and coordination, clumsiness, vision problems, perception difficulties, emotional and behavioral problems, difficulty with reading, writing, and speaking, poor social skills, poor posture, and poor short-term memory. Although individuals with the disorder may be of average or above average intelligence, they may behave immaturely.

Is there any treatment?

Treatment is symptomatic and supportive and may include occupational and speech therapy, and "cueing" or other forms of communication such as using pictures and hand gestures. Many children with the disorder require special education.

What is the prognosis?

Developmental dyspraxia is a lifelong disorder. Many individuals are able to compensate for their disabilities through occupational and speech therapy.

This chapter includes: "Developmental Dyspraxia Information Page," National Institute of Neurological Disorders and Stroke (NINDS), December 11, 2007; and, "Apraxia Information Page," NINDS, June 3, 2008.

Apraxia

Apraxia (called dyspraxia if mild) is a neurological disorder characterized by loss of the ability to execute or carry out skilled movements and gestures, despite having the desire and the physical ability to perform them. Apraxia results from dysfunction of the cerebral hemispheres of the brain, especially the parietal lobe, and can arise from many diseases or damage to the brain.

There are several kinds of apraxia, which may occur alone or together. The most common is buccofacial or orofacial apraxia, which causes the inability to carry out facial movements on command such as licking lips, whistling, coughing, or winking. Other types of apraxia include limb-kinetic apraxia (the inability to make fine, precise movements with an arm or leg), ideomotor apraxia (the inability to make the proper movement in response to a verbal command), ideational apraxia (the inability to coordinate activities with multiple, sequential movements, such as dressing, eating, and bathing), verbal apraxia (difficulty coordinating mouth and speech movements), constructional apraxia (the inability to copy, draw, or construct simple figures), and oculomotor apraxia (difficulty moving the eyes on command). Apraxia may be accompanied by a language disorder called aphasia. Corticobasal ganglionic degeneration is a disease that causes a variety of types of apraxia, especially in elderly adults.

Is there any treatment?

Generally, treatment for individuals with apraxia includes physical, speech, or occupational therapy. If apraxia is a symptom of another disorder, the underlying disorder should be treated.

What is the prognosis?

The prognosis for individuals with apraxia varies and depends partly on the underlying cause. Some individuals improve significantly while others may show very little improvement.

What research is being done?

The National Institute of Neurological Disorders and Stroke (NINDS) supports research on movement disorders and conditions such as dyspraxia and apraxia. The goals of this research are to increase scientific understanding of these disorders, and to find ways to prevent, treat, and cure them.

For More Information

American Speech-Language-Hearing Association (ASHA)
2200 Research Blvd.
Rockville, MD 20850
Toll-Free: 800-638-8255
Toll-Free TTY: 800-498-2071
Fax: 301-296-8580
Website: http://www.asha.org
E-mail: actioncenter@asha.org

National Rehabilitation Information Center (NARIC)
8201 Corporate Drive, Suite 600
Landover, MD 20785
Toll-Free: 800-346-2742
Phone: 301-459-5900
TTY: 301-459-5984
Fax: 301-459-4263
Website: http://www.naric.com
E-mail: naricinfo@heitechservices.com

Chapter 24

Emotional/Behavioral Disorders

Definition

Many terms are used to describe emotional, behavioral, or mental disorders. Currently, students with such disorders are categorized as having an emotional disturbance, which is defined under the Individuals with Disabilities Education Act (IDEA) as "...a condition exhibiting one or more of the following characteristics over a long period of time and to a marked degree that adversely affects a child's educational performance:

(A) An inability to learn that cannot be explained by intellectual, sensory, or health factors.

(B) An inability to build or maintain satisfactory interpersonal relationships with peers and teachers.

(C) Inappropriate types of behavior or feelings under normal circumstances.

(D) A general pervasive mood of unhappiness or depression.

(E) A tendency to develop physical symptoms or fears associated with personal or school problems." [Code of Federal Regulations, Title 34, Section 300.7(c)(4)(i)]

Excerpted from "Emotional Disturbance," National Dissemination Center for Children with Disabilities (NICHCY), Fact Sheet 5, January 2004.

As defined by the IDEA, emotional disturbance includes schizophrenia but does not apply to children who are socially maladjusted, unless it is determined that they have an emotional disturbance. [Code of Federal Regulation, Title 34, Section 300.7(c)(4)(ii)]

Incidence

In the 2000–2001 school year, 473,663 children and youth with an emotional disturbance were provided special education and related services in the public schools (Twenty-Fourth Annual Report to Congress, U.S. Department of Education, 2002).

Characteristics

The causes of emotional disturbance have not been adequately determined. Although various factors such as heredity, brain disorder, diet, stress, and family functioning have been suggested as possible causes, research has not shown any of these factors to be the direct cause of behavior or emotional problems. Some of the characteristics and behaviors seen in children who have emotional disturbances include the following:

- hyperactivity (short attention span, impulsiveness)

- aggression and self-injurious behavior (acting out, fighting)

- withdrawal (failure to initiate interaction with others, retreat from exchanges of social interaction, excessive fear or anxiety)

- immaturity (inappropriate crying, temper tantrums, poor coping skills)

- learning difficulties (academically performing below grade level)

Children with the most serious emotional disturbances may exhibit distorted thinking, excessive anxiety, bizarre motor acts, and abnormal mood swings. Some are identified as children who have a severe psychosis or schizophrenia.

Many children who do not have emotional disturbances may display some of these same behaviors at various times during their development. However, when children have an emotional disturbance, these behaviors continue over long periods of time. Their behavior thus signals that they are not coping with their environment or peers.

Educational Implications

The educational programs for children with an emotional disturbance need to include attention to providing emotional and behavioral support as well as helping them to master academics, develop social skills, and increase self-awareness, self-control, and self-esteem. A large body of research exists regarding methods of providing students with positive behavioral support in the school environment, so that problem behaviors are minimized and positive, appropriate behaviors are fostered. It is also important to know that, within the school setting:

- For a child whose behavior impedes learning (including the learning of others), the team developing the child's individualized education program (IEP) needs to consider, if appropriate, strategies to address that behavior, including positive behavioral interventions, strategies, and supports.

- Students eligible for special education services under the category of emotional disturbance may have psychological or counseling services included in their IEP. These are important related services which are available under law and are to be provided by a qualified social worker, psychologist, guidance counselor, or other qualified personnel.

- Career education (both vocational and academic) is also a major part of secondary education and should be a part of the transition plan included in every adolescent's IEP.

There is growing recognition that families, as well as their children, need support, respite care, intensive case management, and a collaborative, multi-agency approach to services. Many communities are working toward providing these wrap-around services. There are a growing number of agencies and organizations actively involved in establishing support services in the community.

Other Considerations

Families of children with emotional disturbances may need help in understanding their children's condition and in learning how to work effectively with them. Help is available from psychiatrists, psychologists or other mental health professionals in public or private mental health settings. Children should be provided services based on their individual needs, and all persons who are involved with these children should be aware of the care they are receiving. It is important to coordinate all services between home, school, and therapeutic community with open communication.

Chapter 25

Fetal Alcohol Syndrome and Other Mental Retardation

Fetal Alcohol Syndrome

Prenatal exposure to alcohol can cause a range of disorders, known as fetal alcohol spectrum disorders (FASD). One of the most severe effects of drinking during pregnancy is fetal alcohol syndrome (FAS). FAS is one of the leading known preventable causes of mental retardation and birth defects. If a woman drinks alcohol during her pregnancy, her baby can be born with FAS, a lifelong condition that causes physical and mental disabilities. FAS is characterized by abnormal facial features, growth deficiencies, and central nervous system (CNS) problems. People with FAS might have problems with learning, memory, attention span, communication, vision, hearing, or a combination of these. These problems often lead to difficulties in school and problems getting along with others. FAS is a permanent condition. It affects every aspect of an individual's life and the lives of his or her family.

Fetal alcohol spectrum disorders include FAS as well as other conditions in which individuals have some, but not all, of the clinical signs of FAS. Three terms often used are fetal alcohol effects (FAE), alcohol-related neurodevelopmental disorder (ARND), and alcohol-related birth defects (ARBD). The term FAE has been used to describe behavioral and cognitive problems in children who were

This chapter includes text from "Fetal Alcohol Syndrome Information," Centers for Disease Control and Prevention (CDC), May 2, 2006; and excerpts from "Mental Retardation," Fact Sheet 8, National Dissemination Center for Children with Disabilities (NICHCY), January 2004.

prenatally exposed to alcohol, but who do not have all of the typical diagnostic features of FAS. In 1996, the Institute of Medicine (IOM) replaced FAE with the terms ARND and ARBD. Children with ARND might have functional or mental problems linked to prenatal alcohol exposure. These include behavioral or cognitive abnormalities, or a combination of both. Children with ARBD might have problems with the heart, kidneys, bones, or hearing.

How common are FAS and FASD?

The reported rates of FAS vary widely. These different rates depend on the population studied and the surveillance methods used. CDC studies show FAS rates ranging from 0.2 to 1.5 per 1,000 live births in different areas of the United States. Other FASD are believed to occur approximately three times as often as FAS.

What are the characteristics of children with FAS and other FASD?

FAS is the severe end of a spectrum of effects that can occur when a woman drinks during pregnancy. Fetal death is the most extreme outcome. FAS is a disorder characterized by abnormal facial features and growth and central nervous system (CNS) problems. If a pregnant woman drinks alcohol but her child does not have all of the symptoms of FAS, it is possible that her child has another FASD, such as alcohol-related neurodevelopmental disorder (ARND). Children with ARND do not have full FAS but might demonstrate learning and behavioral problems caused by prenatal exposure to alcohol. Examples of these problems are difficulties with mathematical skills, difficulties with memory or attention, poor school performance, and poor impulse control or judgment.

Children with FASD might have the following characteristics or exhibit the following behaviors:

- small size for gestational age or small stature in relation to peers
- facial abnormalities such as small eye openings
- poor coordination
- hyperactive behavior
- learning disabilities
- developmental disabilities (for example, speech and language delays)

- mental retardation or low intelligence quotient (IQ)
- problems with daily living
- poor reasoning and judgment skills
- sleep and sucking disturbances in infancy

Children with FASD are at risk for psychiatric problems, criminal behavior, unemployment, and incomplete education. These are secondary conditions that an individual is not born with but might acquire as a result of FAS or a related disorder. These conditions can be very serious, but there are protective factors that have been found to help individuals with FASD. For example, a child who is diagnosed early in life can be placed in appropriate educational classes and given access to social services that can help the child and his or her family. Children with FASD who receive special education are more likely to achieve their developmental and educational potential. In addition, children with FASD need a loving, nurturing, and stable home life to avoid disruptions, transient lifestyles, or harmful relationships. Children with FASD who live in abusive or unstable homes or who become involved in youth violence are much more likely than those who do not have such negative experiences to develop secondary conditions.

If you think your child might have an FASD, contact your doctor who might be able to refer you to a specialist who can assess your child.

How can we prevent FASD?

Fetal alcohol spectrum disorders are completely preventable—if a woman does not drink alcohol while she is pregnant or could become pregnant. If a woman is drinking during pregnancy, it is never too late for her to stop. The sooner a woman stops drinking, the better it will be for both her baby and herself. If a woman is not able to stop drinking, she should contact her doctor, local Alcoholics Anonymous, or local alcohol treatment center. If a woman is sexually active and is not using an effective form of birth control, she should not drink alcohol. She could become pregnant and not know it for several weeks or more.

Mothers are not the only ones who can prevent FASD. The father's role is also important in helping the mother abstain from drinking alcohol during pregnancy. He can encourage her not drinking alcohol by avoiding social situations that involve drinking and by not drinking alcohol himself. Significant others, family members, schools, health and social service organizations, and communities can also help prevent FASD through education and intervention.

Mental Retardation

Mental retardation is a term used when a person has certain limitations in mental functioning and in skills such as communicating, personal care and social skills. These limitations will cause a child to learn and develop more slowly than a typical child. Children with mental retardation may take longer to learn to speak, walk, and take care of their personal needs such as dressing or eating. They are likely to have trouble learning in school. They will learn, but it will take them longer. There may be some things they cannot learn.

What causes mental retardation?

Doctors have found many causes of mental retardation. The most common include the following:

- **Genetic conditions:** Sometimes mental retardation is caused by abnormal genes inherited from parents, errors when genes combine, or other reasons. Examples of genetic conditions are Down syndrome, fragile X syndrome, and phenylketonuria (PKU).

- **Problems during pregnancy:** Mental retardation can result when the baby does not develop inside the mother properly. For example, there may be a problem with the way the baby's cells divide as it grows. A woman who drinks alcohol or gets an infection like rubella during pregnancy may also have a baby with mental retardation.

- **Problems at birth:** If a baby has problems during labor and birth, such as not getting enough oxygen, he or she may have mental retardation.

- **Health problems:** Diseases like whooping cough, the measles, or meningitis can cause mental retardation. Mental retardation can also be caused by extreme malnutrition (not eating right), not getting enough medical care, or by being exposed to poisons like lead or mercury.

Mental retardation is not a disease. You can't catch mental retardation from anyone. Mental retardation is also not a type of mental illness, like depression. There is no cure for mental retardation. However, most children with mental retardation can learn to do many things. It just takes them more time and effort than other children.

How is mental retardation diagnosed?

Mental retardation is diagnosed by looking at two main things. These are:

- the ability of a person's brain to learn, think, solve problems, and make sense of the world (called IQ or intellectual functioning); and

- whether the person has the skills he or she needs to live independently (called adaptive behavior, or adaptive functioning).

Intellectual functioning, or IQ, is usually measured by a test called an IQ test. The average score is 100. People scoring below 70 to 75 are thought to have mental retardation. To diagnose mental retardation, professionals look at the person's mental abilities (IQ) and his or her adaptive skills. To measure adaptive behavior, professionals look at what a child can do in comparison to other children of his or her age. Certain skills are important to adaptive behavior. These are:

- daily living skills, such as getting dressed, going to the bathroom, and feeding one's self;

- communication skills, such as understanding what is said and being able to answer; and,

- social skills with peers, family members, adults, and others.

Providing services to help individuals with mental retardation has led to a new understanding of how we define mental retardation. After the initial diagnosis of mental retardation is made, we look at a person's strengths and weaknesses. We also look at how much support or help the person needs to get along at home, in school, and in the community. This approach gives a realistic picture of each individual. It also recognizes that the situation can change. As the person grows and learns, his or her ability to get along in the world grows as well.

IDEA defines mental retardation as ". . . significantly subaverage general intellectual functioning, existing concurrently with deficits in adaptive behavior and manifested during the developmental period, that adversely affects a child's educational performance." [34 Code of Federal Regulations §300.7(c)(6)]

How common is mental retardation?

As many as three out of every 100 people in the country have mental retardation (The Arc, 2001). Nearly 613,000 children ages 6–21 have some level of mental retardation and need special education in school (Twenty-Fourth Annual Report to Congress, U.S. Department of Education, 2002). In fact, one out of every ten children who need special education has some form of mental retardation.

What are the signs of mental retardation?

There are many signs of mental retardation. For example, children with mental retardation may:

- sit up, crawl, or walk later than other children;
- learn to talk later, or have trouble speaking;
- find it hard to remember things;
- not understand how to pay for things;
- have trouble understanding social rules;
- have trouble seeing the consequences of their actions;
- have trouble solving problems; or,
- have trouble thinking logically.

About 87% of people with mental retardation will only be a little slower than average in learning new information and skills. When they are children, their limitations may not be obvious. They may not even be diagnosed as having mental retardation until they get to school. As they become adults, many people with mild retardation can live independently. Other people may not even consider them as having mental retardation.

The remaining 13% of people with mental retardation score below 50 on IQ tests. These people will have more difficulty in school, at home, and in the community. A person with more severe retardation will need more intensive support his or her entire life. Every child with mental retardation is able to learn, develop, and grow. With help, all children with mental retardation can live a satisfying life.

What about school?

A child with mental retardation can do well in school but is likely to need individualized help. Fortunately, states are responsible for meeting the educational needs of children with disabilities.

For children up to age three, services are provided through an early intervention system. Staff work with the child's family to develop what is known as an individualized family services plan, or IFSP. The IFSP will describe the child's unique needs. It also describes the services the child will receive to address those needs. The IFSP will emphasize the unique needs of the family, so that parents and other family members will know how to help their young child with mental retardation. Early intervention services may be provided on a sliding-fee basis, meaning that the costs to the family will depend upon their income. In some states, early intervention services may be at no cost to parents.

For eligible school-aged children (including preschoolers), special education and related services are made available through the school system. School staff will work with the child's parents to develop an individualized education program (IEP). The IEP is similar to an IFSP. It describes the child's unique needs and the services that have been designed to meet those needs. Special education and related services are provided at no cost to parents.

Many children with mental retardation need help with adaptive skills, which are skills needed to live, work, and play in the community. Teachers and parents can help a child work on these skills at both school and home. Some of these skills include:

- communicating with others;
- taking care of personal needs (dressing, bathing, going to the bathroom);
- health and safety;
- home living (helping to set the table, cleaning the house, or cooking dinner);
- social skills (manners, knowing the rules of conversation, getting along in a group, playing a game);
- reading, writing, and basic math; and,
- as they get older, skills that will help them in the workplace.

Supports or changes in the classroom (called adaptations) help most students with mental retardation.

Tips for Parents

- Learn about mental retardation. The more you know, the more you can help yourself and your child.
- Encourage independence in your child. For example, help your child learn daily care skills, such as dressing, feeding him or herself, using the bathroom, and grooming.

- Give your child chores. Keep her age, attention span, and abilities in mind. Break down jobs into smaller steps. For example, if your child's job is to set the table, first ask her to get the right number of napkins. Then have her put one at each family member's place at the table. Do the same with the utensils, going one at a time. Tell her what to do, step by step, until the job is done. Demonstrate how to do the job. Help her when she needs assistance. Give your child frequent feedback. Praise your child when he or she does well. Build your child's abilities.

- Find out what skills your child is learning at school. Find ways for your child to apply those skills at home. For example, if the teacher is going over a lesson about money, take your child to the supermarket with you. Help him count out the money to pay for your groceries. Help him count the change.

- Find opportunities in your community for social activities, such as scouts, recreation center activities, sports, and so on. These will help your child build social skills as well as to have fun.

- Talk to other parents whose children have mental retardation. Parents can share practical advice and emotional support. Call NICHCY (800-695-0285) and ask how to find a parent group near you.

- Meet with the school and develop an educational plan to address your child's needs. Keep in touch with your child's teachers. Offer support. Find out how you can support your child's school learning at home.

Tips for Teachers

- Learn as much as you can about mental retardation.

- Recognize that you can make an enormous difference in this student's life. Find out what the student's strengths and interests are, and emphasize them. Create opportunities for success.

- If you are not part of the student's individualized education program (IEP) team, ask for a copy of his or her IEP. The student's educational goals will be listed there, as well as the services and classroom accommodations he or she is to receive. Talk to specialists in your school as necessary. They can help you identify effective methods of teaching this student, ways to adapt the curriculum, and how to address the student's IEP goals in your classroom.

- Be as concrete as possible. Demonstrate what you mean rather than just giving verbal directions. Rather than just relating new information verbally, show a picture. And rather than just showing a picture, provide the student with hands-on materials and experiences and the opportunity to try things out.

- Break longer, new tasks into small steps. Demonstrate the steps. Have the student do the steps, one at a time. Provide assistance, as necessary.

- Give the student immediate feedback.

- Teach the student life skills such as daily living, social skills, and occupational awareness and exploration, as appropriate. Involve the student in group activities or clubs.

- Work together with the student's parents and other school personnel to create and implement an educational plan tailored to meet the student's needs. Regularly share information about how the student is doing at school and at home.

Chapter 26

Gerstmann Syndrome

Gerstmann syndrome is a cognitive impairment that results from damage to a specific area of the brain—the left parietal lobe in the region of the angular gyrus. It may occur after a stroke or in association with damage to the parietal lobe. It is characterized by four primary symptoms: a writing disability (agraphia or dysgraphia), a lack of understanding of the rules for calculation or arithmetic (acalculia or dyscalculia), an inability to distinguish right from left, and an inability to identify fingers (finger agnosia). The disorder should not be confused with Gerstmann-Sträussler-Scheinker disease, a type of transmissible spongiform encephalopathy.

In addition to exhibiting the above symptoms, many adults also experience aphasia, (difficulty in expressing oneself when speaking, in understanding speech, or in reading and writing).

There are few reports of the syndrome, sometimes called developmental Gerstmann syndrome, in children. The cause is not known. Most cases are identified when children reach school age, a time when they are challenged with writing and math exercises. Generally, children with the disorder exhibit poor handwriting and spelling skills, and difficulty with math functions, including adding, subtracting, multiplying, and dividing. An inability to differentiate right from left and to discriminate among individual fingers may also be apparent. In addition to the four primary symptoms, many children also suffer

"Gerstmann Syndrome Information Page," National Institute of Neurological Disorders and Stroke (NINDS), July 2, 2008.

from constructional apraxia, an inability to copy simple drawings. Frequently, there is also reading impairment. Children with a high level of intellectual functioning as well as those with brain damage may be affected with the disorder.

Is there any treatment?

There is no cure for Gerstmann syndrome. Treatment is symptomatic and supportive. Occupational and speech therapies may help diminish the dysgraphia and apraxia. In addition, calculators and word processors may help school children cope with the symptoms of the disorder.

What is the prognosis?

In adults, many of the symptoms diminish over time. Although it has been suggested that in children symptoms may diminish over time, it appears likely that most children probably do not overcome their deficits, but learn to adjust to them.

What research is being done?

The National Institute of Neurological Disorders and Stroke (NINDS) supports research on disorders that result from damage to the brain such as dysgraphia. The NINDS and other components of the National Institutes of Health also support research on learning disabilities. Current research avenues focus on developing techniques to diagnose and treat learning disabilities and increase understanding of the biological basis of them.

Chapter 27

Hearing Impairment

What's Hearing Loss?

You know what hearing is, but what is hearing loss? Hearing loss, or hearing impairment (say: im-pare-ment), happens when there is a problem with one or more parts of the ear or ears. Someone who has hearing loss or impairment may be able to hear some sounds or nothing at all. Impairment means something is not working correctly or as well as it should. People also may use the words deaf, deafness, or hard of hearing when they're talking about hearing loss.

About three in 1,000 babies are born with hearing impairment, making it the most common birth defect. A hearing problem can also develop later in life. To understand how and why hearing loss happens, it helps to know how the ear works.

How Hearing Works

The ear is made up of three different sections: the outer ear, the middle ear, and the inner ear. These parts work together so you can hear

This chapter includes: "What's Hearing Loss?" June 2006, reprinted with permission from www.Kids.Health.org. Copyright © 2006 The Nemours Foundation. This information was provided by KidsHealth, one of the largest resources online for medically reviewed health information written for parents, kids, and teens. For more articles like this one, visit www.KidsHealth.org, or www.TeensHealth.org. Also, excerpts from "Has Your Baby's Hearing Been Screened?" National Institute on Deafness and Other Communication Disorders (NIDCD), December 2007.

and process sounds. The outer ear, or pinna (the part you can see), picks up sound waves and the waves then travel through the outer ear canal.

When the sound waves hit the eardrum in the middle ear, the eardrum starts to vibrate. When the eardrum vibrates, it moves three tiny bones in your ear. These bones are called the hammer (or malleus), anvil (or incus), and stirrup (or stapes). They help sound move along on its journey into the inner ear.

The vibrations then travel to the cochlea, which is filled with liquid and lined with cells that have thousands of tiny hairs on their surfaces. There are two types of hair cells: the outer and inner cells. The sound vibrations make the tiny hairs move. The outer hair cells take the sound information, amplify it (make it louder), and tune it. The inner hair cells send the sound information to your hearing nerve, which then sends it to your brain, allowing you to hear.

Types of Hearing Loss

There are a few different types of hearing loss: conductive, sensory, mixed (conductive and sensory combined), and neural.

- **Conductive (say: kun-duk-tiv) hearing loss:** This happens when there is a problem with a part of the outer or middle ear. Most kids with conductive hearing loss have a mild hearing loss and it is usually temporary because in most cases medical treatment can help.

- **Sensory (say: sen-suh-ree) hearing loss:** This happens when the cochlea is not working correctly because the tiny hair cells are damaged or destroyed. Depending on the loss, a kid may be able to hear most sounds (although they would be muffled); may be able to hear in quiet but not in noise; only some sounds; or no sounds at all. Sensory hearing impairment is almost always permanent and a kid's ability to talk normally may be affected.

- **Neural (say: nur-ul) hearing loss:** This happens when there is a problem with the connection from the cochlea to the brain. Neural means related to nerve, so neural hearing loss means the nerve that carries the messages from the cochlea to the brain is damaged.

What Causes Hearing Loss?

Hearing loss can happen because a person was born with parts of the ear that didn't form correctly and don't work well. Other problems can happen later because of an injury or illness, including:

- middle ear fluid;
- serious infections, such as meningitis;
- head injury;
- listening to very loud music, especially through headphones;
- repeated exposure to loud sounds, such as machinery.

Lots of kids have had ear infections, which also can cause hearing loss. Permanent hearing loss is rare from an ear infection, but you need to visit the doctor if you or your parents suspect you have one.

How Does a Doctor Test for Hearing Loss?

If a doctor thinks that a baby or child may have hearing loss, the doctor will recommend that the parents take him or her to an audiologist. An audiologist (say: awd-ee-ah-luh-jist) is someone who is specially trained to test and help with the problems related to hearing loss.

A pediatric audiologist tests a child's hearing by doing different types of tests. They even have hearing tests for babies. Maybe you've had a hearing test, when you wore headphones and had to raise your left or right hand to show that you could hear in each ear.

If an audiologist finds that a child has hearing loss, he or she will recommend treatment and suggest the family work with a special team. This team can help figure out the best way for the kid to learn and communicate.

How Is Hearing Loss Treated?

The kind of treatment depends on the type of hearing loss, how severe it is, and the child's other needs. Common treatments include medicine, operations, hearing aids, or assistive listening devices, which emphasize voices and help kids hear better in noisy settings. With treatment, most kids will be able to hear normally again.

Hearing aids are kind of like tiny amplifiers. They help someone hear sounds better and can even pick up the sounds so that what kids hear is more clear. Hearing aids deliver amplified sounds (via sound vibrations) from the eardrum and middle ear to the inner ear or cochlea. Hearing aid technology is available that can adjust the volume of sounds automatically.

For some kids who are not able to hear or understand words even with the help of hearing aids, there is a device called a cochlear implant (say: ko-klee-ur im-plant). This is a very tiny piece of electronic equipment that is put into the cochlea during an operation. It takes over the job of the damaged or destroyed hair cells in the cochlea by turning sounds into electrical signals that stimulate the hearing nerve directly.

Learning and Communicating

A kid with hearing loss may attend a special school, special classes within a regular school, or may be part of a regular classroom. Depending on how severe their hearing loss is, some kids may work with audiologists or speech-language pathologists to help them develop their hearing and speaking skills. Some people with hearing loss may need to use special techniques like these to communicate:

- Speechreading, which involves looking closely at a person's lips, facial expressions, and gestures to help figure out spoken words.

- American Sign Language, or ASL, which is a language of hand movements that allows deaf people to communicate with one another without speaking.

What about talking on the phone? Thanks to a telecommunication device, also called a telecommunications device for the deaf (TDD), a conversation can be typed out instead of spoken. The messages appear on a special screen or on a printout.

You might wonder how a hearing-impaired person could see a movie or watch television (TV). Closed-captioned TV shows and movies provide text at the bottom of the screen, so people with hearing loss can read along to follow the action.

So hearing-impaired kids can go to school, talk on the phone, and watch a movie. If that sounds a lot like a typical kid's life, you're right.

Has Your Baby's Hearing Been Screened?

How early should I have my baby's hearing screened?

Your baby should have a hearing screening within the first month of life. If hearing loss is suspected, make sure a hearing expert, called an audiologist tests your baby's hearing by three months of age. If hearing loss is confirmed, it is important to consider the use of hearing devices and other communication options by six months of age.

Where can my baby's hearing be screened?

Many hospitals automatically screen all newborns for hearing loss. Some screen only those newborns at high risk for hearing loss, such as babies with a family history of deafness or hearing problems, low birth weight, or certain other medical conditions. Even if your baby does not have risk factors, being screened is important, because many children with no risk factors have hearing loss. Even children whose parents and grandparents hear normally may be born with a hearing loss. Find out what your hospital does. If you and your baby are already home and you don't know if your baby's hearing was tested, ask the doctor or the clinic where your baby's records are.

Many states have passed early hearing detection and intervention legislation. A few other states regularly screen the hearing of most newborns, but have no legislation that requires screening. To find out what your state does, visit the American Speech-Language-Hearing Association (ASHA) website at http://www.asha.org.

How will my baby's hearing be screened?

Two hearing tests are used to screen babies. In both tests, no activity is required from your child other than lying still.

- **Otoacoustic emissions (OAE):** This test can show whether parts of the ear respond properly to sound. During this test, a sponge earphone is placed into the ear canal. The ear is stimulated with sound, and the "echo" is measured. The echo is found in everyone who hears normally. If there is no echo, it could indicate a hearing loss.

- **Auditory brain stem response (ABR):** This test checks how the brain stem (the part of the nerve that carries sound from the ear to the brain) and the brain respond to sound. During this test, your child wears earphones, and electrodes are placed on the head and ears. A mild sedative may be given to help keep your child calm and quiet during the test. The nurse or doctor sends sounds through the earphones and measures the electrical activity in your child's brain when he or she should be hearing.

If your child doesn't respond consistently to the sounds presented during either of these tests, your doctor may suggest a follow up hearing screening and a referral to an audiologist for a more comprehensive hearing evaluation.

213

Why is it important to have my baby's hearing screened early?

The most important time for a child to be exposed to and learn language is in the first three years of life. In fact, children begin learning speech and language in the first six months of life. Research suggests that those who have hearing impairment and get intervention have better language skills than those who do not. The earlier you know about deafness or hearing loss, the sooner you can make sure your child benefits from strategies that will help him or her learn to communicate.

How can I recognize hearing loss during early childhood?

Even though screening is designed to detect hearing loss as early as possible, some children don't develop hearing loss until later in life. In those instances, parents, caregivers, or grandparents are often the first to notice. Even if you've had your baby's hearing tested, you should look for signs that your baby is hearing well.

For example, during the first year, notice whether your baby reacts to loud noises, imitates sounds, and begins to respond to his or her name. At age two, ask yourself whether or not your child plays with his or her voice, imitates simple words, and enjoys games like peek-a-boo and pat-a-cake. Is he or she using two-word sentences to talk about and ask for things? At age three, notice whether or not he or she begins to understand "not now" and "no more" and follows simple directions. If for any reason you think your child is not hearing well, talk to your doctor.

How can I help my child communicate?

There are a variety of ways to help children with hearing loss express themselves and interact with others. The main options are listed below. The option you choose will depend on how you want your child to learn and communicate. Find out about all of the choices and talk to lots of experts.

- **Oral/auditory options:** Combine hearing, lip-reading, and hearing devices such as hearing aids and cochlear implants. The goals of oral/auditory options are to help children develop speech and English-language skills.

- **American Sign Language (ASL):** A language used by some deaf children and their families. ASL consists of hand signs, body movements, facial expressions, and gestures. It's a language with its own grammar and syntax, which are different from English. ASL has no written form.

- **Cued speech:** A system that uses handshapes in different locations along with the natural mouth movements to represent speech sounds. Watching the mouth movements and the handshapes can help some children learn to speech-read English; this is especially important in discriminating between sounds that sound different but look the same on the lips.

- **Signed English:** A system that uses signs to represent words or phrases in the English language. Signed English is designed to enhance the use of both spoken and written English.

- **Combined options:** Use portions of the various methods listed above. For example, some deaf children who use oral/auditory options also learn sign language. Children who use ASL also learn to read and write in English. Combined options can expose children who are deaf or hard of hearing to many different ways to communicate and express themselves.

Will my child have a tough time in school?

Just like other children, children who are deaf or hard-of-hearing can develop strong academic, social, and emotional skills and succeed in school. You can do a lot to make sure this happens. Find out how your school system helps children with hearing loss. With your input, your child's school will develop an individualized education program (IEP) for your child. Explore programs outside of school that may help you and your child, and talk with other parents who have already dealt with these issues. Remember, the Individuals with Disabilities Education Act (IDEA) ensures that children with hearing loss receive free, appropriate, early intervention programs from birth throughout the school years.

Chapter 28

Pervasive Developmental Disorders

Chapter Contents

Section 28.1

Autism Spectrum Disorders

Text in this section is from: "Autism Spectrum Disorders: Pervasive Developmental Disorders, with February 2007 Addendum," National Institute of Mental Health (NIMH), NIH Publication No. 06–5511, 2007; "Learning to Diagnose Autism Spectrum Disorders," by Vicki Contie, *NIH Research Matters*, National Institutes of Health (NIH), July 16, 2007; and, text under the heading "Autism Spectrum Disorder: Classification and Education," is excerpted from "Autism and Pervasive Developmental Disorder," National Dissemination Center for Children with Disabilities (NICHCY), April 2007.

Autism Spectrum Disorders

The autism spectrum disorders (ASD) are more common in the pediatric population than are some better known disorders such as diabetes, spinal bifida, or Down syndrome. Pediatricians, family physicians, daycare providers, teachers, and parents may initially dismiss signs of ASD, optimistically thinking the child is just a little slow and will catch up. Although early intervention has a dramatic impact on reducing symptoms and increasing a child's ability to grow and learn new skills, it is estimated that only 50% of children are diagnosed before kindergarten.

Children with ASD do not follow the typical patterns of child development. In some children, hints of future problems may be apparent from birth. In most cases, the problems in communication and social skills become more noticeable as the child lags further behind other children the same age. Some other children start off well enough. Oftentimes between 12 and 36 months old, the differences in the way they react to people and other unusual behaviors become apparent. Some parents report the change as being sudden, and that their children start to reject people, act strangely, and lose language and social skills they had previously acquired. In other cases, there is a plateau, or leveling, of progress so that the difference between the child with autism and other children the same age becomes more noticeable.

ASD is defined by a certain set of behaviors that can range from the very mild to the severe. The following are possible indicators of ASD:

- does not babble, point, or make meaningful gestures by one year of age
- does not speak one word by 16 months
- does not combine two words by two years.
- does not respond to name
- loses language or social skills
- poor eye contact
- doesn't seem to know how to play with toys
- excessively lines up toys or other objects
- is attached to one particular toy or object
- doesn't smile
- at times seems to be hearing impaired

Social Symptoms

From the start, typically developing infants are social beings. Early in life, they gaze at people, turn toward voices, grasp a finger, and even smile. In contrast, most children with ASD seem to have tremendous difficulty learning to engage in the give-and-take of everyday human interaction. Even in the first few months of life, many do not interact and they avoid eye contact. They seem indifferent to other people, and often seem to prefer being alone. They may resist attention or passively accept hugs and cuddling. Later, they seldom seek comfort or respond to parents' displays of anger or affection in a typical way. Research has suggested that although children with ASD are attached to their parents, their expression of this attachment is unusual and difficult to read. To parents, it may seem as if their child is not attached at all. Parents who looked forward to the joys of cuddling, teaching, and playing with their child may feel crushed by this lack of the expected and typical attachment behavior.

Children with ASD also are slower in learning to interpret what others are thinking and feeling. Subtle social cues—whether a smile, a wink, or a grimace—may have little meaning. To a child who misses these cues, "come here" always means the same thing, whether the speaker is smiling and extending her arms for a hug, or frowning and planting her fists on her hips. Without the ability to interpret gestures and facial expressions, the social world may seem bewildering.

To compound the problem, people with ASD have difficulty seeing things from another person's perspective. Most five-year-olds understand that other people have different information, feelings, and goals than they have. A person with ASD may lack such understanding. This inability leaves them unable to predict or understand other people's actions.

Although not universal, it is common for people with ASD also to have difficulty regulating their emotions. This can take the form of immature behavior such as crying in class or verbal outbursts that seem inappropriate to those around them. The individual with ASD might also be disruptive and physically aggressive at times, making social relationships still more difficult. They have a tendency to lose control, particularly when they're in a strange or overwhelming environment, or when angry and frustrated. They may at times break things, attack others, or hurt themselves. In their frustration, some bang their heads, pull their hair, or bite their arms.

Communication Difficulties

By age three, most children have passed predictable milestones on the path to learning language; one of the earliest is babbling. By the first birthday, a typical toddler says words, turns when he hears his name, points when he wants a toy, and when offered something distasteful, makes it clear that the answer is no.

Some children diagnosed with ASD remain mute throughout their lives. Some infants who later show signs of ASD coo and babble during the first few months of life, but they soon stop. Others may be delayed, developing language as late as age five to nine. Some children may learn to use communication systems such as pictures or sign language.

Those who do speak often use language in unusual ways. They seem unable to combine words into meaningful sentences. Some speak only single words, while others repeat the same phrase over and over. Some ASD children parrot what they hear, a condition called echolalia. Although many children with no ASD go through a stage where they repeat what they hear, it normally passes by the time they are three.

Some children only mildly affected may exhibit slight delays in language, or even seem to have precocious language and unusually large vocabularies, but have great difficulty in sustaining a conversation. The give and take of normal conversation is hard for them, although they often carry on a monologue on a favorite subject, giving no one else an opportunity to comment. Another difficulty is often the inability to understand body language, tone of voice, or phrases of speech. They might interpret a sarcastic expression such as "oh, that's just great" as meaning it really is great.

While it can be hard to understand what ASD children are saying, their body language is also difficult to understand. Facial expressions, movements, and gestures rarely match what they are saying. Also, their tone of voice fails to reflect their feelings. A high-pitched, sing-song, or flat, robot-like voice is common. Some children with relatively good language skills speak like little adults, failing to pick up on the kid-speak that is common in their peers.

Without meaningful gestures or the language to ask for things, people with ASD are at a loss to let others know what they need. As a result, they may simply scream or grab what they want. Until they are taught better ways to express their needs, ASD children do whatever they can to get through to others. As people with ASD grow up, they can become increasingly aware of their difficulties in understanding others and in being understood. As a result they may become anxious or depressed.

Repetitive Behaviors

Although children with ASD usually appear physically normal and have good muscle control, odd repetitive motions may set them off from other children. These behaviors might be extreme and highly apparent or more subtle. Some children and older individuals spend a lot of time repeatedly flapping their arms or walking on their toes. Some suddenly freeze in position.

As children, they might spend hours lining up their cars and trains in a certain way, rather than using them for pretend play. If someone accidentally moves one of the toys, the child may be tremendously upset. ASD children need, and demand, absolute consistency in their environment. A slight change in any routine—in mealtimes, dressing, taking a bath, going to school at a certain time and by the same route—can be extremely disturbing. Perhaps order and sameness lend some stability in a world of confusion.

Repetitive behavior sometimes takes the form of a persistent, intense preoccupation. For example, the child might be obsessed with learning all about vacuum cleaners, train schedules, or lighthouses. Often there is great interest in numbers, symbols, or science topics.

Problems That May Accompany ASD

Sensory problems: When children's perceptions are accurate, they can learn from what they see, feel, or hear. On the other hand, if sensory information is faulty, the child's experiences of the world can be confusing. Many ASD children are highly attuned or even painfully sensitive to certain sounds, textures, tastes, and smells. Some children find the feel of clothes touching their skin almost unbearable. Some sounds—a vacuum cleaner, a ringing telephone, a sudden storm, even the sound of waves lapping the shoreline—will cause these children to cover their ears and scream.

In ASD, the brain seems unable to balance the senses appropriately. Some ASD children are oblivious to extreme cold or pain. An ASD child may fall and break an arm, yet never cry. Another may bash his head against a wall and not wince, but a light touch may make the child scream with alarm.

Mental retardation: Many children with ASD have some degree of mental impairment. When tested, some areas of ability may be normal, while others may be especially weak. For example, a child with ASD may do well on the parts of the test that measure visual skills but earn low scores on the language subtests.

Seizures: One in four children with ASD develops seizures, often starting either in early childhood or adolescence. Seizures, caused by abnormal electrical activity in the brain, can produce a temporary loss of consciousness (a blackout), a body convulsion, unusual movements, or staring spells. Sometimes a contributing factor is a lack of sleep or a high fever. An EEG (electroencephalogram—a recording of the electric currents developed in the brain by means of electrodes applied to the scalp) can help confirm the seizure's presence.

In most cases, seizures can be controlled by a number of medicines called anticonvulsants. The dosage of the medication is adjusted carefully so that the least possible amount of medication will be used to be effective.

Fragile X syndrome: This disorder is the most common inherited form of mental retardation. It was so named because one part of the X chromosome has a defective piece that appears pinched and fragile when under a microscope. Fragile X syndrome affects about two to five percent of people with ASD. It is important to have a child with ASD checked for fragile X, especially if the parents are considering having another child. For an unknown reason, if a child with ASD also has fragile X, there is a one-in-two chance that boys born to the same parents will have the syndrome. Other members of the family who may be contemplating having a child may also wish to be checked for the syndrome.

Tuberous sclerosis: This is a rare genetic disorder that causes benign tumors to grow in the brain as well as in other vital organs. It has a consistently strong association with ASD. One to four percent of people with ASD also have tuberous sclerosis.

Learning to Diagnose Autism Spectrum Disorders

For children with autism, the sooner the disorder is identified and treated the better the outcome for the child. Now researchers report that it's possible to detect autism in some children as young as 14 months of age, the earliest the disorder has ever been diagnosed. In other children, the scientists didn't see definite signs of autism until later—by about two years old.

Most experts agree that early intervention—including behavioral therapies, specialized teaching and medication—can improve quality of life for years to come. Unfortunately, ASD is rarely diagnosed before age three.

Dr. Rebecca J. Landa at the Kennedy Krieger Institute in Baltimore and her colleagues set out to study the progression of ASD in at-risk children to see if earlier diagnoses could be made. As reported in the July 2007 issue of the *Archives of General Psychiatry*, the scientists studied 107 children considered to be at high risk for ASD because they had a sibling with the disorder. An additional 18 children with no family history of ASD served as the comparison group. The children's social and communication skills were repeatedly assessed beginning at 14 months until about three years of age.

By the end of the study, 30 of the high-risk children had been diagnosed with ASD. These children fell into two distinct groups. Half of them—called the early-diagnosis group—had dramatically lower social and communications abilities at 14 months of age than the other groups. The other half—the later-diagnosis group—were nearly indistinguishable from "normal" children at 14 months of age. However, by the time they were two years old, their social and communication skills declined and approached the lower scores of the early-diagnosis group.

These findings reveal two unique pathways that ASD may take during early childhood. While ASD can be distinguished in some children at just over one year of age, others appear to show only very subtle differences from normal development until after 14 months of age, when their skills begin to backslide.

The researchers note their findings may not be applicable to the general population, in part because all the children with ASD in their study had a familial risk. More research will be needed, with larger groups of children, to better understand the developmental patterns of ASD and to develop reliable tools for early diagnosis.

Autism Spectrum Disorder: Classification and Education

In the diagnostic manual used to classify mental disorders, the *Diagnostic and Statistical Manual of Mental Disorders, Fourth Edition, Text Revision (DSM-IV-TR)*, autistic disorder is listed under the heading of pervasive developmental disorders. A diagnosis of autistic disorder is made when an individual displays six or more of twelve symptoms across three major areas: (a) social interaction, (b) communication, and (c) behavior. When children display similar behaviors but do not meet the specific criteria for autistic disorder, they may receive a diagnosis of pervasive developmental disorder-not otherwise specified (PDD-NOS).

Autism is one of the disabilities specifically defined in the Individuals with Disabilities Education Act (IDEA), the federal legislation under which infants, toddlers, children, and youth with disabilities receive early intervention, special education, and related services. IDEA defines the disorder as "a developmental disability significantly affecting verbal and nonverbal communication and social interaction, generally evident before age three that adversely affects a child's educational performance. Other characteristics often associated with autism are engagement in repetitive activities and stereotyped movements, resistance to environmental change or change in daily routines, and unusual responses to sensory experiences." [See 34 Code of Federal Regulations §300.8(c)(1).]

How common is autism/PDD?

Information from the National Institute of Mental Health and the Centers for Disease Control and Prevention (CDC) indicates that between two to six per 1,000 children (from one in 500 to one in 150) have some form of autism/PDD. These disorders are four times more common in boys than in girls, although Rett syndrome has only been reported and diagnosed in girls.

The causes of autism or PDD are unknown. Currently, researchers are investigating areas such as brain development, structure, genetic factors, and biochemical imbalance in the brain as possible causes. These disorders are not caused by psychological factors.

What about school?

Early diagnosis and intervention are very important for children with autism/PDD. Under the Individuals with Disabilities Education Act, children with autism/PDD may be eligible for early intervention services (birth to three years) and an educational program appropriate to their individual needs. In addition to academic instruction, special education programs for students with autism/PDD (ages 3–22) focus on improving communication, social, academic, behavioral, and daily living skills. Behavior and communication problems that interfere with learning often require the assistance of a professional who is particularly knowledgeable in the autism field to develop and help implement a plan which can be carried out at home and school.

The classroom environment should be structured so that the program is consistent and predictable. Students with autism/PDD learn better and are less confused when information is presented visually as well as verbally. Interaction with non-disabled peers is also important, for these students provide models of appropriate language, social, and behavioral skills. Consistency and continuity are very important for children with autism/PDD, and parents should always be involved in the development of their child's program, so that learning activities, experiences, and approaches will be most effective and can be carried over into the home and community.

With educational programs designed to meet a student's individual needs and specialized adult support services in employment and living arrangements, many children and adults with autism/PDD grow to live, work, and participate fully in their communities.

Tips for Parents

- Learn about autism/PDD. The more you know, the more you can help yourself and your child.

- Be mindful to interact with and teach your child in ways that are most likely to get a positive response. Learn what is likely to trigger melt-downs for your child, so you can try to minimize them. Remember, the earliest years are the toughest, but it does get better.

- Learn from professionals and other parents how to meet your child's special needs, but remember your son or daughter is first and foremost a child; life does not need to become a never-ending round of therapies.

- If you weren't born loving highly structured, consistent schedules, and routines, ask for help from other parents and professionals on how to make it second nature for you. Behavior, communication, and social skills can all be areas of concern for a child with autism and experience tells us that maintaining a solid, loving, and structured approach in caring for your child, can help greatly.

- Learn about assistive technology that can help your child. This may include a simple picture communication board to help your child express needs and desires, or may be as sophisticated as an augmentative communication device.

- Work with professionals in early intervention or in your school to develop an individualized family service plan (IFSP) or an individualized education program (IEP) that reflects your child's needs and abilities. Be sure to include related services, supplementary aids and services, assistive technology, and a positive behavioral support plan, if needed.

- Be patient, and stay optimistic. Your child, like every child, has a whole lifetime to learn and grow.

Tips for Teachers

- Learn more about autism/PDD. Research effective instructional interventions and behavior guidelines for autistic/PDD students.

- Make sure directions are given step-by-step, verbally, visually, and by providing physical supports or prompts, as needed by the student. Students with autism spectrum disorders often have trouble interpreting facial expressions, body language, and tone of voice. Be as concrete and explicit as possible in your instructions and feedback to the student.

- Find out what the student's strengths and interests are and emphasize them. Tap into those avenues and create opportunities for success. Give positive feedback and lots of opportunities for practice.

- Build opportunities for the student to have social/collaborative interactions throughout the regular school day. Provide support, structure, and lots of feedback.

- If behavior is a significant issue for the student, seek help from expert professional resources (including parents) to understand the meanings of the behaviors and to develop a unified, positive approach to resolving them.

- Have consistent routines and schedules. When you know a change in routine will occur (for example, a field trip or assembly) prepare the student for what is going to be different and what to expect or do. Reward students for each small success.

- Work together with the student's parents and other school personnel to create and implement an educational plan tailored to meet the student's needs. Regularly share information about how the student is doing at school and at home.

Section 28.2

Asperger Syndrome

Excerpted from "Asperger Syndrome Fact Sheet," National Institute of Neurological Disorders and Stroke (NINDS), NIH Publication No. 05–5624, April 11, 2008.

Asperger syndrome (AS) is a developmental disorder that is characterized by limited interests or an unusual preoccupation with a particular subject to the exclusion of other activities including the following:

- repetitive routines or rituals

- peculiarities in speech and language, such as speaking in an overly formal manner or in a monotone, or taking figures of speech literally

- socially and emotionally inappropriate behavior and the inability to interact successfully with peers

- problems with non-verbal communication, including the restricted use of gestures, limited or inappropriate facial expressions, or a peculiar, stiff gaze

- clumsy and uncoordinated motor movements

AS is an autism spectrum disorder (ASD), one of a distinct group of neurological conditions characterized by a greater or lesser degree of impairment in language and communication skills, as well as repetitive or restrictive patterns of thought and behavior.

Parents usually sense there is something unusual about a child with AS by the time of his or her third birthday, and some children may exhibit symptoms as early as infancy. Unlike children with autism, children with AS retain their early language skills. Motor development delays—crawling or walking late, clumsiness—are sometimes the first indicator of the disorder.

The incidence of AS is not well established, but experts in population studies conservatively estimate that two out of every 10,000 children have the disorder. Boys are three to four times more likely than girls to have AS.

Studies of children with AS suggest that their problems with socialization and communication continue into adulthood. Some of these children develop additional psychiatric symptoms and disorders in adolescence and adulthood.

Although diagnosed mainly in children, AS is being increasingly diagnosed in adults who seek medical help for mental health conditions such as depression, obsessive-compulsive disorder (OCD), and attention deficit/hyperactivity disorder (AD/HD). No studies have yet been conducted to determine the incidence of AS in adult populations.

What are some common signs or symptoms?

The most distinguishing symptom of AS is a child's obsessive interest in a single object or topic to the exclusion of any other. Some children with AS have become experts on vacuum cleaners, makes and models of cars, even objects as odd as deep fat fryers. Children with AS want to know everything about their topic of interest and their conversations with others will be about little else. Their expertise, high level of vocabulary, and formal speech patterns make them seem like little professors.

Children with AS will gather enormous amounts of factual information about their favorite subject and will talk incessantly about it, but the conversation may seem like a random collection of facts or statistics, with no point or conclusion. Their speech may be marked by a lack of rhythm, an odd inflection, or a monotone pitch. Children with AS often lack the ability to modulate the volume of their voice to match their surroundings. For example, they will have to be reminded to talk softly every time they enter a library or a movie theatre.

Unlike the severe withdrawal from the rest of the world that is characteristic of autism, children with AS are isolated because of their poor social skills and narrow interests. In fact, they may approach other people, but make normal conversation impossible by inappropriate or eccentric behavior, or by wanting only to talk about their singular interest.

Children with AS usually have a history of developmental delays in motor skills such as pedaling a bike, catching a ball, or climbing outdoor play equipment. They are often awkward and poorly coordinated with a walk that can appear either stilted or bouncy.

Many children with AS are highly active in early childhood, and then develop anxiety or depression in young adulthood. Other conditions that often co-exist with AS are AD/HD, tic disorders (such as Tourette syndrome), depression, anxiety disorders, and OCD.

What causes AS? Is it genetic?

Current research points to brain abnormalities as the cause of AS. Using advanced brain imaging techniques, scientists have revealed structural and functional differences in specific regions of the brains of normal versus AS children. These defects are most likely caused by the abnormal migration of embryonic cells during fetal development that affects brain structure and wiring and then goes on to affect the neural circuits that control thought and behavior.

For example, one study found a reduction of brain activity in the frontal lobe of AS children when they were asked to respond to tasks that required them to use their judgment. Another study found differences in activity when children were asked to respond to facial expressions. A different study investigating brain function in adults with AS revealed abnormal levels of specific proteins that correlate with obsessive and repetitive behaviors.

Scientists have always known that there had to be a genetic component to AS and the other ASDs because of their tendency to run in families. Additional evidence for the link between inherited genetic mutations and AS was observed in the higher incidence of family members who have behavioral symptoms similar to AS but in a more limited form. For example, they had slight difficulties with social interaction, language, or reading.

A specific gene for AS, however, has never been identified. Instead, the most recent research indicates that there are most likely a common group of genes whose variations or deletions make an individual vulnerable to developing AS. This combination of genetic variations or deletions will determine the severity and symptoms for each individual with AS.

How is AS diagnosed?

The diagnosis of AS is complicated by the lack of a standardized diagnostic screen or schedule. In fact, because there are several screening instruments in current use, each with different criteria, the same child could receive different diagnoses, depending on the screening tool the doctor uses.

To further complicate the issue, some doctors believe that AS is not a separate and distinct disorder. Instead, they call it high-functioning autism (HFA), and view it as being on the mild end of the ASD spectrum with symptoms that differ—only in degree—from classic autism. Some clinicians use the two diagnoses, AS or HFA, interchangeably. This makes gathering data about the incidence of AS difficult, since some children will be diagnosed with HFA instead of AS, and vice versa.

Most doctors rely on the presence of a core group of behaviors to alert them to the possibility of a diagnosis of AS including the following:

- abnormal eye contact
- aloofness
- the failure to turn when called by name
- the failure to use gestures to point or show
- a lack of interactive play
- a lack of interest in peers

Some of these behaviors may be apparent in the first few months of a child's life, or they may appear later. Problems in at least one of the areas of communication and socialization or repetitive, restricted behavior must be present before the age of three.

The diagnosis of AS is a two-stage process. The first stage begins with developmental screening during a well-child check-up with a family doctor or pediatrician. The second stage is a comprehensive team evaluation to either rule in or rule out AS. This team generally includes a psychologist, neurologist, psychiatrist, speech therapist, and additional professionals who have expertise in diagnosing children with AS.

The comprehensive evaluation includes neurologic and genetic assessment, with in-depth cognitive and language testing to establish intelligence quotient (IQ) and evaluate psychomotor function, verbal and non-verbal strengths and weaknesses, style of learning, and independent living skills. An assessment of communication strengths and weaknesses includes evaluating non-verbal forms of communication (gaze and gestures); the use of non-literal language (metaphor, irony, absurdities, and humor); patterns of inflection, stress and volume modulation; pragmatics (turn-taking and sensitivity to verbal cues); and the content, clarity, and coherence of conversation. The physician will look at the testing results and combine them with the child's developmental history and current symptoms to make a diagnosis.

Are there treatments available for AS?

The ideal treatment for AS coordinates therapies that address the three core symptoms of the disorder: poor communication skills, obsessive or repetitive routines, and physical clumsiness. There is no single best treatment package for all children with AS, but most professionals agree that the earlier the intervention, the better.

An effective treatment program builds on the child's interests, offers a predictable schedule, teaches tasks as a series of simple steps, actively engages the child's attention in highly structured activities, and provides regular reinforcement of behavior. This kind of program generally includes:

• social skills training, a form of group therapy that teaches children with AS the skills they need to interact more successfully with other children;

• cognitive behavioral therapy, a type of talk therapy that can help the more explosive or anxious children to manage their emotions better and cut back on obsessive interests and repetitive routines;

• medication for co-existing conditions such as depression and anxiety;

• occupational or physical therapy for children with sensory integration problems or poor motor coordination;

• specialized speech/language therapy to help children who have trouble with the pragmatics of speech—the give and take of normal conversation; and,

• parent training and support to teach parents behavioral techniques to use at home.

Do children with AS get better? What happens when they become adults?

With effective treatment, children with AS can learn to cope with their disabilities, but they may still find social situations and personal relationships challenging. Many adults with AS are able to work successfully in mainstream jobs, although they may continue to need encouragement and moral support to maintain an independent life.

Chapter 29

Traumatic Brain Injury

Susan was seven years old when she was hit by a car while riding her bike. She broke her arm and leg. She also hit her head very hard. The doctors say she sustained a traumatic brain injury. When she came home from the hospital, she needed lots of help, but now she looks fine.

In fact, that's part of the problem, especially at school. Her friends and teachers think her brain has healed because her broken bones have. But there are changes in Susan that are hard to understand. It takes Susan longer to do things. She has trouble remembering things. She can't always find the words she wants to use. Reading is hard for her now. It's going to take time before people really understand the changes they see in her.

What is traumatic brain injury?

A traumatic brain injury (TBI) is an injury to the brain caused by the head being hit by something or shaken violently. This injury can change how the person acts, moves, and thinks. A traumatic brain injury can also change how a student learns and acts in school. The term TBI is used for head injuries that can cause changes in one or more areas, such as:

- thinking and reasoning,
- understanding words,

Excerpted from "Traumatic Brain Injury," Fact Sheet 18, National Dissemination Center for Children with Disabilities (NICHCY), May 2006.

- remembering things,
- paying attention,
- solving problems,
- thinking abstractly,
- talking,
- behaving,
- walking and other physical activities,
- seeing or hearing, and
- learning.

The term TBI is not used for a person who is born with a brain injury. It also is not used for brain injuries that happen during birth.

IDEA's Definition of Traumatic Brain Injury

The Individuals with Disabilities Education Act (IDEA) is the federal law that guides how schools provide special education and related services to children and youth with disabilities. IDEA defines traumatic brain injury as "...an acquired injury to the brain caused by an external physical force, resulting in total or partial functional disability or psychosocial impairment, or both, that adversely affects a child's educational performance. The term applies to open or closed head injuries resulting in impairments in one or more areas, such as cognition; language; memory; attention; reasoning; abstract thinking; judgment; problem-solving; sensory, perceptual, and motor abilities; psycho-social behavior; physical functions; information processing; and speech. The term does not apply to brain injuries that are congenital or degenerative, or to brain injuries induced by birth trauma." [34 Code of Federal Regulations §300.7(c)(12)]

How common is traumatic brain injury?

More than one million children receive brain injuries each year. More than 30,000 of these children have lifelong disabilities as a result of the brain injury.

What are the signs of traumatic brain injury?

The signs of brain injury can be very different depending on where the brain is injured and how severely. Children with TBI may have one or more of the following difficulties:

- **Physical disabilities:** Individuals with TBI may have problems speaking, seeing, hearing, and using their other senses. They may have headaches and feel tired a lot. They may also have trouble with skills such as writing or drawing. Their muscles may suddenly contract or tighten (this is called spasticity). They may also have seizures. Their balance and walking may also be affected. They may be partly or completely paralyzed on one side of the body, or both sides.

- **Difficulties with thinking:** Because the brain has been injured, it is common that the person's ability to use the brain changes. For example, children with TBI may have trouble with short-term memory (being able to remember something from one minute to the next, like what the teacher just said). They may also have trouble with their long-term memory (being able to remember information from a while ago, like facts learned last month). People with TBI may have trouble concentrating and only be able to focus their attention for a short time. They may think slowly. They may have trouble talking and listening to others. They may also have difficulty with reading and writing, planning, understanding the order in which events happen (called sequencing), and judgment.

- **Social, behavioral, or emotional problems:** These difficulties may include sudden changes in mood, anxiety, and depression. Children with TBI may have trouble relating to others. They may be restless and may laugh or cry a lot. They may not have much motivation or much control over their emotions.

A child with TBI may not have all of the mentioned difficulties: Brain injuries can range from mild to severe, and so can the changes that result from the injury. This means that it is hard to predict how an individual will recover from the injury. Early and ongoing help can make a big difference in how the child recovers. This help can include physical or occupational therapy, counseling, and special education.

It is also important to know that, as the child grows and develops, parents and teachers may notice new problems. This is because, as students grow, they are expected to use their brain in new and different ways. The damage to the brain from the earlier injury can make it hard for the student to learn new skills that come with getting older. Sometimes parents and educators may not even realize that the student's difficulty comes from the earlier injury.

What about school?

Although TBI is very common, many medical and education professionals may not realize that some difficulties can be caused by a childhood brain injury. Often, students with TBI are thought to have a learning disability, emotional disturbance, or mental retardation. As a result, they do not receive the type of educational help and support they really need.

When children with TBI return to school, their educational and emotional needs are often very different than before the injury. Their disability has happened suddenly and traumatically. They can often remember how they were before the brain injury. This can bring on many emotional and social changes. The child's family, friends, and teachers also recall what the child was like before the injury. These other people in the child's life may have trouble changing or adjusting their expectations of the child.

Therefore, it is extremely important to plan carefully for the child's return to school. Parents will want to find out ahead of time about special education services at the school. This information is usually available from the school's principal or special education teacher. The school will need to evaluate the child thoroughly. This evaluation will determine the student's educational needs. The school and parents will then develop an individualized education program (IEP) that addresses those educational needs.

It is important to remember that the IEP is a flexible plan. It can be changed as the parents, the school, and the student learn more about what the student needs at school.

Tips for Parents

- Learn about TBI. The more you know, the more you can help yourself and your child.

- Work with the medical team to understand your child's injury and treatment plan. Do not be shy about asking questions. Tell them what you know or think. Make suggestions.

- Keep track of your child's treatment. A binder or a box can help you store this history. As your child recovers, you may meet with many doctors, nurses, and others. Write down what they say. Put any paperwork they give you in the notebook or throw it in the box. You cannot remember all this. Also, if you need to share any of this paperwork with someone else, make a copy. Do not give away your original.

- Talk to other parents whose children have TBI. There are parent groups all over the U.S. Parents can share practical advice and emotional support. To locate parent groups near you, call the National Dissemination Center for Children with Disabilities (NICHCY) at 800-695-0285, or visit online at http://www.nichcy.org/states.htm.

- If your child was in school before the injury, plan for his or her return to school. Get in touch with the school. Ask the principal about special education services. Have the medical team share information with the school.

- When your child returns to school, ask the school to test your child as soon as possible to identify his or her special education needs. Meet with the school and help develop a plan for your child called an individualized education program (IEP).

- Keep in touch with your child's teacher. Tell the teacher about how your child is doing at home. Ask how your child is doing in school.

Tips for Teachers

- Find out as much as you can about the child's injury and his or her present needs.

- Give the student more time to finish schoolwork and tests.

- Give directions one step at a time. For tasks with many steps, it helps to give the student written directions.

- Show the student how to perform new tasks. Give examples to go with new ideas and concepts.

- Have consistent routines. This helps the student know what to expect. If the routine is going to change, let the student know ahead of time.

- Check to make sure that the student has actually learned the new skill. Give the student lots of opportunities to practice the new skill.

- Show the student how to use an assignment book and a daily schedule. This helps the student get organized.

- Realize that the student may get tired quickly. Let the student rest as needed.

- Reduce distractions.

- Keep in touch with the student's parents. Share information about how the student is doing at home and at school.

- Be flexible about expectations. Be patient. Maximize the student's chances for success.

For More Information

Brain Injury Association (formerly the National Head Injury Foundation)
1608 Spring Hill Road, Suite 110
Vienna, VA 22182
Toll-Free: 800-444-6443
Phone: 703-761-0750
Fax: 703-761-0755
Website: http://www.biausa.org
E-mail: FamilyHelpline@biausa.org

Brain Injury Resource Center
P.O. Box 84151
Seattle, WA 98124
Phone: 206-621-8558
Website: http://www.headinjury.com
E-mail: brain@headinjury.com

National Resource Center for Traumatic Brain Injury
Department of Physical Medicine and Rehabilitation
P.O. Box 980542
Richmond, VA 23298-0542
Phone: 804-828-9055
Fax: 804-828-2378
Website: http://www.neuro.pmr.vcu.edu
E-mail: mbking@vcu.edu

Chapter 30

Visual Impairment

The human eye is like a camera that collects, focuses, and transmits light through a lens to create an image of its surroundings. In a camera, the image is created on film or an image sensor. In the eye, the image is created on the retina, a thin layer of light-sensitive tissue at the back of the eye.

Like a camera, the human eye controls the amount of light that enters the eye. The iris (the colored circular part of the eye) controls the amount of light passing through the pupil. It closes up the pupil in bright light and opens it wider in dim light. The cornea is the transparent, protective surface of the eye. It helps focus light, as does the lens, which sits just behind the iris.

When light enters the eye, the retina changes the light into nerve signals. The retina then sends these signals along the optic nerve (a cable of more than 1,000,000 nerve fibers) to the brain. Without a retina, the eye can't communicate with the brain, making vision impossible.

This chapter includes: "Visual Impairment," January 2007, reprinted with permission from www.kidshealth.org. Copyright © 2007 The Nemours Foundation. This information was provided by KidsHealth, one of the largest resources online for medically reviewed health information written for parents, kids, and teens. For more articles like this one, visit www.KidsHealth.org, or www.TeensHealth.org. Text under the heading "Visual Impairments Disability Information," is excerpted from "Visual Impairments," Fact Sheet 13, National Dissemination Center for Children with Disabilities (NICHCY), January 2004.

What Is Visual Impairment?

Many people have some type of visual problem at some point in their life. Some can no longer see objects far away. Others have problems reading small print. These types of conditions are often easily treated with eyeglasses or contact lenses.

But when one or more parts of the eye or brain that are needed to process images become diseased or damaged, severe or total loss of vision can occur. In these cases, vision can't be fully restored with medical treatment, surgery, or corrective lenses like glasses or contacts.

The American Foundation for the Blind estimates that ten million people in the United States are visually impaired. Visual impairment is a term experts use to describe any kind of vision loss, whether it's someone who cannot see at all or someone who has partial vision loss.

Some people are completely blind, but many others have what's called legal blindness. They haven't lost their sight completely but have lost enough vision that they'd have to stand 20 feet from an object to see it as well as someone with perfect vision could from 200 feet away.

What Causes Visual Impairment?

People rarely lose their eyesight during their teen years. When they do, it's usually caused by an injury like getting hit in the eye or head with a baseball or having an automobile or motorcycle accident.

Some babies have congenital blindness, which means they are visually impaired at birth. Congenital blindness can be caused by a number of things—it can be inherited, for instance, or caused by an infection (like German measles) that's transmitted from the mother to the developing fetus during pregnancy.

Conditions that may cause vision loss after birth include:

- **Amblyopia** (pronounced: am-blee-oh-pee-uh) is reduced vision in an eye caused by lack of use of that eye in early childhood. Some conditions cause a child's eyes to send different messages to the brain (for example, one eye might focus better than the other). The brain may then turn off or suppress images from the weaker eye and vision from that eye then stops developing normally. This is also known as a "lazy eye." Strabismus (misaligned or crossed eyes) is a common cause of amblyopia, since the brain will start to ignore messages sent by one of the misaligned eyes.

- **Cataracts** are cloudy areas in part or all of the lens of the eye. In people without cataracts, the lens is crystal clear and allows light to pass through and focus on the retina. Cataracts prevent light from easily passing through the lens, and this causes loss of vision. Cataracts often form slowly and usually affect people in their 60s and 70s, but sometimes babies are born with congenital cataracts. Symptoms include double vision, cloudy or blurry vision, difficulty seeing in poorly lit spaces, and colors that seem faded.

- **Diabetic retinopathy** (pronounced: reh-ton-ah-pa-thee) occurs when the tiny blood vessels in the retina are damaged due to diabetes. People with retinopathy may not have any problems seeing at first. But if the condition gets worse, they can become blind. Teens who have diabetes should be sure to get regular eye exams because there are no early warning signs for this condition. To help prevent retinopathy, people with diabetes should also avoid smoking, keep their blood pressure under control, and keep their blood sugar at an even level.

- **Glaucoma** is an increase in pressure inside the eye. The increased pressure impairs vision by damaging the optic nerve. Glaucoma is mostly seen in older adults, although babies may be born with the condition and children and teens can sometimes develop it as well.

- **Macular degeneration** (pronounced: mah-kyoo-lur dih-jeh-nuh-ray-shun) is a gradual and progressive deterioration of the macula, the most sensitive region of the retina. The condition leads to progressive loss of central vision (the ability to see fine details directly in front). Macular degeneration is often age related (it occurs in older people, especially older than 60), but sometimes it can occur in younger people. Excessive exposure to sunlight and smoking can increase the risk for age-related macular degeneration. Symptoms may include increased difficulty reading or watching television, or distorted vision in which straight lines appear wavy or objects look larger or smaller than normal.

- **Trachoma** (pronounced: truh-ko-muh) occurs when a very contagious microorganism called *Chlamydia trachomatis* causes inflammation in the eye. It's often found in poor rural countries that have overcrowded living conditions and limited access to

241

water and sanitation. Blindness due to trachoma has been virtually eliminated from the USA.

What Do Doctors Do?

If you, your parent, or your doctor suspects a visual problem, you'll probably pay a visit to an ophthalmologist (pronounced: af-thal-mah-luh-jist), a medical doctor who specializes in examining, diagnosing, and treating eyes and eye diseases. When someone goes for an examination, the ophthalmologist will look at the structure of that person's eye.

Other simple tests an ophthalmologist may perform include:

- **Visual acuity test:** A person reads an eye chart to measure how well he or she sees at various distances.

- **Visual field test:** Ophthalmologists use this test to measure side, or peripheral, vision.

- **Tonometry test:** This test determines the fluid pressure inside the eye to evaluate for glaucoma.

If your doctor determines that you have an eye condition that is likely to cause visual impairment, many treatments are available. Options may include eyeglasses, contact lenses, and eye drops or other medicines. In some cases, surgery may be required. For instance, cataracts are often treated by removing the clouded lens and replacing it with an intraocular lens (an artificial plastic lens that requires no special care and restores vision).

Other methods can compensate for vision loss. Guide dogs can help people get from place to place independently. Braille allows those with visual impairment to read and write. Special equipment such as microscopic and telescopic glasses and voice-recognition software can make school and homework easier.

What's It Like to Be Visually Impaired?

Just as you don't think about your eye color every day, people with visual impairment don't always think about their condition every day either.

Someone with sight problems can become isolated from others more easily, though. If a visually impaired person asks for assistance, don't hesitate to help. But someone who uses a cane or a guide dog is probably self-sufficient and may not need help.

Visual Impairments Disability Information

Incidence

The rate at which visual impairments occur in individuals under the age of 18 is 12.2 per 1,000. Severe visual impairments (legally or totally blind) occur at a rate of .06 per 1,000.

Characteristics

The effect of visual problems on a child's development depends on the severity, type of loss, age at which the condition appears, and overall functioning level of the child. Many children who have multiple disabilities may also have visual impairments resulting in motor, cognitive, or social developmental delays.

A young child with visual impairments has little reason to explore interesting objects in the environment, and thus, may miss opportunities to have experiences and to learn. This lack of exploration may continue until learning becomes motivating or until intervention begins. Because the child cannot see parents or peers, he or she may be unable to imitate social behavior or understand nonverbal cues. Visual handicaps can create obstacles to a growing child's independence.

Educational Implications

Children with visual impairments should be assessed early to benefit from early intervention programs, when applicable. Technology in the form of computers and low-vision optical and video aids enable many partially sighted, low vision, and blind children to participate in regular class activities. Large print materials, books on tape, and braille books are available.

Students with visual impairments may need additional help with special equipment and modifications in the regular curriculum to emphasize listening skills, communication, orientation and mobility, vocation and career options, and daily living skills. Students with low vision or those who are legally blind may need help in using their residual vision more efficiently and in working with special aids and materials. Students who have visual impairments combined with other types of disabilities have a greater need for an interdisciplinary approach and may require greater emphasis on self care and daily living skills.

For More Information

National Association for Parents of the Visually Impaired, Inc.
P.O. Box 317
Watertown, MA 02472-0317
Toll-Free: 800-562-6265
Phone: 617-972-7441
Fax: 617-972-7441
Website: http://www.napvi.org
E-mail: napvi@perkins.org

National Association for Visually Handicapped
22 West 21st Street, 6th Floor
New York, NY 10010
Phone: 212-889-3141
Fax: 212-727-2931
Website: http://www.navh.org
E-mail: navh@navh.org

National Braille Association, Inc. (NBA)
3 Townline Circle
Rochester, NY 14623-2513
Phone: 585-427-8260
Fax: 585-427-0263
Website: http://www.nationalbraille.org
E-mail: nbaoffice@nationalbraille.org

National Braille Press
88 Saint Stephen St.
Boston, MA 02115
Toll-Free: 800-548-7323
Phone: 617-266-6160
Website: http://www.nbp.org
E-mail: orders@nbp.org

National Eye Institute
31 Center Drive, MSC 2510
Bethesda, MD 20892-2510
Phone: 301-496-5248
Website: http://www.nei.nih.gov
E-mail: 2020@nei.nih.gov

National Library Service for the Blind and Physically Handicapped

Library of Congress
Toll-Free: 800-424-8567
Phone: 202-707-5100
TTY: 202-707-0744
Website: http://www.loc.gov/nls
E-mail: nls@loc.gov

Prevent Blindness America

211 W. Wacker Dr., Suite 1700
Chicago, IL 60606
Toll-Free: 800-331-2020
Website: http://www.preventblindness.org
E-mail: info@preventblindness.org

Part Five

Assessment, Accommodations, and Therapies for Learning Disabilities

Chapter 31

Assessing Individuals for Learning Disabilities

Chapter Contents

Section 31.1

Young Children with Disabilities (Birth–Five Years): Identification and Intervention

Excerpted from "Learning Disabilities and Young Children: Identification and Intervention," © 2006 National Joint Committee on Learning Disabilities. Reprinted with permission.

Early Identification

The purpose of early identification is to determine which children have developmental problems that may be obstacles to learning or that place children at risk. Development in infants, toddlers, and preschoolers is characterized by broad variability in rates and patterns of maturation. For some children, differences and delays in abilities are temporary and are resolved during the normal course of development. For other children, delays may persist in different domains of functioning, necessitating the child's referral for targeted screening and/or comprehensive evaluation. At present, no clear distinction can be made in the early years between the children whose problems may persist from those who will make adequate progress with time. Therefore, young children who demonstrate difficulties in early development may or may not be at risk for learning disabilities (LD); nevertheless, screening, evaluation, enhanced learning opportunities, and possibly intervention services should be provided. It is not in the child's best interest to wait and see, or hope that the child will grow out of his or her problems. Conversely, it is important to guard against the premature identification of a disability, especially if high quality learning opportunities have not been provided.

It is often during the early years that families and caregivers first suspect a problem and may share their concerns with qualified professionals. However, some families initially may deny the existence of a problem because they are fearful of, or threatened by, its possibilities and consequences. Family cooperation is critical to early identification. Thus, professionals must recognize and be sensitive to differences in family responses, including cultural differences in viewing and addressing a disability, and provide appropriate support.

The identification process includes (1) screening, (2) examination for the presence of risk indicators and protective factors, (3) systematic observations, and if indicated, (4) a comprehensive evaluation. An effective early identification program must take into account the numerous biological, environmental, and cultural factors that may influence the course of a child's development. Information from the identification process is the basis for making decisions about the need for further services and supports.

Screening: The purpose of screening is to determine if additional evaluation is required and in what developmental domains. Examples of large scale state-wide screening programs include Universal Newborn and Infant Hearing Screening, and Child Find, a component of Individuals with Disabilities Education Act 2004 (IDEA '04) that requires states to have a system to identify, locate, and evaluate all children with disabilities (birth–21 years), who need early intervention or special education services. Screening tools are not intended for diagnosis, placement, and educational planning. Careful consideration of reliability, validity, standardization, cultural and linguistic sensitivity, and relevance of screening instruments and procedures is required for appropriate selection, use, and interpretation. The National Joint Committee on Learning Disabilities (NJCLD) supports the recommendations by the *Learning Disabilities Roundtable* in 2002 that "all preschoolers should be screened to assess early language and reading skill development just as they are for vision and hearing" (p. 1).

Risk indicators and protective factors: A range of environmental, biological, genetic, and perinatal conditions may be associated with adverse developmental outcomes and may be risk indicators (warning signs) for LD. Also, advances in medical technology have kept an increasing number of fragile children alive, and these children often are at risk for developmental and later educational problems. Such risk indicators, especially when several are present, warrant careful monitoring of a child's development and signal the need to ensure high quality learning opportunities for this population. Children who do not respond adequately to these opportunities may be at increased risk for LD. Furthermore, young children with identified disabilities (for example, cerebral palsy) also may be at risk for LD. However, risk indicators do not always predict which children will have future learning problems. Risk indicators must be considered within the context of typical developmental expectations. For example, an inability to follow one-step directions is not a risk indicator for a six-month-old, but is for a four-year-old, especially in combination with other risk indicators, such as poor fine motor coordination.

Protective factors that reduce risk and foster resilience can buffer children and families from circumstances that place them at risk. Risk indicators interact with protective factors in unique ways for each child. For example, some children with a history of birth complications may exhibit typical developmental patterns and require few if any special services, whereas other children without such histories may struggle to learn and may require formal assessment and intervention. Likewise, children who may have multiple risk indicators may not demonstrate learning problems if they receive strong culturally and developmentally appropriate early learning experiences. The two lists that follow, though not all-inclusive, identify possible risk indicators and protective factors for LD among infants, toddlers, and preschoolers.

Risk Indicators

Perinatal Conditions

- Low Apgar scores
- Low birth weight and/or preterm birth
- Hospitalization for longer than 24 hours in a neonatal intensive care unit
- Difficulty with suckling, sucking, and swallowing
- Chronic otitis media that may result in intermittent hearing loss

Genetic or Environmental Conditions

- Family history of LD
- Adopted child status
- Family history of spoken and/or written language problems
- Exposure to environmental toxins or other harmful substances
- Limited language exposure in home, childcare, and other settings
- Poverty

Developmental Milestones

- Delay in cognitive skills
  - Not demonstrating object permanence

- Limited understanding of means-ends relationships (using a stool to reach a cookie jar)
- Lack of symbolic play behavior
- Delay in comprehension and/or expression of spoken language
  - Limited receptive vocabulary
  - Reduced expressive vocabulary (late talkers)
  - Difficulty understanding simple (for example, one-step) directions
  - Monotone or other unusual prosodic features of speech
  - Reduced intelligibility
  - Infrequent or inappropriate spontaneous communication (vocal, verbal, or nonverbal)
  - Immature syntax
- Delay in emergent literacy skills
  - Slow speed for naming objects and colors
  - Limited phonological awareness (rhyming, syllable blending)
  - Minimal interest in print
  - Limited print awareness (for example: book handling, recognizing environmental print)
- Delay in perceptual-motor skills
  - Problems in gross or fine motor coordination (for example: hopping, dressing, cutting, stringing beads)
  - Difficulty coloring, copying, and drawing

Attention and Behavior

- Distractibility/inattention
- Impulsivity
- Hyperactivity
- Difficulty changing activities or handling disruptions to routines
- Perseveration (constant repetition of an idea)

Protective Factors

- Access to quality pre-, peri-, and postnatal care

- Maternal education
- High quality learning opportunities
  - Exposure to rich and varied vocabulary, syntax, and discourse patterns
  - Responsive learning environments sensitive to all cultural and linguistic backgrounds
  - Access to printed materials
  - Involvement in structured and unstructured individual/ group play interactions and conversations
  - Engagement in gross and fine motor activities
- Multiple supports
  - Assistance adapted to the child's responsiveness to instruction or intervention
  - Access to adaptive and assistive technology (AT) and services
  - Transition planning between early intervention services (birth to age three years) and preschool programs (ages 3–5 years), and between preschool and elementary school
  - Service coordination

In summary, risk indicators do not necessarily predict later learning problems or indicate the existence of a disability, particularly when only a single indicator is present. Similarly, protective factors do not rule out the presence of a disability. However, the presence of risk indicators warrants substantial and serious efforts to facilitate early learning success, because many children at risk respond positively to high quality instruction and support. Therefore, children at risk, who may or may not have LD, need to receive carefully planned and responsive services and supports to enhance their opportunities for learning.

Systematic observations: Systematic observations of a child's behavior and abilities over time are an important addition to examining the presence of risk indicators and protective factors. Observations may be informal or may follow a standard observation protocol; in either case, they should be conducted multiple times and in varying contexts (for example: home, diagnostic preschool, Head Start classroom, playgroup) to increase the reliability and validity of the hypotheses made regarding a child's behavior. In many cases, an extended period of observations will be necessary. Observations should provide a description of the frequency, consistency, and severity of the behaviors causing concerns in relation to contextual demands.

The child's family should be involved throughout the entire process. When professionals raise a question about the course of the child's development as a result of systematic observation, they should discuss the findings with the caregivers and family. When indicated, a referral should be made to appropriate professionals for further evaluation and, if warranted, provision of supports and services should be recommended.

Comprehensive evaluation: When a screening, a review of risk indicators and protective factors, and systematic observations suggest that a child is at risk for LD, professionals should conduct periodic evaluations to ascertain whether development follows expected patterns. The major goal of a comprehensive evaluation is to determine the individual child's specific pattern of abilities and needs and to identify strategies and resources to address learning and behavioral problems as soon as possible. These evaluations should occur across different settings and should consider multiple perspectives offered by caregivers and professionals. An interdisciplinary approach is especially valuable in obtaining and interpreting evaluation information derived from a variety of sources. Evaluations should focus on developmental norms across domains (for example: cognition, communication, emergent literacy, motor and sensory abilities, and/or social-emotional adjustment); however, it is important to recognize that there is a wide range of individual differences, both within and between children, some of which may fall within the normal range of expected behaviors.

A comprehensive evaluation involves the use of multiple instruments and procedures, including norm- and criterion-referenced tests, teacher/parent rating scales, and developmental checklists. The use of a single instrument or procedure does not constitute a comprehensive evaluation. Practitioners should use culturally and linguistically sensitive instruments to ensure appropriate assessment of children with potential LD. Evaluation of the child's status and needs depends on an integrated assessment of the child's functioning in the following domains:

- Cognition, including perceptual organization, memory, concept formation, attention, and problem solving

- Communication, including speech/language form, content, and use for receptive and expressive purposes

255

- Emergent literacy, including phonological awareness, awareness of print; and numeracy, including number recognition, and number concepts

- Motor functions, including gross, fine, and oral motor abilities

- Sensory functions, including auditory, haptic, kinesthetic, and visual systems

- Social-emotional adjustment, including behavior, temperament, affect, self-regulation, play, and social interaction

Time-limited placement in a diagnostic preschool setting can be a useful part of the comprehensive evaluation for addressing diagnostic questions and determining the effectiveness of various evidence-based interventions for the child.

Early Services and Supports

If a learning problem or delay in development has been suggested based on screening, review of risk indicators and protective factors, systematic observation, and if indicated, comprehensive evaluation, then the priority should be to ensure that services and supports based on individual needs and strengths are available. Such services and supports may include: (a) providing special education interventions that meet the child's developmental, behavioral, and pre-academic learning needs; (b) offering strong preschool programs; and (c) enhancing the home language and literacy environment. Services and supports for young children should be evidence-based, developmentally appropriate, family-centered, and culturally and linguistically sensitive. Professionals must ensure that their findings and recommendations for services and supports are sensitive to all cultural and linguistic backgrounds, such as those for English language learners. Likewise, professionals must ensure that caregivers and family members have access to a range of supports such as:

- helping families and caregivers to recognize, understand, and accept the child's problems;

- selecting programs that meet the child's individual needs;

- locating parent support networks and programs;

- finding a service provider or agency whose treatment philosophy is congruent with the family's preferences;

- identifying appropriate interventions and resources available within public or private preschool programs; and

- facilitating the child's development in the home and childcare environment.

A variety of professionals, in collaboration with families and caregivers, is involved in the selection and delivery of services and supports. Collectively, the professionals should possess knowledge of typical and atypical patterns of development in the domains of cognition, communication, emergent literacy, pre-academic interventions, and motor, sensory, and social-emotional functioning, as well as the capacity to collaborate effectively. The following is a list of the roles of some of the professionals in addition to the child's pediatrician who typically are involved with infants, toddlers, and preschoolers:

- **Audiologist:** Specializes in the nonmedical management of hearing and related problems (balance).

- **Early childhood general and special education teachers:** Plan and provide educationally relevant interventions and other services based on the individualized education program (IEP) or individualized family service plan (IFSP).

- **Occupational therapist:** Helps children improve their ability to perform fine motor skills and daily activities and to achieve independence.

- **Physical therapist:** Helps children develop gross motor skills and coordination; they also provide services aimed at preventing or slowing the progression of conditions resulting from injury, disease, and other causes.

- **School psychologist:** Collaborates with educators, parents, and other professionals to create safe, healthy, and supportive learning environments that strengthen connections between home and school.

- **Speech-language pathologist:** Assesses, diagnoses, and provides intervention services and supports for individuals with speech, language, literacy, cognitive-communication, social communication, and swallowing problems.

Other professionals may be involved, such as childcare providers, educational diagnosticians, educational therapists, reading specialists, social workers, English as a second language (ESL) teachers, child/developmental psychologists, pediatric neurologists, and child psychiatrists. The specific needs of the child should determine the mix of professionals who will assist the family and caregivers at home, in the preschool, and in the special education setting.

The provision of services and supports may enhance the learning opportunities for young children who may be at risk for LD but who have not been identified with a specific disability. The services and supports required by children and their families and caregivers vary along a continuum of intensity and may be provided in different settings. Providing a continuum of services and supports is consistent with a response to intervention (RTI) model, which is a framework that may be used for identifying school-age students with LD. The application of RTI principles has been proposed for preschool-age children, with its characteristic use of different levels of instructional intensity, collaborative problem-solving, early response, and data to inform instruction and monitor progress.

Less intensive services and supports: The initial level of early services and supports for young children at risk for LD would be less intensive and would revolve around daily experiences generally available in any strong preschool program. Such services and supports may involve assisting caregivers and families in increasing interactions with their children. Experiences like shared book reading, conversations about current and past events, and family trips to the zoo, market, library, and playground provide opportunities for such interactions and also stimulate conceptual and linguistic development. It is important to provide activities that develop perceptual, coordination, and fine and gross motor skills such as use of scissors, crayons, finger paints, beads, balls, and puzzles. Emergent literacy can be encouraged by having books, magazines, and other literacy artifacts available in home, childcare, preschool, and other settings, and by engaging in activities such as word play, drawing, and storytelling. Literacy activities at home, in the preschool, and in other settings can develop print concepts, story sense, phonological awareness, and matching speech to print, and offer opportunities for practicing beginning reading and writing skills.

More intensive services and supports: More intensive services and supports may add ongoing, regular consultation with one or more service providers and participation in more structured programs. For preschool-age children, for example, such support might mean an increased emphasis on activities focusing on the acquisition of emergent literacy skills and enrollment in a high quality preschool program that includes more individualized activities. In fact, Head Start programs are now required to document children's progress in early development, particularly literacy. This has resulted from an increased recognition of the importance of early development to later school success and an increased awareness of the discrepancies in development for young children due to differences in socioeconomic, sociolinguistic, and sociocultural factors.

Most intensive services and supports: If young children do not respond to the earlier levels, more specialized and individualized instruction and intervention strategies may be needed. Such services would be provided to children with identified disabilities who are eligible to receive special education. Some of these children with disabilities, such as those with developmental delay or speech and language impairment, may be identified later as having LD. Because no single instructional approach or intervention strategy can be expected to serve the different needs presented by young children with disabilities, it is essential that selection of an instructional strategies and program be based on a clear understanding of a child's specific strengths and needs. The selection of the service delivery system, including the setting (inclusive or non-inclusive), models (pull-out, classroom-based, collaborative-consultation), and supports can then proceed. The least restrictive environment (LRE) provision in IDEA '04 requires that young children with disabilities receive services in settings that best match their education needs. State and local agencies need to ensure the availability of a continuum of service delivery options for students with disabilities, provide funding, and promote interagency cooperation among public and private sectors.

Instruction/Intervention Strategies

An effective instructional program is based on a child's individual strengths and needs and includes well-defined goals, objectives, content, materials, and support (for example: occupational and physical therapy, assistive technology [AT]). Careful development of the individual instructional program is especially important due to the increased recognition that the pre-kindergarten years are a critical period during which intervention efforts are most effective. A summary of research suggests that decisions about instructional programming should be guided by five quality indicators of successful programs for young children:

1. Have a philosophy of individualized programming based on specific needs with a preference for inclusive practices.

2. Rely on relevant research to design service delivery models that meet the individual, changing needs of a child over time and that provide opportunities for interactions in natural environments.

3. Form collaborative partnerships that select and achieve goals for each child.

4. Provide ongoing professional development.

5. Conduct program evaluation and research.

Decisions regarding which instructional approach or intervention strategy to use should be determined with interdisciplinary, family, and caregiver input on the basis of individual learner characteristics and needs and incorporated within the IFSP or IEP. The family and caregivers have an important responsibility for the application of learned skills in the home environment—direct family and caregiver involvement is a major determinant of intervention effectiveness. The interventions selected should be based on current research, principles of evidence-based practice (for example: an integration of theory, research, professional judgment, and family preferences), and progress-monitoring data. In summary, appropriate evidence-based intervention practices should be a collaborative effort that:

- focuses on the child's needs while capitalizing on the child's existing strengths;

- is explicit, systematic, and comprehensive;

- links intervention activities to family activities;

- integrates intervention with the preschool curriculum and makes curricular adaptations as necessary; and,

- results in functional and meaningful progress that can be sustained over time and across settings.

Once an instructional program has been planned, determining the setting in which special education services are provided is an important decision. For children from birth to three years, IDEA '04 Part C mandates that services be delivered in a "natural environment." The home often is considered to be the ideal setting for providing services to these young children; however, childcare centers also may be considered natural environments.

Also influencing decisions about the service setting is the clear preference in IDEA '04 for inclusive settings, where children with disabilities are served with typically developing children. The two main types of inclusive settings are (a) full inclusion, where the child with disabilities is placed in a classroom in which the majority of the children exhibit typical developmental patterns, and less frequently, (b) reverse inclusion, where a few children who exhibit typical developmental patterns are placed in a classroom of children with disabilities. An advantage of inclusive settings is that typically developing young children can serve as appropriate models for their peers with disabilities. One barrier to placement in either type of inclusive setting is the fact that public preschool programs are not available in all states for children without disabilities. Head Start programs provide access to inclusive settings for young children from low-income families. The national pre-kindergarten movement in the United States may be one response to the challenge of creating more inclusive preschool programs because more young children without disabilities will be attending public preschools.

Different types of service delivery models may be used across settings and also should be selected based on individual child needs. While home-based, classroom-based, and collaborative consultation models are most compatible with the characteristics of inclusive settings (for example: encouraging peer interactions, providing services in the natural environment, integrating services within the ongoing home or classroom routine), pull-out services may be appropriate at times for some children. When the child makes a transition from one service setting or service delivery model to another, coordination and orderly, timely transfer of information among professionals is essential to ensure continuity of services.

Another consideration to the provision of effective instructional programs is the use of supportive services such as AT when needed. Technological advances have improved intervention programming for young children at risk for or with identified disabilities. The use of AT and augmentative and alternative communication (AAC) systems, a subset of AT, can foster access, interaction, and integration in daily communication and classroom activities for young children. Since the late 1980s, AAC systems have been used to enhance communication and literacy skills for young children who do not speak or whose speech is unintelligible. Instructional approaches for teaching communication skills, whether through AAC or more conventional speech modes, have moved from one-on-one, discrete and repetitive skills training to teaching more contextually based (home, community, classroom) communication functions (requesting, commenting, rejecting) in everyday situations and with a child's regular communication partners.

A number of instructional software programs has been designed specifically for young children. Software may enhance children's concept development, develop emergent literacy skills, and increase attention. However, there is little empirical evidence of the efficacy of many software programs for accomplishing these aims, and computer-assisted instruction should not replace interactions with families, peers, and professionals.

Section 31.2

Detecting Learning Disabilities in Children

Excerpted from "Reading and Learning Disabilities," National Dissemination Center for Children with Disabilities (NICHCY), 2004.

Learning disabilities are lifelong conditions that may require special understanding and help throughout grade school, high school, and beyond. They are also life disabilities that have important effects outside of the classroom, interfering not only with academic work but also with children's games, daily activities, and even friendships. Therefore, help for these children means more than classroom special education.

Types of Learning Disabilities

Learning disabilities can be classified by their effects at one or more of the following stages. Each child has individual strengths and weaknesses at each stage.

Input

The first major type of problem at the input stage is a visual perception disability. Some students have difficulty in recognizing the position and shape of what they see. Letters may be reversed or rotated; for example, the letters d, b, p, q, and g might be confused. The child might also have difficulty distinguishing a significant form from its background. People with this disability often have reading problems. They may jump over words, read the same line twice, or skip lines. Other students have poor depth perception or poor distance judgement. They might bump into things, fall over chairs, or knock over drinks.

The other major input disability is in auditory perception. Students may have difficulty understanding because they do not distinguish subtle differences in sounds. They confuse words and phrases that sound alike—for example, "blue" with "blow" or "ball" with "bell." Some children find it hard to pick out an auditory figure from its background; they may not respond to the sound of a parent's or teacher's voice, and it may seem that they are not listening or paying attention. Others process sound slowly and therefore cannot keep up with the flow of conversation, inside or outside the classroom. Suppose a parent says, "It's getting late. Go upstairs, wash your face, and get into your pajamas. Then come back down for a snack." A child with this disability might hear only the first part and stay upstairs.

Integration

Integration disabilities take several forms, corresponding to the three stages of sequencing, abstraction, and organization.

A student with a sequencing disability might recount a story by starting in the middle, going to the beginning, and then proceeding to the end. The child might also reverse the order of letters in words, seeing "dog" and reading "god." Such children are often unable to use single units of a memorized sequence correctly. If asked what comes after Wednesday, they have to start counting from Sunday to get the answer. In using a dictionary, they must start with "A" each time.

The second type of integration disability involves abstraction. Students with this problem have difficulty in inferring meaning. They may read a story but not be able to generalize from it. They may confuse different meanings of the same word used in different ways. They find it difficult to understand jokes, puns, or idioms.

Once recorded, sequenced, and understood, information must be organized—integrated into a constant flow and related to what has previously been learned. Students with an organization disability find it difficult to make bits of information cohere into concepts. They may learn a series of facts without being able to answer general questions that require the use of these facts. Their lives in and outside of the classroom reflect this disorganization.

263

Memory

Disabilities also develop at the third stage of information processing, memory. Short-term memory retains information briefly while we attend to it or concentrate upon it. For example, most of us can retain the ten digits of a long distance telephone number long enough to dial, but we forget it if we are interrupted. When information is repeated often enough, it enters long-term memory, where it is stored and can be retrieved later. Most memory disabilities affect short-term memory only; students with these disabilities need many more repetitions than usual to retain information.

Output

At the fourth stage, output, there are both language and motor disabilities. Language disabilities almost always involve what is called demand language rather than spontaneous language. Spontaneous language occurs when we initiate speaking—select the subject, organize our thoughts, and find the correct words before opening our mouths. Demand language occurs when someone else creates the circumstances in which communication is required. A question is asked, and we must simultaneously organize our thoughts, find the right words, and answer. A child with a language disability may speak normally when initiating conversation but respond hesitantly in demand situations—pause, ask for the question to be repeated, give a confused answer, or fail to find the right words.

Motor disabilities are of two types: poor coordination of large muscle groups, which is called gross motor disability; and poor coordination of small muscle groups, which is called fine motor disability. Gross motor disabilities make children clumsy. They stumble, fall, and bump into things; they may have difficulty in running, climbing, riding a bicycle, buttoning shirts, or tying shoelaces. The most common type of fine motor disability is difficulty in coordinating the muscles needed for writing. Children with this problem write slowly, and their handwriting is often unreadable. They may also make spelling, grammar, and punctuation errors.

Detecting Learning Disabilities in Children

There are several early clues to the presence of a learning disability. In preschool children, we look for failure to use language in communication by age three, or inadequate motor skills (buttoning, tying, climbing) by age five. In school-age children, we observe whether they are learning the skills appropriate to their grade. Schools and families should always consider the possibility of a learning disability before assuming that a child who has been doing poorly in school is lazy or emotionally disturbed. The Individuals with Disabilities Education Act (IDEA), Public Law (P.L.) 105–17—formerly known as the Education for All Handicapped Children Act (EHA), P.L. 94–142—requires public school systems to evaluate children who are at risk for a learning disability. Evaluations can also be performed by professionals in private practice, beginning with family doctors. Attention deficit disorder (ADD), attention deficit/hyperactivity disorder (AD/HD), and other problems should always be considered as well and evaluated by qualified professionals with expertise with these conditions. It is important to distinguish between emotional, social, and family problems that are causes and those that are consequences of academic difficulties, because they require different treatments.

The psychological assessment may include a neuropsychological or a clinical psychological evaluation. The intelligence of the child should be determined to learn whether the child is performing below potential. Discrepancies in performance between different sections of the IQ (intelligence quotient) test will help to clarify learning strengths and weaknesses. Other tests may be used to assess perception, cognition, memory, and language abilities. Current academic skills are judged by achievement tests. Both IQ and achievement tests help to clarify discrepancies between potential and actual ability. There are also specific tests that help to uncover learning disabilities. A speech pathologist, occupational therapist, or other professional may contribute further information, as can parents.

Treating Learning Disabilities in Children

Special education is the treatment of choice for learning disabilities in school. The Individuals with Disabilities Education Act requires that school personnel, in conjunction with the child's parents, develop an individualized education program (IEP) for each student with learning disabilities who is eligible for special education. This plan is revised every year to take into account each eligible student's present skills and learning disabilities and abilities. The specific instruction students receive will vary depending upon their needs and capabilities. Some children need specific related services as well: a note taker (for a student with a fine motor disability), word processors, laptop computers, books on tape, or extra time for tests. The IDEA requires schools to provide these special education and related services at no cost to families.

It's encouraging to know that a lot of research has been done to find out how to help students with learning disabilities succeed at school and elsewhere. Parents must also try to understand the nature of their children's problems. Like classroom teachers, they must build on the child's strengths while compensating for or adjusting to the child's needs without exposing them unnecessarily. A child with a visual motor disability, for example, might find it hard to load a dishwasher but could carry out the trash. The same child might have difficulty catching or throwing a ball, but no trouble swimming. Parents must think ahead about these matters to minimize their child's stress and to maximize his or her chance to experience success, make friends, and develop self-esteem. Treatment that affects only school work will not succeed, because learning disabilities are life disabilities.

It is essential to recognize learning disabilities and related problems as early as possible. Without recognition and help, children may become increasingly frustrated and distressed as they persistently fail. By the time they reach high school, they may give up. On the other hand, children whose special needs are recognized early and treated appropriately can overcome or learn to compensate for their disabilities.

Section 31.3

Adults with Learning Disabilities: Assessing the Problem

Introduction

When adults suspect they have a learning disability, or that someone they care about does, they need information. They often have
questions such as: What can I do? Whom can I call? How can I obtain
information? Where are available services?

Assessing the Problem

Those adults who suspect they may have a learning disability can
begin to find assistance by having an assessment conducted by qualified professionals. Qualified professionals are individuals trained to
conduct assessments. Often the professionals have been certified to
select, administer, and interpret a variety of neurological, psychological, educational, and vocational assessment instruments.

Different assessment procedures may be appropriate in various settings such as community colleges, adult basic education programs, and
through vocational rehabilitation agencies. It is important for the adult
not only to be actively involved in the assessment process, but also to
have confidence in the professional with whom he or she is working.

An assessment refers to the gathering of relevant information that
can be used to help an adult make decisions, and provides a means
for assisting an adult to live more fully. An adult is assessed because
of problems in employment, education, and/or life situations. An assessment involves more than just taking tests. An assessment includes
an evaluation, a diagnosis, and recommendations.

The first stage of an evaluation is usually a screening. Screening tools
use abbreviated, informal methods to determine if an individual is at
risk for a learning disability. Examples of informal methods include, but

are not limited to: an interview; reviews of medical, school, or employment histories; written answers to a few questions; or a brief test. It is important to understand, however, that being screened for a learning disability is different from undergoing a thorough evaluation. When conducting a thorough evaluation, qualified professionals may first refer to the results of the screening in order to plan which tests to administer. Such tests may include, but are not limited to, those that provide information on intelligence, aptitude, achievement, and vocational interests. During the evaluation stage of the assessment process, all relevant information about an individual should be gathered.

A diagnosis is a statement of the specific type of learning disability that an individual may have, based on an interpretation of the information gathered during the evaluation. A diagnosis serves a useful purpose if it explains an individual's particular strengths and weaknesses, as well as determines eligibility for resources or support services that have not been otherwise available. Through a careful examination and analysis of all the information gathered during the evaluation, qualified professionals use the diagnostic stage of the assessment process to explain the information gathered and to offer recommendations.

Recommendations should provide direction in employment, education, and daily living. Specific recommendations may be made regarding the instructional strategies which an individual will find most successful, as well as other ways to compensate for and/or overcome some of the effects of the disability. Based on specific strengths and areas for development identified during the evaluation and diagnostic stages of the assessment process, recommendations should also suggest possible accommodations that an individual can use to be more successful and feel less frustrated in everyday life.

Adults should be assessed according to their age, experience, and career objectives. This is the only way appropriate, helpful, and conclusive information can be provided to adults. As a result of an assessment, adults will have new information that can help them plan how to obtain the assistance they need. Regardless of their diagnosis, individuals will know more about themselves, have a greater understanding of their strengths and weaknesses, and feel better about themselves.

Locating a Qualified Professional

In addition to the resources listed here, there are agencies in most areas that can refer inquirers to diagnosticians or professionals qualified to conduct assessments appropriate for adults. Check your telephone directory for the following:

- Learning Disabilities Association of America, often listed with the name of the city or county first
- adult education in the public school system
- adult literacy programs or literacy councils
- community mental health agencies
- counseling or study skills center at a local college or university
- educational therapists or learning specialists in private practice
- guidance counselors in high schools
- International Dyslexia Association
- private schools or institutions specializing in learning disabilities
- special education departments and/or disability support service offices in colleges or universities
- state vocational rehabilitation agency
- university-affiliated hospitals

Questions to Ask Qualified Professionals

- Have you tested many adults with learning disabilities?
- How long will the assessment take?
- What will the assessment cover?
- Will there be a written and an oral report of the assessment?
- Will our discussion give me more information regarding why I am having trouble with my job or job training, school, or daily life?
- Will you also give me ideas on how to improve my skills and how to compensate for my disability?
- Will the report make recommendations about where to go for immediate help?
- What is the cost? What does the cost cover?
- What are possibilities and costs for additional consultation?
- Can insurance cover the costs? Are there other funding sources? Can a payment plan be worked out?

A Learning Disabilities Checklist

A checklist is a guide. It is a list of characteristics. It is difficult to provide a checklist of typical characteristics of adults with learning disabilities because their most common characteristics are their unique differences. In addition, most adults exhibit or have exhibited some of these characteristics. In other words, saying yes to any one item on this checklist does not mean you are a person with a learning disability. Even if a number of the following items sound familiar to you, you are not necessarily an individual with a learning disability. However, if you say that's me for most of the items, and if you experience these difficulties to such a degree that they cause problems in employment, education, and/or daily living, it might be useful for you to obtain an assessment by qualified professionals experienced in working with adults with learning disabilities.

There are many worthwhile checklists available from a number of organizations. The following checklist was adapted from lists of learning disabilities' characteristics developed by the following organizations: Learning Disabilities Association of America, *For Employers... A Look at Learning Disabilities*, ERIC Clearinghouse on Disabilities and Gifted Education, *Examples of Learning Disability Characteristics*; The International Dyslexia Association's *Annals of Dyslexia*; and the Council for Learning Disabilities, *Infosheet*.

While individuals with learning disabilities have average or above average intelligence, they do not excel in employment, education, and/or life situations at the same level as their peers. Identified characteristics are as follows:

- May perform similar tasks differently from day to day

- May read well but not write well, or write well but not read well

- May be able to learn information presented in one way, but not in another

- May have a short attention span, be impulsive, and/or be easily distracted

- May have difficulty telling or understanding jokes

- May misinterpret language, have poor comprehension of what is said

- May have difficulty with social skills, may misinterpret social cues

- May find it difficult to memorize information

- May have difficulty following a schedule, being on time, or meeting deadlines
- May get lost easily, either driving or in large buildings
- May have trouble reading maps
- May often misread or miscopy
- May confuse similar letters or numbers, reverse them, or confuse their order
- May have difficulty reading the newspaper, following small print, or following columns
- May be able to explain things orally, but not in writing
- May have difficulty writing ideas on paper
- May reverse or omit letters, words, or phrases when writing
- May have difficulty completing job applications correctly
- May have persistent problems with sentence structure, writing mechanics, and organizing written work
- May experience continuous problems with spelling the same word differently in one document
- May have trouble dialing phone numbers and reading addresses
- May have difficulty with math, math language, and math concepts
- May reverse numbers in checkbook and have difficulty balancing a checkbook
- May confuse right and left, up and down
- May have difficulty following directions, especially multiple directions
- May be poorly coordinated
- May be unable to tell you what has just been said
- May hear sounds, words, or sentences imperfectly or incorrectly

As mentioned previously, an adult with learning disabilities may exhibit some of these characteristics, but not necessarily all of them. If an individual exhibits several or many of these characteristics to such a degree that they cause problems in work, school, or everyday life, he or she might benefit from an assessment by a qualified professional.

Section 31.4

Specialists in the Learning Disabilities Field

"Specialists in the Learning Disabilities Field," Jan Baumel, M.S., excerpted from *LD Basics: A Parent's Guide*, © 2008 GreatSchools, Inc. All Rights Reserved. Reprinted with permission. For additional information, visit http://www.schwablearning.org.

Being a parent isn't easy. Parenting a child with learning disabilities (LD) is even more challenging because you may be involved with a variety of professionals during your child's education. Here's a brief list of some of them and an explanation of the services they provide.

Attorney: Provides legal assistance to parents about issues pertaining to federal and state special education laws and regulations.

Advocate: Represents parents in legal issues related to special education but may not have legal training.

Audiologist: Assesses for degree of hearing loss and advises on devices for hearing amplification.

Child psychiatrist: Specializes in the assessment and treatment of behavior and emotional aspects of infants, children, and adolescents; medical doctor who can prescribe medication.

Clinical psychologist: Provides non-medical diagnosis and therapeutic treatment of emotional and behavioral problems for individuals or groups.

Developmental behavioral pediatrician: Focuses on the diagnosis and treatment of developmental disorders in children; medical doctor who can prescribe medication.

Educational psychologist: Administers psychological and educational assessments, prepares written report that interprets test results and behavior, and consults regarding education and behavior.

Educational therapist: Assesses educational needs; develops and carries out programs for school-related behavior and learning problems, especially LD.

Neurologist: Specializes in diagnosis and treatment of disorders of the brain and nervous system; medical doctor who can prescribe medication.

Neuropsychologist: Assesses brain functioning and its relationship to learning and behavior through psychological tests.

Occupational therapist: Assesses for and provides training to improve muscular strength, motor, or sensory coordination and functioning.

Ophthalmologist: A medical doctor who specializes in the diagnosis and treatment of eye defects and disease. Can prescribe corrective lenses and perform eye surgery.

Optometrist: A licensed doctor who is trained to examine the eyes for visual defects and impairments, and to prescribe corrective lenses and provide other types of treatment.

Pediatrician: Specializes in the primary care of infants, children, and adolescents; medical doctor who can prescribe medication.

Resource teacher/resource specialist: Job title used in some states or school districts for a special education teacher who is trained to provide educational assessments, instructional planning, ongoing evaluation of students, and to consult with general educational teachers regarding the needs of special education students.

School psychologist: A psychologist who is specially trained to address students' needs in the public school setting, including psychoeducational evaluations, planning and evaluating services, and acting as liaison between students, parents, teachers, and administrators.

Social worker: Provides counseling for individuals and families.

Special education teacher: A teacher trained to provide specially designed instruction to students with disabilities, and to adapt and develop materials to match the special needs of each student.

Speech and language therapist: Provides assessment and training to improve communication skills.

Tutor: Provides instructional support in academic areas; no specific training requirements; may or may not be a teacher with credentials.

Chapter 32

Responsiveness to Intervention (RTI): An Emerging Method for Learning Disabilities Identification

What Is Responsiveness to Intervention?

Responsiveness to intervention (RTI) is an education model that promotes early identification of students who may be at risk for learning difficulties. RTI is addressed through federal law and refers to a tiered approach to instruction. Students who do not make adequate academic progress and who are at risk for reading and other learning disabilities receive increasingly intensive instructional services.

In many schools today, when a student can't keep up in class, that student's only option for help is to qualify for special education services. However, if a student struggles at a school that uses the responsiveness to intervention (RTI) model, the school staff's first thought is: Maybe this child isn't getting the instruction that he or she needs to succeed. In other words, the student isn't being responsive to the instruction. This doesn't mean that the student isn't trying, but most generally he or she isn't understanding what is being taught by the teacher.

These schools don't wait for students to fail for an extended period. They want to act immediately to get the student the help needed. They regularly screen all students to make sure classroom instruction is on target for the students. Each child is compared to others of the same age and in the same grade and same class.

This chapter includes text from: National Research Center on Learning Disabilities (2007). What is responsiveness to intervention? [Brochure], and How can early intervening services and responsiveness to intervention work together? [Brochure]. Lawrence, KS.

School-wide screenings and progress monitoring focus on all students' achievements in class. For those students who score lowest on in-class subjects and don't seem to be mastering classroom lessons, the school uses a step-by-step teaching process using scientifically proven teaching techniques and frequent brief assessments to monitor progress—that is, to determine whether the teaching techniques are helping. Results from progress monitoring, usually given at least once a week, show what planning and methods to use for academic success. This process, when done according to effective teaching practices, helps to determine whether a student's low achievement is due to instructional or behavioral factors or whether the child has a possible learning disability.

Think of responsiveness to intervention as a series of steps:

1. The first step is instruction in the general classroom. Screening tests given in the classroom reveal students at risk for reading and other learning difficulties. For example, testing may show that a student who has difficulty reading needs additional instruction in phonics.

2. In the second step, the classroom teacher might handle the instruction. In other cases, someone who has expertise in reading and phonics might instruct the student and other students who have the same difficulty.

3. Students who fail to respond to this instruction may then be considered for more specialized instruction in step three, where instruction may occur with greater frequency or duration. If the achievement difficulties persist, a team of educators from different fields (for example, reading or counseling) completes a comprehensive evaluation to determine eligibility for special education and related services. That's because responsiveness to intervention alone is not sufficient to identify a learning disability. All in all, the goal is to provide the type of instruction and educational assistance the student needs to be successful in the general education classroom.

In the responsiveness to intervention model, one of the benefits for parents is that they get to see how their child is doing, compared to peers, and how the child's class measures up to other classes of the same grade. They can get these results on a regular basis from their school. If class scores are down, for instance, questions will be raised about the quality of teaching in that class; thus, classroom teachers are more accountable for their instruction.

Responsiveness to intervention, with its increased instructional precision, is now used more to prevent academic failure than to specifically determine which students have learning disabilities. Also, it has been used mostly for reading in elementary schools. Almost no research results yet exist on how it works in middle schools or high schools; practical application of it in math instruction, too, needs to be further documented.

Although unanswered questions need further research, RTI thus far has compelling benefits. When RTI is implemented with rigor and fidelity, all students receive high-quality instruction in their general education setting. All students are screened for academics and behavior and have their progress monitored to pinpoint specific difficulties.

A continuing advantage for all students is the opportunity to be identified as at risk for learning difficulties early in their education instead of having to fail—sometimes for years—before getting additional services. And, all students have the opportunity to get assistance at the level needed, reducing the number of students referred for special education services.

For a long time, special education has been the instructional solution for struggling learners even when they didn't have learning disabilities. Because an abundance of research has shown that well-designed instructional programs and strategies significantly improve learning when carefully monitored, the responsiveness to intervention approach may be a method to improve learning in general education and reduce referrals to special education.

How Can Early Intervening Services and Responsiveness to Intervention Work Together?

One of the hallmark changes in the Individuals with Disabilities Education Improvement Act of 2004 (IDEA 2004), which was signed into law in December 2004, allows for the use of special education funds (Part B) for at-risk students. These are students who may need additional academic or behavioral support but who do not qualify for special education services. This change is referred to as early intervening services.

"A local educational agency (LEA) may not use more than 15% of the amount such agency receives under this part (Part B)...to develop and implement coordinated, early intervening services ... for students in kindergarten through grade 12 (with particular emphasis on students in kindergarten through grade three) who do not meet the definition of a child with a disability... but who need additional academic and behavioral support to succeed in a general education environment." IDEA 2004 Section 613(f)(1)

These funds, which cannot exceed 15 percent of the Part B funds, have a restriction: They have to be used to deliver scientifically based academic and behavioral interventions within the general education environment. This additional instruction can't be a little bit of this and that, or simply what a teacher thinks might be of value; the interventions have to be based on proven research and delivered with fidelity, that is, according to specified parameters to get desired results. This "fidelity of instruction" (an assurance that the instruction is delivered in exactly the way it was designed to be delivered) requires that teachers and other staff be well-versed in the instructional program and that there is a way to verify whether they have followed its methods correctly.

The fact that to intervene with children who are having difficulties in learning requires that students be screened to see which ones need assistance brings up questions: What tool or method can schools use to accurately assess student progress and determine need for additional assistance? And, once students have received early intervening services, what accurate method can schools use to judge student progress in relation to their peers and to make instructional decisions?

IDEA says "... a local educational agency may use a process that determines if the child responds to scientific, research-based intervention as a part of the evaluation procedures...." however, IDEA doesn't name one specific process. In special education research literature, from which policy makers drew to update IDEA, the process mentioned is typically responsiveness to intervention (RTI).

The RTI process uses school-wide procedures, including whole-class interventions, screening, and progress monitoring to assess an entire class as well as individual student progress. RTI promotes early identification of students at risk for academic failure and uses multiple performance measures rather than measurement at a single point in time.

Using a tiered approach, responsiveness to intervention is applied on a school-wide basis, in which the majority of students receive instruction in the general classroom (tier one). Students at risk for reading and other learning disabilities are identified through screening to receive more intense support in tier two. Here, specialists, tutors, or special education teachers provide additional instruction in small groups, (for example, one teacher to up to five students).

At the end of this small group instructional period, if a student has made sufficient progress, he or she might return to the general education classroom (tier one), continue in the tier two intervention, or be considered for a more intensive intervention in tier three. In tier three, often considered "special education," instruction in a specified area of need is individualized or delivered in small groups of one teacher to no more than three students. Students who meet tier three targets return to tier one but also may re-enter tier two, or, if needed, stay in tier three until they are able to maintain progress in tier one. This system is enhanced if procedures are in place for parental involvement.

When designing an early intervening services and responsiveness to intervention system, the focus is on positive behavior support— introducing, modeling, and reinforcing positive social behavior—and academics with school-wide screening, tiered levels of intervention, and progress monitoring that guides decision-making.

Chapter 33

Functional Behavior Assessment and Positive Interventions: What Parents Need to Know

Many children have inappropriate behaviors that are part of their disability. These behaviors may make it difficult to learn, cause harm to the child or others, or isolate a child from his or her peers. Some children have behaviors that they can't control, such as tics for a child with Tourette syndrome or self-harming behaviors for some children with developmental disabilities. Some children may be sad or anxious. Others simply have not learned positive ways to have their needs met. In any of these instances, the behaviors interfere with the children's ability to learn the skills they need to be successful.

We can teach appropriate behavior skills to children. To do so, we need to understand problem behaviors, such as where they occur and what purpose they serve for a child. The process of learning about how children develop problem behaviors is called functional behavioral assessment (FBA). If we learn about the behaviors and know when and where they are likely to happen, we can plan positive strategies to teach new behaviors. These strategies are called positive behavioral interventions. Teachers and parents will use the information from an FBA to help a child learn new skills. The goal is to teach children how to manage their own behaviors.

This chapter will help parents understand functional behavioral assessment and positive interventions. You have a very important role in this assessment, because you have information about your child that no one else has. When you understand the process, you can work effectively with the rest of the team. You will have the tools to make decisions when functional behavioral assessment is proposed for your child. What you know about your child will be used to help develop effective instruction.

Thinking about Behavior

Adults often have two different approaches to dealing with problem behaviors. These different approaches are based on different beliefs. One belief is that the child is a problem, and the other is that the child has a problem.

The Child Is a Problem

Billy is a 12-year-old sixth-grade student. He refuses to do his schoolwork, and then his teacher does not know what to do. He becomes angry when the teacher reminds him to get to work. He screams, swears, and even throws his work on the floor so the teacher will leave him alone. The teacher may think Billy is lazy, mean, or disrespectful. The teacher may feel angry or threatened. Adults who are angry often use punishment or threats: "Do it or else." We do not always realize that children do not think about their problem behaviors the way we do.

When we punish often, children may see us as uncaring. Some may come to fear or avoid us. Others may become even louder and angrier because of the punishment. Children who do not back down when arguing with adults often receive increasingly harsh punishments. Many adults think children should not be permitted to win disagreements. Children, on the other hand, often say things they do not really mean because they are angry. They may refuse to give up even if they lose privileges or are suspended from school.

When a child is suspended from school for problem behaviors, some people think of it as "good medicine for bad behavior." They think the removal teaches the child a lesson and that the child will change the problem behaviors as a result. But what if that child does not like going to school? He or she may learn that using problem behaviors is a good way to earn a vacation from school. The child may actually want what we think is a punishment.

The Child Has a Problem

Billy, the 12-year-old described earlier, has behaviors that need to change. Let's assume we have assessment data that give a clearer picture of Billy. We find that he reads at a second-grade level. He was sexually abused at age three by a neighbor. Billy is angry over his parents' recent divorce and continuing custody battle. He is worried about where he will live.

Clearly Billy's problem behaviors must change. They are serious and interfere with learning. What we decide to do about the behavior, however, comes from how we feel about it and whether we believe it is willful. That is where functional behavioral assessment comes in. It can help us to identify why Billy is frustrated and angry, so we can help him to learn the skills he needs. A reasonable person would have a hard time believing that punishment alone could help Billy succeed.

Positive Behavioral Interventions

Positive: Characterized by or displaying approval, acceptance, or affirmation.

Behavior: What we do.

Intervention: An action that changes a course of events.

(Adapted from *Merriam Webster's Tenth Collegiate Dictionary*.)

The 1997 Individuals with Disabilities Education Act (IDEA) Regulations

IDEA states that the individualized education program (IEP) team shall, in the case of a child whose behavior impedes his or her learning or that of others, consider, where appropriate, strategies, including positive behavioral interventions, strategies, and supports that address that behavior. IDEA 300.346(2)(i)

Positive behavioral interventions are used before problem behaviors occur. To develop positive interventions, the team must understand why a child has problem behaviors and what strategies might be helpful. Many different strategies can be used to reduce problem behaviors in school: changing where a child sits in the classroom, adjusting the schoolwork, or rewarding the child for positive behaviors. The child's teacher may speak in a different tone of voice to help the child remain calm. Adults may try to keep calm when the child is angry. The goal is to stop or reduce the problem behaviors so that punishment does not become necessary.

Here is an example: The teacher knows that Mary is more likely to argue with the teacher when she sits next to Mark. If the teacher thinks Mary argues because she wants Mark to notice her, there are several things the teacher can do. She can separate Mary and Mark so that Mary does not try so hard to get his attention. She can also teach Mary more positive ways to gain Mark's attention and provide positive reinforcement for using the new behaviors.

Behaviors Are Governed by Their Consequences

John has a fight (behavior) and is suspended from school (consequence). If John loves school and can control the behavior, the consequence is negative because he has to give up something he wants (school). If John dislikes school, however, he may see that same consequence as positive. He may learn that fighting is a good way to be sent home. The next time John does not want to be in school, what behavior is he likely to use?

Many of us have learned to deal with problem behaviors by doing nothing until they occur. After a child uses the behaviors, we punish. Punishment does not teach new skills, though. Its goal is to stop problem behaviors from continuing. If we do not teach a child what to do instead, the child will probably continue to misbehave. Any time a child uses a behavior that is successful in meeting a need, the behavior is likely to be repeated. The behavior serves a function for the child.

Most people agree that we need to have consequences for problem behaviors. We must also focus on teaching the positive behavior skills we would like to see. If we can understand the function of problem behaviors, we can teach a child more positive behaviors that serve the same function, and the problem behaviors are no longer needed.

Functional Behavioral Assessment

Functional behavioral assessment (FBA) is a process for collecting information. The data the team collects are used to help determine why problem behaviors occur. The data will also help identify ways to address the behaviors. Functional behavioral assessment data are used to develop a positive behavioral intervention plan. The Individuals with Disabilities Education Act specifically requires an FBA whenever a child with a disability has his or her current placement changed for disciplinary reasons. This does not mean that we should not think about FBA at other times, too.

The evaluation requirements of IDEA make it clear that children must be evaluated in "all areas related to the suspected disability."

This means that if your child has problem behaviors that are not improving, your child may need an evaluation to examine the behaviors more closely. You may request an FBA at any time if your child's problem behaviors are becoming worse, or when the team cannot explain to you why the problem behaviors occur.

There are many reasons a child might misbehave. Some have to do with the nature of the child, such as allergies to dust, foods, or plants. A sinus infection, headache, or toothache can also lead to problem behaviors. Some children have a medical diagnosis, such as bipolar disorder or attention-deficit/hyperactivity disorder that affects behavior. The team's responsibility is to collect data to help it understand why a child has problem behaviors.

The people who complete the functional behavioral assessment use different ways to collect data. School staff may interview you and your child. They observe your child in different settings, such as the lunchroom or classroom, or on the playground. They gather reports from teachers and others. The team reviews your child's records, including any assessments you would like to share.

The results of this process should lead to a hypothesis about why problem behaviors occur. A hypothesis is an educated guess, based on the data the team has gathered. Assessment results are used to develop a positive behavior intervention plan.

Behaviors Are Context-Related

Most behaviors are related to their context. This means that behaviors often result from what is happening in the child's world or environment. These are just a few of the factors that may lead to problem behaviors:

- a disagreement between children
- the number of children in a classroom
- the quality of peer relationships
- the size of the classroom
- medicine changes
- the difficulty of schoolwork

Other things, such as who is present and what their expectations are, also affect behaviors. Behaviors may also be a problem when a child is emotionally upset and cannot handle the demands of the environment.

Behaviors Serve a Function

Problem behaviors usually serve a function, or purpose, for the child. Sometimes we see problem behaviors when a substitute teacher is in the classroom. In this case, we must be careful not to assume that the child doesn't like the teacher or that the child wants to show off for friends. Perhaps the child likes his or her regular teacher and is upset when she is not there. Or the child may be anxious about what to expect with a new teacher. A child who is upset about having a new teacher may use problem behaviors in order to be placed in a less stressful setting. Some children would rather be in a time-out space than in their classroom.

Unfortunately, consequences that improve the behaviors of most students do not work with all. Sending a child to the principal's office, for example, can be ineffective if the consequence does not address the complex function of a child's behavior.

What a child does (the behavior) and why a child does it (the function) may be unrelated. Skipping school and getting good grades are two very different behaviors. Yet they may serve the same function for different children—gaining adult attention. Two children may both want to be noticed by their parents; one may study hard to have good grades while the other skips class. They do very different things to get the attention they want. While the function of both behaviors is positive (parent attention), skipping class is not an acceptable way to be noticed.

Behaviors Are Influenced by Events in the Environment (Antecedents)

What happens in an environment affects behavior. The size of a classroom, the number of students, transitions, or early morning bus incidents are all antecedents that might affect a child's behavior.

It is important to know what leads to both positive and negative behaviors. If teachers and parents understand the conditions that lead to problem behaviors, then changing the conditions may reduce the need for the behaviors. Positive teaching strategies such as providing structure, routine, and rewards for appropriate behaviors help to increase positive behavior skills.

Steps in Conducting a Functional Behavioral Assessment

The Individuals with Disabilities Education Act does not define how a functional behavioral assessment is done. The process may vary with the needs of each child. However, several specific steps are always part of this kind of assessment. The process begins with identifying the specific behaviors that must change. If a child has many problem behaviors, it will be important to focus on the most serious one or two behaviors. The problem behaviors are described in a way that helps everyone to understand exactly what the behaviors are. These are typical steps:

1. Identify and agree on the behavior(s) that most need to change.

2. Determine where the behaviors occur and where they do not. Identify what may contribute to the behaviors. The team will ask these kinds of questions:

   - What is unique about the environments where behaviors are not a concern?

   - What is different in the places where the problem behaviors do occur? Could they be related to how the child and teacher get along? Does the number of other students or the work a child is asked to do cause the problem? Could the time of day or a child's mood affect the behaviors? Was there a bus problem or a disagreement in the hallway?

   - Are the behaviors likely to occur in a specific set of circumstances or a specific setting? What events seem to support the problem behaviors?

3. Collect data on the child's performance from as many sources as possible.

4. Develop a hypothesis about why problem behaviors occur (the function of the behaviors). A hypothesis is an educated guess, based on data. It helps predict where and why problem behaviors are most likely to occur, and where and why they are least likely to occur.

5. Identify other behaviors that can be taught that will serve the same function for the child.

6. Test the hypothesis. The team develops and uses positive behavioral interventions that are written into the child's IEP or behavior intervention plan.

7. Evaluate the success of the interventions. Change or fine-tune as needed.

If children have behaviors that place them or others in danger, they may need a crisis intervention plan. Crisis interventions should be developed before they are needed. The team should decide what behaviors are crises and what they (and the child) will do in a crisis. By having a plan that guides actions, teachers can help children through difficult emotional situations.

Behavior Intervention Plan

An effective behavior intervention plan (often called a behavior support plan or positive intervention plan) is used to teach or reinforce positive behaviors. Typically, a child's team develops the plan. It usually includes:

- skills training to increase appropriate behavior;
- changes that will be made in classrooms or other environments to reduce or eliminate problem behaviors;
- strategies to replace problem behaviors with appropriate behaviors that serve the same function for the child; and,
- supports for the child to use the appropriate behaviors.

A positive behavior intervention plan is not a plan to determine what happens to a student who violates a rule or code of conduct. That would be more appropriately called a discipline plan or a punishment plan.

School Discipline Policies

The IEP team determines whether the school discipline policies need to be amended for a child, or whether the consequences need to be different from those written into the policy. This decision should be based on evaluation and a review of the records, including the discipline records or any manifestation determination review(s) that have been completed by the school. A child's IEP or behavior intervention plan should focus on teaching skills.

Sometimes school discipline policies are not successful in correcting problem behaviors. That is, the child does not learn what the school staff intended through the use of punishments such as suspension. The child may learn instead that problem behaviors are useful in meeting a need, such as being noticed by peers. When this is true, it is difficult to defend punishment, by itself, as effective in changing problem behaviors.

One of the most useful questions parents can ask when they have concerns about the discipline recommendations for their child is: "Where are the data that support the recommendations?" Special education decisions are based on data. If school staff wants to use a specific discipline procedure, they should check for data that support the use of the procedure. For instance, if your child has been repeatedly suspended from school for a problem behavior, has suspension taught your child the skills he or she needs to learn?

Zero-Tolerance Policies

Many school districts have zero-tolerance policies that provide immediate negative consequences for specific behaviors. Such policies simply do not provide effective consequences for all children who violate them. If a child with a disability violates a zero-tolerance policy, the consequence may or may not be effective, given that child's needs. Consequences for problem behaviors must not discriminate against a child based on his or her disability. The IEP team is responsible for determining whether exceptions need to be made to the written school district discipline policy for a student, or whether the student needs a different consequence for misbehaviors than is written into the school discipline policies. Instructional goals may need to be written into the IEP to help remediate the problems a child is having in following school discipline policies.

While some administrators may not want to make exceptions to school-wide discipline policies established for all students, exceptions are sometimes necessary. Some students who are unable to conform their behavior to the school expectations may need to have individualized consequences that will be more effective in supporting positive behaviors.

In the U.S. legal system, the consequences for breaking a law are generally based on an evaluation of the events around the violation. Yet schools often have one discipline standard for all students regardless of individual needs. They may use the same consequences for all students. Parents must carefully examine school policies to help determine whether modifications need to be made to meet the needs of their child.

Examples of Behavioral Intervention Strategies

Schools use the following common strategies to help reduce problem behaviors and teach children positive behavioral skills.

Stop, relax, and think: Teaches children how to think about the problem they are having and find a solution. Children learn these steps:

1. Define the problem.

2. Decide who "owns" the problem.

3. Think of as many solutions as possible to solve the problem.

4. Select a solution to try.

5. Use the solution.

6. Evaluate its success.

After children understand the steps, role-play and practice can help the process become habit. Helping children to recognize their own response to stress (clenched hands, voice tone, etc.) may become part of the instruction needed to use this strategy effectively.

Planned ignoring: Is useful in stopping behaviors that are annoying. For example, it is useful for students who yell or interrupt the class to attract the teacher's attention or that of students who are not prepared for class. Planned ignoring acknowledges that children's problem behaviors serve a function. If the purpose of a problem behavior is to gain adult attention, then not providing attention means that the behavior does not work. The behavior lessens over time and eventually disappears. Ignoring behavior which is not serious is especially useful for parents when their child is having a tantrum for attention. Many adults find it difficult to ignore behaviors, however, especially if the behaviors interrupt what the adult is doing. Also, attention-seeking behaviors often get worse before they eventually go away.

Planned ignoring is not suitable for behaviors that are extremely disruptive. It also may not work if other children laugh at the problem behaviors the adult is trying to ignore. Some behaviors including those that are unsafe or those that include peer issues such as arguing can grow quickly into more serious behaviors. It may not be possible to ignore these kinds of behaviors. Planned ignoring should never be used for unsafe behaviors. As children grow older and want attention more from their friends than from adults, planned ignoring is less useful.

Preventive cueing (also called signal interference): Lets a child know when he or she is doing something that is not acceptable.

Teachers or parents can frown, shake their head, make eye contact, point to a seat for a wandering child, or snap their fingers, to let the child know he or she needs to pay attention or to stop the problem behaviors. When using preventive cueing it is important not to smile or look pleased with a child. Preventive cueing may be used in steps, depending on the behaviors and how often they occur or how serious they are. For instance, a hand motion may work the first time or two, but it may need to be combined with eye contact or a shake of the head for the next offense.

Proximity control: Means that a teacher or adult moves closer to the child in a gentle way. If the teacher does not get the child's attention by using cues, then he or she may move closer to the student or give the lesson while standing near the child's desk.

Touch control: Meaning touch that is not resisted, is a nonverbal guided intervention. It is used to direct a student toward positive behavior. For example, a teacher may gently place a hand on a child's shoulder to steer the child back to his or her desk. Touch control should never be used with children who react angrily or when school policy does not permit its use. If a child's records show that he or she has a history of violence, has been abused or maltreated, is anxious, or has a mental illness or psychosis, touch control should not be used, unless specifically agreed to by a physician or psychologist.

Humor: Directed either at the teacher or the situation—never at the child—can defuse tensions as well as redirect children. Humor must never be used to demean a child or be used in a manner that might encourage others in the class to ridicule the child.

Nonverbal warning: Gives a child the opportunity to regain control without being singled out for a verbal reprimand. For example, a teacher might place a colored warning cue card or a note on a desk as he or she moves through the room, or hold up the number of fingers that corresponds to the rule being challenged.

Discipline privately: Many children see it as a challenge when teachers attempt to discipline them in front of their peers. Children rarely lose these challenges, even when adults use negative consequences. Young people can gain stature from peers by publicly refusing to obey a teacher. A child is more likely to accept discipline if his or her peers are not watching the process.

Positive phrasing: Lets children know the positive results for using appropriate behaviors. As simple as it sounds, this can be difficult. Teachers and parents are used to focusing on misbehavior. Warning children about a negative response to problem behaviors often seems easier than describing the positive impact of positive behaviors. Compare the difference between positive phrasing and negative phrasing:

- Positive phrasing: "If you finish your reading by recess, we can all go outside together and play a game."

- Negative phrasing: "If you do not finish your reading by recess, you will have to stay inside until it's done."

Positive phrasing helps children learn that positive behaviors lead to positive outcomes. This, in turn, can help them gain control of their behaviors.

I-messages: Described by Thomas Gordon in his 1974 book *Teacher Effectiveness Training*, helps children learn about how their problem behaviors affect others. It also demonstrates the importance of taking responsibility for one's own behavior. For example, parents or teachers will use language like "I'm upset when . . ." not "You are bad when . . ."

When a child has a good relationship with parents and teachers, I-messages can help him or her to understand how the problem behaviors affect adults. If the child dislikes the teacher, though, using I-statements can be a problem. It may even help the child to more effectively annoy the teacher.

Behavior shaping: Acknowledges that not all children can do everything at 100 percent. If a child does not turn in papers daily, expecting that papers will be turned in 100 percent of the time is not realistic. By rewarding small gains and reinforcing the gains as they occur, children learn how to stick with a task and to improve the skill.

Clear routines and expectations: Let children know what comes next in their school day, reducing anxiety or fear. Teachers who post and review the rules daily establish expectations for behavior during the day.

For Additional Information

PACER Center
8161 Normandale Boulevard
Minneapolis, MN 55437-1044
Phone: 952-838-9000
Fax: 952-838-0199
TTY: 952-838-0190
Toll-Free in MN: 800-537-2237
Websites: http://www.pacer.org;
http://www.fape.org;
http://www.taalliance.org
E-mail: pacer@pacer.org

Chapter 34

Individualized Education Plans (IEP)

Kids with delayed skills or other disabilities might be eligible for special services that provide individualized education programs in public schools, free of charge to families. Understanding how to access these services can help parents be effective advocates for their kids.

The passage of the updated version of the Individuals with Disabilities Education Act (IDEA 2004) made parents of kids with special needs even more crucial members of their child's education team. Parents can now work with educators to develop a plan—the individualized education plan (IEP)—to help kids succeed in school. The IEP describes the goals the team sets for a child during the school year, as well as any special support needed to help achieve them.

Who Needs an IEP?

A child who has difficulty learning and functioning and has been identified as a special needs student is the perfect candidate for an IEP. Kids struggling in school may qualify for support services, allowing them to be taught in a special way, for reasons such as:

"Individualized Education Plans (IEPs)," January 2008, reprinted with permission from www.kidshealth.org. Copyright © 2008 The Nemours Foundation. This information was provided by KidsHealth, one of the largest resources online for medically reviewed health information written for parents, kids, and teens. For more articles like this one, visit www.KidsHealth.org, or www.TeensHealth. org.

- learning disabilities,
- attention deficit/hyperactivity disorder (AD/HD),
- emotional disorders,
- mental retardation,
- autism,
- hearing impairment,
- visual impairment,
- speech or language impairment,
- developmental delay.

In most cases, the services and goals outlined in an IEP can be provided in a standard school environment. This can be done in the regular classroom (for example, a reading teacher helping a small group of children who need extra assistance while the other kids in the class work on reading with the regular teacher) or in a special resource room in the regular school. The resource room can serve a group of kids with similar needs who are brought together for help.

However, kids who need intense intervention may be taught in a special school environment. These classes have fewer students per teacher, allowing for more individualized attention. In addition, the teacher usually has specific training in helping kids with special educational needs. The children spend most of their day in a special classroom and join the regular classes for nonacademic activities (like music and gym) or in academic activities in which they don't need extra help.

Because the goal of IDEA is to ensure that each child is educated in the least restrictive environment possible, effort is made to help kids stay in a regular classroom. However, when needs are best met in a special class, then kids might be placed in one.

The Referral and Evaluation Process

The referral process generally begins when a teacher, parent, or doctor is concerned that a child may be having trouble in the classroom, and the teacher notifies the school counselor or psychologist. The first step is to gather specific data regarding the student's progress or academic problems. This may be done through:

- a conference with parents;
- a conference with the student;

- observation of the student;
- analysis of the student's performance (attention, behavior, work completion, tests, class work, homework, and so forth).

This information helps school personnel determine the next step. At this point, strategies specific to the student could be implemented to help the child become more successful in school. If this doesn't work, the child would be tested for a specific learning disability or other impairment to help determine qualification for special services. It's important to note, though, that the presence of a disability doesn't automatically guarantee a child will receive services. To be eligible, the disability must affect the child's functioning at school.

To determine eligibility, a multidisciplinary team of professionals will evaluate the child based on their observations; the child's performance on standardized tests; and daily work such as tests, quizzes, class work, and homework. The professionals on the evaluation team can include:

- a psychologist;
- a physical therapist;
- an occupational therapist;
- a speech therapist;
- a special educator;
- a vision or hearing specialist;
- others, depending on the child's specific needs.

As a parent, you can decide whether to have your child assessed. If you choose to do so, you'll be asked to sign a permission form that will detail who is involved in the process and the types of tests they use. These tests might include measures of specific school skills, such as reading or math, as well as more general developmental skills, such as speech and language. Testing does not necessarily mean that a child will receive services.

Once the team members complete their individual assessments, they develop a comprehensive evaluation report (CER) that compiles their findings, offers an educational classification, and outlines the skills and support the child will need. The parents then have a chance to review the report before the IEP is developed. Some parents will disagree with the report, but they will have the opportunity to work together with the school to come up with a plan that best meets the child's needs.

Developing an IEP

The next step is an IEP meeting at which the team and parents decide what will go into the plan. In addition to the evaluation team, a regular teacher should be present to offer suggestions about how the plan can help the child's progress in the standard education curriculum.

At the meeting, the team will discuss your child's educational needs—as described in the CER—and come up with specific, measurable short-term and annual goals for each of those needs. If you attend this meeting, you can take an active role in developing the goals and determining which skills or areas will receive the most attention.

The cover page of the IEP outlines the support services your child will receive and how often they will be provided (for example, occupational therapy twice a week). Support services might include special education, speech therapy, occupational or physical therapy, counseling, audiology, medical services, nursing, vision or hearing therapy, and many others.

If the team recommends several services, the amount of time they take in the child's school schedule can seem overwhelming. To ease that load, some services may be provided on a consultative basis. In these cases, the professional consults with the teacher to come up with strategies to help the child but doesn't offer any hands-on instruction. For instance, an occupational therapist may suggest accommodations for a child with fine-motor problems that affect handwriting, and the classroom teacher would incorporate these suggestions into the handwriting lessons taught to the entire class.

Other services can be delivered right in the classroom, so the child's day isn't interrupted by therapy. The child who has difficulty with handwriting might work one on one with an occupational therapist while everyone else practices their handwriting skills. When deciding how and where services are offered, the child's comfort and dignity should be a top priority.

The IEP will be reviewed annually to update the goals and make sure the levels of service meet your child's needs. However, IEPs can be changed at any time on an as-needed basis. If you think your child needs more, fewer, or different services, you can request a meeting and bring the team together to discuss your concerns.

What Are Your Legal Rights?

Specific timelines ensure that the development of an IEP moves from referral to providing services as quickly as possible. Be sure to ask about this timeframe and get a copy of your parents' rights when your child is referred. These guidelines (sometimes called procedural safeguards) outline your rights as a parent to control what happens to your child during each step of the process.

The parents' rights also describe how you can proceed if you disagree with any part of the CER or the IEP—mediation and hearings both are options. You can get information about low-cost or free legal representation from the school district or, if your child is in Early Intervention (for kids ages three to five), through that program. Attorneys and paid advocates familiar with the IEP process will provide representation if you need it. You also may invite anyone who knows or works with your child whose input you feel would be helpful to join the IEP team.

A Final Word

Parents have the right to choose where their kids will be educated. This choice includes public or private elementary schools and secondary schools, including religious schools. It also includes charter schools and home schools. It is important to understand that the rights of children with disabilities who are placed by their parents in private elementary schools and secondary schools are not the same as those of children with disabilities who are enrolled in public schools or placed by public agencies in private schools when the public school is unable to provide a free appropriate public education (FAPE).

Two major differences that parents, teachers, other school staff, private school representatives, and the child need to know about are:

1. Children with disabilities who are placed by their parents in private schools may not get the same services they would receive if they attended a public school.

2. Not all children with disabilities placed by their parents in private schools will receive services.

The IEP process is complex, but it's also an effective way to address how your child learns and functions. If you have concerns, don't hesitate to ask questions about the evaluation findings or the goals recommended by the team. You know your child best and should play a central role in creating a learning plan tailored to your child's specific needs.

For more information, the government has a website to educate anyone about IDEA: http://idea.ed.gov.

Chapter 35

IEP Evaluation and Reevaluation: Questions and Answers

The final regulations for the reauthorized Individuals with Disabilities Education Act (IDEA) were published in the *Federal Register* on August 14, 2006, and became effective on October 13, 2006. Since publication of the final regulations, the Office of Special Education and Rehabilitative Services (OSERS) in the U.S. Department of Education has received requests for clarification of some of these regulations. This chapter is one in a series of question and answer documents prepared by OSERS to address some of the most important issues raised by requests for clarification on a variety of high-interest topics. Generally, the questions, and corresponding answers, presented in this chapter required interpretation of IDEA and the regulations and the answers are not simply a restatement of the statutory or regulatory requirements. The responses presented generally are informal guidance representing the interpretation of the Department of Education of the applicable statutory or regulatory requirements in the context of the specific facts presented and are not legally binding. This information is not intended to be a replacement for careful study of IDEA and the regulations. The statute, regulations, and other important documents related to IDEA and the regulations are found at http://idea.ed.gov.

The development and implementation of an individualized education program (IEP) that addresses the unique needs of each child

Excerpts from "Questions and Answers on Individualized Education Programs (IEPs), Evaluations, and Reevaluations," U.S. Department of Education, January 2007.

with a disability and that assists schools and parents in focusing instruction are at the core of the IDEA. IDEA and the final Part B regulations include significant changes related to the content of IEPs (including content related to secondary transition and state and districtwide assessments), IEPs for children with disabilities who transfer from one public agency to another public agency within the same school year, IEP meetings and participants in those meetings, and changes to IEPs following the annual IEP meeting. The reauthorized IDEA also includes significant changes related to parental consent for initial evaluations and reevaluations.

Secondary Transition

Authority: The requirements for the content of the IEP related to secondary transition are found in the regulations at 34 CFR §300.320(b).

Must an IEP include measurable postsecondary goals based on age appropriate transition assessments for every 16-year-old student with a disability regardless of the student's skill levels relating to education, employment and training?

Yes. Under 34 CFR §300.320(b), the IEP for each child with a disability, must, beginning not later than the first IEP to be in effect when the child turns 16, or younger if determined appropriate by the IEP team, and updated annually thereafter, include:

1. Appropriate measurable postsecondary goals based upon age appropriate transition assessments related to training, education, employment, and where appropriate, independent living skills.

2. The transition services (including courses of study) needed to assist the child in reaching those goals.

This requirement applies, whether or not the child's skill levels related to training, education, and employment are age appropriate. The IEP team must, however, develop the specific postsecondary goals for the child, in light of the unique needs of the child as determined based on age appropriate transition assessments of the child's skills in these areas.

May community access skills be included in the IEP as independent living skills?

It depends. The IEP team must determine whether it is necessary to include appropriate measurable postsecondary goals related to independent living skills in the IEP for a particular child, and, if so, what transition services are needed to assist the child in reaching those goals. Under 34 CFR §300.43, "transition services" are defined as "a coordinated set of activities for a child with a disability" "to facilitate movement from school to post-school activities," and include among other activities, "independent living, or community participation." Based on the assessment of the student's independent living skills, the IEP team would need to determine whether transition services in the form of community access skills are necessary for the child to receive a free appropriate public education (FAPE). If so, those skills must be reflected in the transition services in the child's IEP.

If an IEP team chooses to address transition before age 16 (for example, at age 14) are the same standards required?

Yes. The regulations provide, at 34 CFR §300.320(b), that beginning not later than the first IEP to be in effect when the child turns 16, or younger if determined appropriate by the IEP Team, and updated annually, thereafter, the IEP must include the following:

1. Appropriate measurable postsecondary goals based upon age appropriate transition assessments related to training, education, employment, and, where appropriate, independent living skills.

2. The transition services (including courses of study) needed to assist the child in reaching those goals.

If the IEP team for a particular child with a disability determines that it is appropriate to address the requirements of 34 CFR §300.320(b) for a child who is younger than age 16, then the IEP for that child must meet the requirements of 34 CFR §300.320(b).

Section 300.320(b)(1) requires that appropriate postsecondary transition goals be measurable. Must we measure goals once a student has graduated or has aged out?

There is no requirement for public agencies to measure postsecondary goals once a child is no longer eligible for FAPE under Part

303

B of the Act. Under 34 CFR §300.101, FAPE must be made available to all children residing in the state in mandatory age ranges. However, the obligation to make FAPE available does not apply to children who have graduated from high school with a regular high school diploma (34 CFR §300.102(a)(3)) or to children who have exceeded the mandatory age range for provision of FAPE under state law (34 CFR §300.102(a)(2)). When a child's eligibility for FAPE pursuant to Part B terminates under these circumstances, in accordance with 34 CFR §300.305(e)(3), the local educational agency (LEA) must provide a "summary of the child's academic achievement and functional performance, which shall include recommendations on how to assist the child in meeting the child's postsecondary goals." However, this provision does not require the LEA to provide services to the child to meet these goals.

Transfer of Students with IEPs from One Public Agency to a New Public Agency

Authority: The requirements for IEPs for students who transfer from one public agency to another public agency within the same school year are found in the regulations at 34 CFR §300.323(e), (f), and (g).

What if a student whose IEP has not been subject to a timely annual review, but who continues to receive services under that IEP, transfers to another public agency in the same state? Is the new public agency required to provide FAPE from the time the student arrives?

If a child with a disability was receiving special education and related services pursuant to an IEP in a previous public agency (even if that public agency failed to meet the annual review requirements at 34 CFR §300.324(b)(1)(i)), and transfers to a new public agency in the same state and enrolls in a new school within the same school year, the new public agency (in consultation with the parents) must, pursuant to 34 CFR §300.323(e) provide FAPE to the child (including services comparable to those described in the child's IEP from the previous public agency), until the new public agency either:

- adopts the child's IEP from the previous public agency; or

- develops, adopts, and implements a new IEP that meets the applicable requirements in 34 CFR §§300.320 through 300.324.

What options are available when an out-of-state transfer student cannot produce an IEP, and the parent is the source for identifying "comparable" services?

The regulations require, at 34 CFR §300.323(g), that, to facilitate the transition for a child described in 34 CFR §300.323(e) and (f):

1. The new public agency in which the child enrolls must take reasonable steps to promptly obtain the child's records, including the IEP and supporting documents and any other records relating to the provision of special education or related services to the child, from the previous public agency in which the child was enrolled, pursuant to 34 CFR §99.31(a)(2).

2. The previous public agency in which the child was enrolled must take reasonable steps to promptly respond to the request from the new public agency.

If, after taking reasonable steps to obtain the child's records from the public agency in which the child was previously enrolled, including the IEP and any other records relating to the provision of special education or related services to the child, the new public agency is not able to obtain the IEP from the previous public agency or from the parent, the new public agency is not required to provide services to the child pursuant to 34 CFR §300.323(f). This is because the new public agency, in consultation with the parents, would be unable to determine what constitutes comparable services for the child, since that determination must be based on the services contained in the child's IEP from the previous public agency. However, the new public agency must place the child in the regular school program and conduct an evaluation pursuant to 34 CFR §§300.304 through 300.306, if determined to be necessary by the new public agency. If there is a dispute between the parent and the new public agency regarding whether an evaluation is necessary or regarding what special education and related services are needed to provide FAPE to the child, the dispute could be resolved through the mediation procedures in 34 CFR §300.506 or, as appropriate, the due process procedures in 34 CFR §§300.507 through 300.516. Once a due process complaint notice requesting a due process hearing is filed, under 34 CFR §300.518(b), the child would remain in the regular school program during the pendency of the due process proceedings.

Is it permissible for a public agency to require that a student with a disability who transfers from another state with a current IEP that is provided to the new public agency remain at home without receiving services until a new IEP is developed by the public agency?

Under 34 CFR §300.323(f), if a child with a disability (who had an IEP that was in effect in a previous public agency in another state) transfers to a public agency in a new state, and enrolls in a new school within the same school year, the new public agency (in consultation with the parents) must provide the child with FAPE (including services comparable to those described in the child's IEP from the previous public agency), until the new public agency:

1. Conducts an evaluation pursuant to 34 CFR §§300.304 through 300.306 (if determined to be necessary by the new public agency).

2. Develops, adopts, and implements a new IEP, if appropriate, that meets the applicable requirements in 34 CFR §§300.320 through 300.324.

Thus, the public agency must provide FAPE to the child when the child enrolls in the school in the public agency in the new state, and may not deny services to the child pending the development of a new IEP.

What is the timeline for the receiving public agency to adopt an IEP from a previous public agency or to develop and implement a new IEP?

Neither the Act nor the regulations establish timelines for the new public agency to adopt the child's IEP from the previous public agency; or to develop, adopt, and implement a new IEP. However, consistent with 34 CFR §300.323(e) and (f), the new public agency must take these steps within a reasonable period of time to avoid any undue interruption in the provision of required services.

IEP Team Membership and IEP Meetings

Authority: The requirements for IEP team membership are found in the regulations at 34 CFR §300.321. The requirements for IEP meetings are found in the regulations at 34 CFR §300.323(c)(1), and §300.324(a), (b) and (c).

May the representative of the public agency be excused from an IEP team meeting?

Under 34 CFR §300.321(e)(1), the public agency representative is not required to attend an IEP team meeting in whole or in part, if the parent of the child with a disability and the public agency agree, in writing, that the attendance of the member is not necessary because the meeting will not be dealing with curriculum or related services about which this member is knowledgeable.

As provided at 34 CFR §300.321(e)(2) (see also §300.321(a)(4)), a representative of the public agency may be excused from an IEP meeting, in whole or in part, when the meeting does involve a modification to or discussion of the member's area of the curriculum or related services, if:

- the parent, in writing, and the public agency consent to the excuse; and

- the member submits, in writing to the parent and the IEP team, input into the development of the IEP prior to the meeting.

Allowing IEP team members to be excused from attending an IEP team meeting is intended to provide additional flexibility to parents in scheduling IEP team meetings and to avoid delays in holding an IEP team meeting when an IEP team member cannot attend due to a scheduling conflict. Although the public agency, not the parent, determines the specific personnel to fill the roles of the public agency's required participants at the IEP team meeting, the public agency remains responsible for conducting IEP meetings that are consistent with the IEP requirements of the Act and the regulations. Accordingly, it may not be reasonable for a public agency to agree or consent to the excuse of the public agency representative if that individual is needed to ensure that decisions can be made at the meeting about commitment of agency resources that are necessary to implement the child's IEP that would be developed, reviewed, or revised at the IEP team meeting.

Must the public agency receive consent from a parent to excuse multiple regular education teachers if at least one regular education teacher will be in attendance?

No. As provided in 34 CFR §300.321(a)(2), the public agency must ensure that the IEP team includes "[n]ot less than one regular education teacher of the child (if the child is, or may be, participating in the regular education environment) ..." Neither the Act nor the regulations require that an IEP team include more than one regular education teacher. Therefore, if the IEP team includes not less than one regular education teacher of the child, the excuse provisions of 34 CFR §300.321(e)(2) would not apply to additional regular education teachers.

If the regular education teacher were excused from attending the IEP meeting, would an alternate regular education teacher be required to attend?

If the public agency designates a particular regular education teacher as the person who will participate in the IEP team meeting pursuant to 34 CFR §300.321(a)(2), and that individual is excused from the meeting consistent with the requirements of 34 CFR §300 .321(e)(1)-(2), the public agency is not required to include a different regular education teacher in the IEP team meeting.

May a state establish additional regulations to ensure parents' rights are protected with regard to excuse of IEP team members?

Yes, but with certain caveats. A state may establish additional requirements to ensure that parents' rights are protected with regard to excuse of IEP team members, so long as those additional requirements are consistent with the requirements of 34 CFR §300 .321(e)(1) and (2), and do not diminish the right of parents to agree in writing or consent in writing to such excuse. Further, if a state establishes requirements that exceed those required by Part B of the Act and the federal regulations, the state would be required by 34 CFR §300.199(a)(2), to identify in writing to the local educational agencies (LEAs) located in the state and to the secretary that such rule, regulation, or policy is a state-imposed requirement, which is not required by Part B of the Act and federal regulations. However, a state must allow a parent and a public agency to agree in writing or consent in writing to excuse a member of the IEP team, and this provision cannot be made optional for states. A state may not restrict, or otherwise determine, when an IEP team member can be excused from attending an IEP team meeting, or prohibit the excuse of an IEP team member when the public agency and parent agree or consent to the excuse.

May state law or regulations regarding IEP team membership and IEP team meeting attendance requirements exceed those of IDEA?

Yes, but with certain caveats. A state may establish laws or regulations for IEP team membership and IEP team meeting attendance, but must ensure that in doing so it does not establish provisions that reduce parent rights or are otherwise in conflict with the requirements of Part B of the Act and the federal regulations. Further, as required by 34 CFR §300.199(a), each state that receives funds under Part B of the Act must:

1. Ensure that any state rules, regulations, and policies conform to the purposes of this part.

2. Identify in writing to LEAs located in the state and the secretary any such rule, regulation, or policy as a state-imposed requirement that is not required by Part B of the Act and federal regulations.

3. Minimize the number of rules, regulations, and policies to which the LEAs and schools located in the state are subject under Part B of the Act.

Must an IEP team document in writing that they considered all of the requirements of 34 CFR §300.324, regarding the development, review, and revision of IEPs?

Section 300.112 requires that the state ensure that an IEP, or an individualized family service plan (IFSP) that meets the requirements of section 636(d) of the Act, is developed, reviewed, and revised for each child with a disability. Section 300.201 requires public agencies to have in effect policies and procedures established under 34 CFR §§300.101 through 300.163 and §§300.165 through 300.174, which include the requirements related to developing, reviewing, and revising an IEP for each child with a disability in 34 CFR §300.324. While the Act and these regulations generally do not specify what documentation must be maintained consistent with the requirements of 34 CFR §300.324, states and public agencies are required to maintain records to show compliance with the Act and the regulations, in accordance with 34 CFR §76.731 of the Education Department General Administrative Regulations (EDGAR).

How must a public agency document that IEP team members have been informed of changes to the IEP?

The regulations provide, at 34 CFR §300.324(a)(4)(i), that, in making changes to a child's IEP after the annual IEP team meeting for a school year, the parent of a child with a disability and the public agency may agree not to convene an IEP team meeting for the purposes of making those changes, and instead may develop a written document to amend or modify the child's current IEP. The regulations require, at 34 CFR §300.324(a)(4)(ii), that if changes are made to the child's IEP in accordance with 34 CFR §300.324(a)(4)(i), the public agency must ensure that the child's IEP team is informed of those changes. While the Act and the regulations do not specify the manner in which public agencies must document compliance with the requirements of 34 CFR §300.324(a)(4)(ii), they must maintain records to show compliance with the requirements of the Act and regulations, in accordance with 34 CFR §76.731 of EDGAR.

Who must participate when an IEP is amended without convening the IEP team?

The regulations provide, at 34 CFR §300.324(a)(4)(i) that, in making changes to a child's IEP after the annual IEP team meeting for a school year, the parent of a child with a disability and the public agency may agree not to convene an IEP team meeting for the purposes of making those changes, and instead may develop a written document to amend or modify the child's current IEP. The Act and the regulations are silent as to which individuals must participate in making changes to the IEP where there is agreement between the parent and the public agency not to convene a meeting for the purpose of making the changes.

Must a public agency provide a parent with written notice prior to amending an IEP without convening the IEP team?

The regulations require, at 34 CFR §300.503(a), that written notice that meets the requirements of 34 CFR §300.503(b) must be given to the parents of a child with a disability a reasonable time before the public agency:

- proposes to initiate or change the identification, evaluation, or educational placement of the child or the provision of FAPE to the child; or

310

- refuses to initiate or change the identification, evaluation, or educational placement of the child or the provision of FAPE to the child.

This provision applies, even if the IEP is revised without convening an IEP team meeting, pursuant to 34 CFR §300.324(a)(4).

Consent for Initial Evaluation and Reevaluation

Authority: The requirements for consent for initial evaluations and reevaluations are found in the regulations at 34 CFR §300.300(a), (c), and (d)(4). The requirements for reevaluations are found in the regulations at 34 CFR §300.303.

What may a public agency do if a parent does not respond to the public agency's request for the parent's consent to a reevaluation?

Under 34 CFR §300.300(c)(2), the public agency need not obtain informed parent consent for the reevaluation if the public agency can demonstrate that it made reasonable efforts to obtain consent for the reevaluation, and the child's parent has failed to respond to the request for such consent. Thus, under this regulation, a public agency may conduct a reevaluation of a child with a disability if the public agency can demonstrate that it made reasonable efforts to obtain parent consent for the reevaluation, and the child's parent has failed to respond to the request for consent.

The regulations provide, at 34 CFR §300.303(b)(2), that a reevaluation must occur at least once every three years, unless the parent and the public agency agree that a reevaluation is unnecessary. What options are available to a public agency if a parent refuses to consent to a three-year reevaluation under 34 CFR §300.303(b)(2)?

The regulations provide, at 34 CFR §300.300(c)(1), that subject to 34 CFR §300.300(c)(2), each public agency:

1. Must obtain informed parental consent, in accordance with 34 CFR §300.300(a)(1), prior to conducting any reevaluation of a child with a disability.

2. If the parent refuses to consent to the reevaluation, the public agency may, but is not required to, pursue the reevaluation by

using the consent override procedures described in 34 CFR §300.300(a)(3).

3. The public agency does not violate its obligation under 34 CFR §300.111 and §§300.301 through 300.311 if it declines to pursue the evaluation or reevaluation.

If a parent refuses to consent to a three-year reevaluation under 34 CFR §300.303(b)(2), the public agency has the following options:

1. The public agency and the parent may, as provided at 34 CFR §300.303(b)(2), agree that the reevaluation is unnecessary. If such an agreement is reached, the three-year reevaluation need not be conducted. However, the public agency must continue to provide FAPE to the child.

2. If the public agency and the parent do not agree that the reevaluation is unnecessary, and the parent refuses to consent to the reevaluation, the public agency may, but is not required to, pursue the reevaluation by using the consent override procedures described in 34 CFR §300.300(a)(3) (the procedural safeguards in subpart E of Part B, including the mediation procedures under 34 CFR §300.506 or the due process procedures under 34 CFR §§300.507 through 300.516), if appropriate, except to the extent inconsistent with state law relating to such parental consent.

3. If the public agency chooses not to pursue the reevaluation by using the consent override procedures described in 34 CFR §300.300(a)(3), and the public agency believes based on existing data that the child does not continue to have a disability or does not continue to need special education and related services, the public agency may determine that it will not continue to provide special education and related services to the child. If the public agency determines that it will not continue to provide special education and related services to the child, the public agency must provide the parent with prior written notice of its proposal to discontinue the provision of FAPE to the child consistent with 34 CFR §300.503(a)(2).

At an initial IEP meeting, may a parent give consent to provide some or all of the services in the IEP?

If a public agency has provided prior written notice, consistent with 34 CFR §300.503(a)(1), of its proposal to initiate the provision of FAPE, the parent may provide informed consent to the initial provision of special education and related services, consistent with 34 CFR §300 .300(b).

May a foster parent provide consent for an initial evaluation even if the biological parent refuses to provide such consent?

If the biological parent of the child refuses consent for an initial evaluation of the child, and the parental rights of the biological parent have not been terminated in accordance with state law or a court has not designated a foster parent to make educational decisions for the child in accordance with state law, a foster parent may not provide consent for an initial evaluation. See 34 CFR §300.30(b)(1).

Chapter 36

Progress Monitoring: Assessing Students' Performance

On Monday, the teacher assigns her class a list of 20 spelling words to learn. On Friday, she tests the students on how well they learned to spell these words. This mastery measurement is the traditional way of determining student progress. The next spelling mastery test will indicate mastery of the next week's 20 new words, a new skill. Throughout the year, the teacher will test for different skills in different academic areas. When a math test in November covers one set of skills and a math test the next May covers a different set of skills, these test scores can't be compared. Thus, teachers and parents may be uncertain whether students have maintained the skills taught earlier in the year, and the student's rate of progress can't be described.

Another method of determining student progress, more recently researched, checks how well students are doing through a process called progress monitoring. Teachers do this monitoring regularly—weekly or monthly—for two reasons. One is to determine whether the students are learning what is being taught. And secondly, if the students are not learning, then test results will show what instruction is needed to pinpoint and address problem areas.

Research findings suggest that the best method of progress monitoring is curriculum-based measurement (CBM). Each CBM test is based on all of the skills that are going to be taught in one school year. For example, a fourth-grader would take a mathematics test in September that

National Research Center on Learning Disabilities (2007). What is progress monitoring? [Brochure]. Lawrence, KS.

contains all of the math concepts he or she should know by the end of the fourth-grade year. This test might include fractions, division, charts, and problem-solving skills. The next month, and in all of the following months, the student would take the same type of test but with different (yet similar) items. The student's scores should be getting higher. If they aren't, teachers will know what instruction needs more focus.

If a teacher, for instance, is testing a student's reading fluency, the teacher will ask a student to read a passage aloud for a certain length of time, often just one minute. The score will be the number of words read correctly. A teacher won't count as correct mispronunciations, substitutions, and missed words. With the resulting information, the teacher will have insight into that student's reading roadblocks.

These CBM tests—often one to five minutes each—are brief. This is so they can be given often and so they don't take valuable time away from instruction. Initially, a student may not be able to finish within the time limit. As more knowledge is acquired, he or she will be able to finish the tests sooner.

Each CBM test is administered to all the students in the same grade. The teacher knows what knowledge is being assessed by these CBM measures and teaches accordingly.

Students' scores are usually displayed in a graph to easily indicate each student's skill progression in the annual curriculum. If scores keep going up, then the student is learning what he or she needs to know. If the graph line stays the same or goes down, then the student is not benefiting from the instructional program.

Studies have been done that estimate typical student progress. A teacher can use those to compare her or his class to large numbers of students. Besides discovering which individual students need additional help, the teacher can compare individual student's class scores to the scores of large numbers of students to measure teaching success or needed adjustments.

So, not only can student scores be used to compare how one student has done on similar class-wide screenings and individual progression to year-end goals, but continuous progress monitoring also shows how a student has benefited from modified instruction and how the student compares to other students in the class or grade level. The scores, too, show teachers how to improve their instruction. Teachers can adjust their methods and use the scores to see what works best for students.

CBM is typically used in the elementary grades to monitor skills such as pre-reading, reading, spelling, mathematics, and written expression. It also has been used to monitor the basic skills of students at the secondary-school level and to measure their mastery of content in subjects such as social studies and science.

Curriculum-Based Measurement Benefits

- It is based on the curriculum taught.
- It is easy to administer and grade.
- It does not take much time.
- Results can guide instruction
- Teachers make decisions based on numbers, not guesses.
- Results can be used to custom-tailor an individual student's learning plan.
- Research has shown it to be both reliable and valid. Students, for instance, who score high or low on annual state-wide screenings have similar scores on progress monitoring measures.

Chapter 37

Assessing and Selecting Accommodations

The world is full of examples of accommodations that permit people with disabilities to perform specific tasks they might not otherwise be able to do. Drivers with poor vision wear glasses or contacts, elevators mark the buttons in Braille, and voters with disabilities may be given assistance by the person of their choice.

Accommodations play an important role in educational settings, too, particularly for students whose disabilities interfere with performing learning tasks (such as reading a book, taking notes in class, or writing an essay) or testing tasks (such as getting through the items within the time limit or filling in the circles on a multiple-choice test). A critical part of teaching and assessing students with disabilities, then, is providing them with accommodations that support learning and that support their ability to show what they know and can do.

But what accommodations are appropriate for which students? How do accommodations affect students' learning and their performance on tests? This chapter addresses these and other questions and explores the research base in this area.

The Big Picture: Expectations, Content, and Testing

Assessment in school is not a casual affair—not for the school, district, or state that must demonstrate adequate yearly progress (AYP)

Excerpted from "Assessment and Accommodations," by Stephen D. Luke, Ed.D. and Amanda Schwartz, Ph.D., in *Evidence for Education, Volume II, Issue 1*, National Dissemination Center for Children with Disabilities (NICHCY), 2007.

as part of public accountability—and not for students working to meet high performance standards. More than ever before, students with disabilities are included in the high performance standards states establish and in the required testing they conduct. In fact, federal law mandates it. Both the Individuals with Disabilities Education Improvement Act (IDEA) of 2004 and No Child Left Behind (NCLB) call for students with disabilities to participate in the general education curriculum and in testing programs to the maximum extent possible for each student. Because of these laws, schools have become accountable in new and significant ways for the education of all students with disabilities.

Three critical elements come together in this new world of accountability. Schools must now carefully consider these areas:

- **What students with disabilities are studying:** In the past— the recent past, in fact—many students with disabilities did not study the same curriculum as their peers without disabilities. This changed with the reauthorization of IDEA in 1997, which greatly emphasized the involvement of students with disabilities in the general education curriculum. IDEA 2004 has further strengthened this requirement.

- **What students with disabilities are expected to know:** Previously, performance standards for students with disabilities were not aligned with the standards established for those without disabilities. Now it is important that all students with disabilities be held to the highest possible academic standards. States have scrambled in recent years to introduce grade-level content standards into the curriculum for students with disabilities.

- **How well students with disabilities are learning:** Including students with disabilities in state and district assessments is not only required by NCLB and IDEA, it also is a logical and essential element in improving results for them. Without testing students, how will we know if they are actually learning what they need to know, or what they may still need to master?

Not surprisingly, what is becoming evident is that "raised expectations can lead to increased participation supported appropriately with individualized accommodations, improved instruction, and, thus, performance." Melissa Fincher, Assistant Director of Georgia's Department of Education's Testing Division, sums up the emerging reality this way: "Prior to IDEA and NCLB, students were not necessarily included to the fullest extent in instruction based on the curriculum or on grade-level content, or in assessments. Now, with both of these laws indicating that students have to be assessed—that all students have to be assessed, and all students have the right to quality instruction on the same curriculum—we're seeing that, if we expose the kids to the curriculum, they can rise to the occasion."

The role that accommodations play in helping students "rise to the occasion"—both in the classroom and in testing situations—is the focus of this chapter. The plain truth is that disability can pose a serious challenge to learning and to demonstrating knowledge and abilities fully. Accommodations can help students overcome or minimize the barriers presented by their disabilities—which is why federal law requires their use when necessary and why the U.S. Department of Education has issued numerous policy guidances for the field.

Deciding Which Accommodations a Student Needs

The challenge for educators and families is to decide which accommodations will help students learn new skills and knowledge—and which will help them demonstrate what they've learned. The Online Accommodations Bibliography at the National Center on Educational Outcomes (NCEO) is an excellent source of information on the range of possible accommodations (http://cehd.umn.edu/nceo/AccomStudies .htm) as well as the effects of various testing accommodations for students with disabilities. What accommodations are "allowable," however, may vary from state to state. Moreover, what helps one student may not address another's needs at all. Decisions about accommodations must be made on an individualized basis, student by student.

Who's responsible for making such decisions for a given student? The team that develops that student's individualized education program (IEP), otherwise known as the IEP team, is responsible. A thoughtful and customized IEP serves as the foundation for providing each student with a disability access to a free appropriate public education (FAPE), as required under federal legislation (IDEA, 2004a). The IEP team is also responsible for listing in the IEP all the accommodations to be provided to the student in the classroom and in statewide or district-wide testing.

When an IEP team gathers to decide whether or not a student needs accommodations in the classroom or in testing, team members must consider the specific strengths, challenges, and routines of that student. This will help the team determine which accommodations will support the student across a range of school situations and activities, as well as help the student access instruction designed to meet educational

321

standards established by the district and state. Further, the team must also know what types of accommodations their state or locale allows, especially in testing situations. Many states make a distinction between standard accommodations, those that don't alter the nature of what a test is designed to measure, and nonstandard accommodations, those with the potential to significantly change what is being tested.

In the end, the team may determine that no accommodations are needed or that a combination of individualized accommodations is necessary to meet the student's specific needs. Students can also help inform these decisions by talking with the team about what works best for them. Involving students in the process of determining goals and respecting their voices about which accommodations might best help them achieve those goals recognizes them as valued participants and can ultimately lead to feelings of increased control and responsibility in their education.

When taken alone, accommodations themselves may not result in much of an impact, but when thoughtfully integrated with other components in the IEP and implemented in the classroom, they can help students reach and demonstrate their full potential. It is also important to note that accommodations are most effective when they are based on individual strengths and needs rather than disability type. Further, accommodations chosen for testing situations can be most effective when they are adopted as an integral part of day-to-day instruction, to ensure that students have ample opportunity to practice their use prior to a mandated testing situation. This sentiment is reflected in the comment from Dr. Lynn Boyer, Executive Director of West Virginia's Office of Special Education, "There certainly is an expectation that the accommodations that are used on our state assessment are also used daily in the classroom. You would not have a student introduced for the first time to a scribe, for instance, or a calculator on a state assessment, when such an accommodation has not been used during instruction."

What Do States Allow?

IDEA 2004 mandates that all students with disabilities participate in statewide and districtwide testing "with appropriate accommodations and alternate assessments where necessary and as indicated in their respective individualized education programs" (IDEA, 2004b).

As part of implementing this requirement, state education agencies have been working to establish policies to guide IEP teams and schools in making accommodation decisions for students with disabilities, especially with respect to their participation in large-scale testing programs and the types of accommodations that are allowed.

The National Center on Educational Outcomes (NCEO) has been tracking and analyzing these state policies since 1992 and reports that considerable variability exists from state to state (and even within states and individual schools) in the ways in which accommodations are selected and applied, making it imperative that IEP teams know their current state and local accommodation policies. Fortunately, an increasing number of documents, training manuals, and guidelines are available online for teams to consult. You can find out more about accommodations in your state by visiting these websites:

- The National Center on Educational Outcomes (NCEO) at http://cehd.umn.edu/nceo/TopicAreas/Accommodations/ StatesAccomm.htm

- Your state education agency's website, identified on NICHCY's state resource sheets at http://www.nichcy.org/states.htm

Types of Accommodations

There are many ways in which accommodations can be used to support students with disabilities in the classroom and when they are taking a mandated state or district assessment.

Accommodations in presentation: Affect the way directions and content are delivered to students. Students with visual, hearing, and learning disabilities are much more able to engage in the content when it is presented in a form they can understand. Some examples of accommodations in presentation include:

- oral reading (either by an adult or on audiotape);
- large print;
- magnification devices;
- sign language;
- Braille and Nemeth code (a specific type of Braille used for math and science notations);
- tactile graphics (3-D topographical maps, 2-D raised line drawings);
- manipulatives (geometric solids, real coins and currency, abacus);
- audio amplification devices (hearing aids); or a
- screen reader. (adapted from Special Connections, 2005b)

Accommodations in response: Offer different ways for students to respond to assessment questions. They help students with visual and hearing impairments, physical disabilities, and organizational problems to structure, monitor, or directly put words to paper. Examples of these accommodations include:

- using a computer/typewriter or a scribe to record answers (directly or through tape recorder);

- using an augmentative communication device or other assistive technology (AT);

- using a brailler;

- responding directly in the test booklet rather than on an answer sheet;

- using organizational devices, including calculation devices, spelling and grammar assistive devices, visual organizers, or graphic organizers. (adapted from Special Connections, 2005c)

Accommodations in setting: Affect either where a test is taken or the way in which the environment is set up. Changing the environment is especially helpful to students who are easily distracted. Some examples include:

- administering the test individually (to the student alone);

- testing in a separate room;

- testing in a small group;

- adjusting the lighting;

- providing noise buffers such as headphones, earphones, or earplugs. (adapted from Special Connections, 2005d)

Accommodations in timing and scheduling: Allow flexibility in the timing of an assessment. Generally, these are chosen for students who may need more time to process information or need breaks throughout the testing process to regroup and refocus. Timing and scheduling accommodations include:

- extended time,

- multiple or frequent breaks,

- change in testing schedule or order of subjects, or

- testing over multiple days. (adapted from Special Connections, 2005e)

When determining accommodations, particular attention should be paid to ensure that they do not give one student an unfair advantage over another, or alter or compromise the test's ability to assess particular knowledge or skills. For example, providing a test in Braille to a student with a significant visual impairment would not seem to provide an unfair advantage over a sighted peer participating in a standard administration of the test. Having an adult read aloud questions on a math assessment may not necessarily alter the math concepts being assessed, but having the same adult read aloud on a test of reading comprehension does have the effect of changing the assessment from one of reading comprehension to one of listening comprehension and, in effect, results in the assessment of a different skill altogether.

How is the IEP team to judge whether an accommodation represents an unfair advantage for a student or is going to inappropriately alter the nature of the test? Conventional wisdom holds that, if non-disabled students also make gains when given the same accommodation (for example, extra time on a test) as students with disabilities, then there are questions about fairness and integrity in the testing situation. As researchers and policy makers continue to wrestle with these complex issues, IEP teams will need to stay current as policies and recommended practices evolve.

Choosing and Using Accommodations: IEP Team Considerations

The following questions are from *Special Connections* (2005a) at the University of Kansas (available at www.specialconnections.ku.edu) and are designed to serve as a tool to help the IEP team discuss and determine what accommodations a student needs in the classroom or in assessment.

- What kinds of instructional strategies (visual, tactile, auditory, combination) work best for the student?

- What learning strategies will help the student overcome challenges?

- What accommodations increase the student's access to instruction and assessment?

- What accommodations has the student tried in the past?

- What has worked well and in what situations?

- What does the student prefer?

- Are there ways to improve the student's use of the accommodation?

- Does the student still need the accommodation?

- What are the challenges of providing the student's preferred accommodations and how can these be overcome?

- Are there other accommodations that the student should try?

- Are there ways the student can use preferred accommodations outside of school (at home, on the job, in the community)?

- Are preferred accommodations allowed on state and district assessments of accountability?

- How can the student learn to request preferred accommodations (self-advocacy)?

- Are there opportunities for the student to use preferred accommodations on practice tests?

- What arrangements need to be made to make sure the student's preferred accommodations are available in assessment situations?

- How can actual use of accommodations be documented?

What Does the Research Say?

Looking to the research evidence, unfortunately, does not provide definitive answers to guide thoughtful policy and practice in this area. Considering the very real implications related to the use of accommodations and their extensive application across testing environments, the lack of conclusive direction from the research base is both disappointing and frustrating. That is not to say that a long look at the research base cannot be instructive. In fact, doing just that can lead to a better understanding of the complexities at play, for both researchers and practitioners alike, and more informed decision making about accommodations may indeed follow.

What we do know is that research has been able to suggest the following:

- Accommodation policies vary considerably from state to state. Interestingly, 12 states even extend eligibility for accommodations to all students.

- Approximately two-thirds of special education students have been afforded accommodations in statewide assessments, the most common being extended time, alternative setting, and read-aloud accommodations.

- Accommodations affect test scores for students with disabilities, lowering scores in some cases, raising scores in most others. Lowered scores appear to result when accommodations are poorly matched to student need or when the student has not had sufficient opportunity to practice using an accommodation in day-to-day settings prior to the testing situation.

- The use of read-aloud accommodations on assessments of mathematics for students with low reading skills and the use of Braille for blind students were found to be the most effective accommodations in a meta-analytic synthesis by Tindal and Fuchs (1999).

However, because of inconclusive and contradictory findings, we cannot automatically say with confidence that accommodations provide an accurate picture of a student's ability. Introducing an unfamiliar accommodation for the first time during a required testing situation may not necessarily help a student who has not had the opportunity to practice its use. Similarly, while providing a one-on-one administration of a test to a student with severe attention problems may help to reduce some distractible elements, it may not necessarily remove them all.

Neither can we automatically say with confidence that scores obtained by students with disabilities in accommodated situations can always be compared fairly to scores obtained by non-disabled students in situations without accommodations.

These last two points in particular make the important task of choosing appropriate accommodations for individual students all the more challenging. Students with disabilities bring an extremely broad range of strengths and weaknesses with them to testing environments. It is quite possible, in fact, for two students with very similar disabilities to require very different accommodations. Teacher training and practical guidance in selecting appropriate accommodations for individual students would clearly go a long way toward improving and informing decision making, but the availability of these valuable commodities can vary even in the same district or school.

Conclusion

The goal of school is learning. Assessments are just one way—albeit a very important way—in which we find out whether students have learned or not. For many students, especially those with disabilities, being able to show what's been learned is greatly improved when teachers provide individualized instruction and appropriate accommodations in the classroom and in testing situations.

The sheer variety of accommodations and assessments allows IEP teams a range of tools by which to understand and maximize student ability. Progress monitoring along the way adds an extra and powerful tool for continually checking on student growth and adjusting instruction to match student need. Carefully selecting accommodations to address student strengths, challenges, and experiences means that students with disabilities have the supports they need to access classroom instruction and then demonstrate what they've learned.

Investigating and providing strategies such as accommodations that support student success can have obviously beneficial results for students, which is reason enough to provide them—plus it's the law—but they can be beneficial for our schools as well. Schools and educational systems as a whole are accountable for the results they achieve and must demonstrate that their students are learning. Providing students with disabilities with the tools necessary for success in the classroom and to show their knowledge and skills in a regular assessment format means that they are truly included in the world of education.

Chapter 38

Evaluating Whether an Educational Program Is Research Based

How Can You Be Involved in School Improvement?

The Individuals with Disabilities Education Improvement Act of 2004 (IDEA 2004), signed into law in December 2004, cited low expectations for student success and a lack of solid research practices in teaching and learning for children with disabilities as roadblocks in fulfilling the hopes expressed in previous IDEA legislation. Important changes have been made in IDEA 2004 that can help your child's success in school. It's important to know how you can be involved.

With IDEA 2004, Congress is attempting to raise expectations and the use of scientifically proven educational research methods to remove these two roadblocks. Will they? That would be great, but that's down the road. What you can do now is enhance your knowledge about what changes are or should be happening at your school.

"When the music changes, so does the dance." That's an African proverb to heed because the music—IDEA—has changed and so should educational practices at your child's school. Within your child's school, you should anticipate higher expectations for all students. Those high expectations should be shared by school district staff, school administration, the classroom teacher, you, and the student. Since administrators and teachers are being held more accountable

This chapter includes text from: National Research Center on Learning Disabilities (2007). How can you be involved in school improvement? [Brochure]; and, How can you evaluate whether a program is research based? [Brochure]. Lawrence, KS.

for student success, you should expect to see research-based education methods that can be measured.

These education methods should include scientifically based instruction and more school-wide screening to make sure students receive the instruction they need to achieve in their learning programs. This focus on knowledge gained in the classroom rather than scores on a state or national test given once a year carries more weight in assessing and guiding student progress. For example, if a student fails to achieve, in spite of appropriate scientifically based instruction (such as that in the responsiveness to intervention method), then a disability may be suspected.

Parents can ask educators these questions:

- What scientifically based practices are used in core academic areas?

- What school-wide screening measures are in place?

- What measures are used to monitor students' progress in core academic areas?

- What early intervening services are available for students who may be at risk for learning difficulties?

- What method does this school use to determine whether a student has a learning disability?

This school-wide screening should reduce the numbers of students classified as having a disability or learning disability. In the past, only those students who qualified as having a disability were able to receive special educational and behavioral services. However, some experts found too many students unnecessarily got this label. Also, too many students of certain races or ethnic backgrounds were determined to have disabilities in comparison to the whole student population.

Although the definition of specific learning disability has not changed from IDEA 1997 to IDEA 2004, how a student is identified—the school's eligibility and evaluation process—may change. Knowing that IDEA 2004 does allow for more flexible learning disability assessments, measurable goals, more support in the general education classroom, continuous progress monitoring, scientifically proven instructional methods, and early intervening services for at-risk students helps you understand what to expect and request.

Stay informed, too, of your child's progress, the school's educational methods, and IDEA 2004 required practices by talking with other parents and parent advocacy groups. You also can learn more from national educational organizations and research organizations, including the National Research Center on Learning Disabilities, which conducts research on the identification of learning disabilities and makes recommendations on putting educational research methods into practice.

If changes are not going on at your school, then you may need to start asking questions. The more you know about IDEA 2004, the better prepared you will be to ask these questions and to understand your rights and responsibilities.

Maybe the biggest preparation you can do in this time of change is to raise your own expectations about your child's academic and behavioral success. Having higher expectations will help you get through the coming changes because any change, even one for the better, comes with some discomforts and issues to resolve.

How Can You Evaluate Whether a Program Is Research Based?

Bell bottoms, the Macarena dance, Beanie Babies—each is a fad that has come and gone and may even turn up again. School program development, too, can be subject to fads; unfortunately, educational fads do not necessarily deliver improved teaching and student achievement.

The benefit of selecting educational programs based on proven research is that they can deliver what is promised if they are implemented as intended. These research-based educational programs are like the medicine that your physician prescribes. Improvement in the medical condition requires that the medicine be taken as prescribed. These educational programs have been tested, have produced desirable results, and then have been retested to make sure the same results happen again. The term research-based appears in connection with many practices and programs. The questions that have to be asked about these research-based claims are, first, "Are they really based on scientific principles?" and second, "How well were these studies done?"

To better equip yourself to answer these questions, you will need to understand some of the terminology associated with scientific research. Research studies vary widely in how scientifically they were conducted. You need to understand research methodology before giving support and making any commitment to instructional changes.

Methodology

Quality research design starts with a review of what other experts have done in the field. Then, researchers decide the study's methodology—how the study will be done, who is going to participate, where the study will be conducted, what procedures will take place, what questions will be answered, and how the results will be judged.

Variables

Researchers focus on variables, those factors that change on purpose within a research study and those factors that the researcher hopes will not change or affect the results of the study.

The independent variable is the one that is changed on purpose by the researcher. An independent variable might be a learning program, a new intervention, or a way of teaching. The independent variable is also known as the cause.

The effect, or the part of the study that appears, disappears, or changes as a result of the intervention (independent variable) is the dependent variable, often a measure of performance. The effect may be contaminated when a third, typically unmeasured and unwanted, variable enters the process. This confounding variable could be age, interest, motivation, teacher experience, time of day, or other factors. Researchers try to recognize and control for these confounding variables to the greatest extent possible.

Experimental Control

Experimental control, identifying what caused change in the dependent variable, is another often-used term. For example, if students participating in a study designed to teach them a reading skill do well on this skill when, and only when, they had received instruction on it, this is a demonstration of experimental control.

Quality Results

After results of the study are produced, observed, and recorded, researchers analyze them to see whether any predictable patterns, associations, or differences appear and what the results actually mean. The quality of this interpretation depends on the adequacy and appropriateness of the evidence.

Some of the results' quality stems from reliability. For example, a student tested with a reliable assessment would get a similar score if the same or similar test were given again under the same conditions. Interobserver reliability refers to how similarly two people separately rate the same behaviors. If one observer records a certain behavior as occurring, the second observer also should record that as happening. The higher the level of interobserver reliability that a study has, the more believable the study results.

Another aspect of evidence quality is validity. Validity, or the degree to which a score represents what it was intended to measure, can be assessed by answering the following two questions: "Did the measurement system accurately measure what it claimed to measure?" and "Did the results provide an answer to the research question?"

Other Quality Measures

How else can you determine the quality of a research-based claim? Journals, the publications in which researchers publish, typically are peer-reviewed, meaning that each submitted article is examined by fellow researchers who analyze the scientific progress. If research lacks the necessary rigor, the journal will not publish the study. So, if a study appears in a peer-reviewed journal, most of the judging has been done for you.

Another way to examine the research quality is to talk to researchers directly and question them, especially on how their approach would work in your school. You also can talk to other researchers and ask them their opinion of a study's promised results.

Replication

One of the best ways to check a study's validity is to have it done again—replication. If you or others follow the same process and produce similar results, then the study results are more likely valid. One way to do this is to test how well the innovation can be replicated in the school. It is not enough to think of the innovation as a framework or an approach or to use just parts of it. The replication should be done using the same methods, because if they are changed much, then the results will change.

Although understanding how research is done well involves much more than this quick summary, this brief provides a good start. Knowing the basic process and some of the terms used in scientific studies will help you better analyze interventions used in your son's or daughter's school.

Chapter 39

Language Development and Speech Therapy

Chapter Contents

Section 39.1

Delayed Speech or Language Development

Your son is two years old and still isn't talking. He says a few words, but compared with his peers you think he's way behind. You remember that his sister could put whole sentences together at the same age. Hoping he will catch up, you postpone seeking professional advice. Some kids are early walkers and some are early talkers, you tell yourself. Nothing to worry about...

This scenario is common among parents of kids who are slow to speak. Unless they observe other areas of "slowness" during early development, parents may hesitate to seek advice. Some may excuse the lack of talking by reassuring themselves that "he'll outgrow it" or "she's just more interested in physical things."

Knowing what's "normal" and what's not in speech and language development can help you figure out if you should be concerned or if your child is right on schedule.

Understanding Normal Speech and Language Development

It's important to discuss early speech and language development, as well as other developmental concerns, with your doctor at every routine well-child visit. It can be difficult to tell whether a child is just immature in his or her ability to communicate or has a problem that requires professional attention. These developmental norms may provide clues:

Before 12 Months

It's important for kids this age to be watched for signs that they're using their voices to relate to their environment. Cooing and babbling are early stages of speech development. As babies get older (often around nine months), they begin to string sounds together, incorporate the different tones of speech, and say words like "mama" and "dada" (without really understanding what those words mean). Before 12 months, children should also be attentive to sound. Babies who watch intently but don't react to sound may be showing signs of hearing loss.

By 12 to 15 Months

Kids this age should have a wide range of speech sounds in their babbling and at least one or more true words (not including "mama" and "dada"). Nouns usually come first, like "baby" and "ball." Your child should also be able to understand and follow single directions ("Please give me the toy," for example).

From 18 to 24 Months

Kids should have a vocabulary of about 20 words by 18 months and 50 or more partial words by the time they turn two. By age two, kids should be learning to combine two words, such as "baby crying" or "Daddy big." A two-year-old should also be able to follow two-step commands (such as "Please pick up the toy and bring me your cup").

From Two to Three Years

Parents often witness an "explosion" in their child's speech. Your child's vocabulary should increase (to too many words to count) and he or she should routinely combine three or more words into sentences. Comprehension should also increase—by three years of age, a child should begin to understand what it means to "put it on the table" or "put it under the bed." Your child should also begin to identify colors and comprehend descriptive concepts (big versus little, for example).

The Difference Between Speech and Language

Speech and language are often confused, but there is a distinction between the two:

- Speech is the verbal expression of language and includes articulation, which is the way words are formed.

- Language is much broader and refers to the entire system of expressing and receiving information in a way that's meaningful.

It's understanding and being understood through communication—verbal, nonverbal, and written.

Although problems in speech and language differ, they frequently overlap. A child with a language problem may be able to pronounce words well but be unable to put more than two words together. Another child's speech may be difficult to understand, but he or she may use words and phrases to express ideas. And another child may speak well but have difficulty following directions.

Warning Signs of a Possible Problem

If you're concerned about your child's speech and language development, there are some things to watch for.

An infant who isn't responding to sound or who isn't vocalizing is of particular concern. Between 12 and 24 months, reasons for concern include a child who:

- isn't using gestures, such as pointing or waving bye-bye by 12 months;
- prefers gestures over vocalizations to communicate by 18 months;
- has trouble imitating sounds by 18 months.

Seek an evaluation if a child over two years old:

- can only imitate speech or actions and doesn't produce words or phrases spontaneously;
- says only certain sounds or words repeatedly and can't use oral language to communicate more than his or her immediate needs;
- can't follow simple directions;
- has an unusual tone of voice (such as raspy or nasal sounding);
- is more difficult to understand than expected for his or her age. Parents and regular caregivers should understand about half of a child's speech at two years and about three quarters at three years. By four years old, a child should be mostly understood, even by people who don't know the child.

Causes of Delayed Speech or Language

Many things can cause delays in speech and language development. Speech delays in an otherwise normally developing child are rarely caused by oral impairments, such as problems with the tongue or palate (the roof of the mouth). Being "tongue-tied" (when the frenulum—the fold beneath the tongue—is too tight) is almost never a cause of delayed speech.

Many kids with speech delays have oral-motor problems, meaning there's inefficient communication in the areas of the brain responsible for speech production. The child encounters difficulty using the lips, tongue, and jaw to produce speech sounds. Speech may be the only problem or may be accompanied by other oral-motor problems such as feeding difficulties. A speech delay may also indicate a more "global" (or general) developmental delay.

Hearing problems are also commonly related to delayed speech, which is why a child's hearing should be tested by an audiologist whenever there's a speech concern. A child who has trouble hearing may have trouble understanding, imitating, and using language.

Ear infections, especially chronic infections, can affect hearing ability. Simple ear infections that have been adequately treated, though, should have no effect on speech.

What Speech-Language Pathologists Do

If you or your doctor suspect that your child has a problem, early evaluation by a speech-language pathologist is crucial. Of course, if there turns out to be no problem after all, an evaluation can ease your fears.

Although you can seek out a speech-language pathologist on your own, your primary care doctor can refer you to one.

In conducting an evaluation, a speech-language pathologist will look at a child's speech and language skills within the context of total development. Besides observing your child, the speech-language pathologist will conduct standardized tests and scales, and look for milestones in speech and language development.

The speech-language pathologist will also assess:

- what your child understands (called receptive language);
- what your child can say (called expressive language);
- if your child is attempting to communicate in other ways, such as pointing, head shaking, gesturing, etc.;
- your child's oral-motor status (how a child's mouth, tongue, palate, etc., work together for speech as well as eating and swallowing).

If the speech-language pathologist finds that your child needs speech therapy, your involvement will be very important. You can observe therapy sessions and learn to participate in the process. The speech therapist will show you how you can work with your child at home to improve speech and language skills.

Evaluation by a speech-language pathologist may find that your expectations are simply too high. Educational materials that outline developmental stages and milestones may help you look at your child more realistically.

What Parents Can Do

Like so many other things, speech development is a mixture of nature and nurture. Genetic makeup will, in part, determine intelligence and speech and language development. However, a lot of it depends on environment. Is a child adequately stimulated at home or at childcare? Are there opportunities for communication exchange and participation? What kind of feedback does the child get?

When speech, language, hearing, or developmental problems do exist, early intervention can provide the help a child needs. And when you have a better understanding of why your child isn't talking, you can learn ways to encourage speech development.

Here are a few general tips you can employ at home:

- Spend a lot of time communicating with your child, even during infancy—talk, sing, and encourage imitation of sounds and gestures.

- Read to your child, starting as early as six months. You don't have to finish a whole book, but look for age-appropriate soft or board books or picture books that encourage kids to look while you name the pictures. Try starting with a classic book such as *Pat the Bunny*, in which the child imitates the patting motion, or books with textures that kids can touch. Later, let your child point to recognizable pictures and try to name them. Then move on to nursery rhymes, which have rhythmic appeal. Progress to predictable books, such as Eric Carle's *Brown Bear, Brown Bear*, in which your child can anticipate what happens. Your little one may even start to memorize favorite stories.

- Use everyday situations to reinforce your child's speech and language. In other words, talk your way through the day. For example, name foods at the grocery store, explain what you're doing as you cook a meal or clean a room, point out objects around the house, and as you drive, point out sounds you hear. Ask questions and acknowledge your child's responses (even when they're hard to understand). Keep things simple, but never use "baby talk."

Whatever your child's age, recognizing and treating problems early on is the best approach to help with speech and language delays. With proper therapy and time, your child will likely be better able to communicate with you and the rest of the world.

Section 39.2

Speech-Language Therapy

"Speech-Language Therapy," June 2005, reprinted with permission from www.kidshealth.org. Copyright © 2005 The Nemours Foundation. This information was provided by KidsHealth, one of the largest resources online for medically reviewed health information written for parents, kids, and teens. For more articles like this one, visit www.KidsHealth.org, or www.TeensHealth.org.

In a recent parent-teacher conference, your child's teacher expressed concern that your child may have a problem with certain speech or language skills. Or perhaps while talking to your child, you noticed an occasional stutter. You're not sure that your child has a problem—what should you do?

Whatever your particular circumstances, it's wise to intervene quickly. A speech-language evaluation conducted by a certified speech-language pathologist can help you determine the nature of your child's difficulties.

What Is Speech-Language Therapy?

Speech-language therapy is the treatment for most children with speech and/or language disorders. A speech disorder refers to a problem with the actual production of sounds, whereas a language disorder refers to a difficulty understanding or putting words together to communicate ideas.

Speech Disorders and Language Disorders

Speech disorders include the following problems, according to Diane Paul-Brown, Ph.D., director of clinical issues in speech-language pathology at the American Speech-Language-Hearing Association (ASHA):

- Articulation disorders include difficulties producing sounds in syllables or saying words incorrectly to the point that other people can't understand what's being said.

- Fluency disorders include problems such as stuttering, the condition in which the flow of speech is interrupted by abnormal stoppages, repetitions (st-st-stuttering), or prolonging sounds and syllables (sssssstuttering).

- Resonance or voice disorders include problems with the pitch, volume, or quality of a child's voice that distract listeners from what's being said. These types of disorders may also cause pain or discomfort for the child when speaking.

Language disorders can be either receptive or expressive. Receptive disorders refer to difficulties understanding or processing language. Expressive disorders include difficulty putting words together, limited vocabulary, or inability to use language in a socially appropriate way.

Specialists in Speech-Language Therapy

Speech-language pathologists (SLP), who are often informally known as speech therapists, are professionals educated in the study of human communication, its development, and its disorders. They hold at least a master's degree and state certification/licensure in the field, as well as a certificate of clinical competency from the American Speech-Hearing-Association.

By assessing the speech, language, cognitive-communication, and swallowing skills of children and adults, speech-language pathologists can determine what types of communication problems exist and the best way to treat these challenges.

Speech-language pathologists typically treat problems in the areas of articulation; disfluency; oral-motor, speech, and voice; and receptive and expressive language disorders.

Remediation

Speech-language therapy involves having a speech-language specialist work with a child on a one-to-one basis, in a small group or directly in a classroom, to overcome difficulties involved with a specific disorder. Speech-language therapy uses a variety of therapeutic strategies, including:

- Language intervention activities—These exercises involve having a speech-language specialist interact with a child by playing and talking to him. The therapist may use pictures, books, objects, or ongoing events to stimulate language development. The therapist may also model correct pronunciation and use repetition exercises to build speech and language skills.

- Articulation therapy—Articulation, or sound production, exercises involve having the therapist model correct sounds and syllables for a child, often during play activities. The level of play is age-appropriate and related to the child's specific needs. Articulation therapy involves physically showing a child how to make certain sounds, such as the "r" sound. A speech-language therapist may demonstrate how a child should move his tongue to produce specific sounds.

When Is Therapy Needed?

Children require speech-language therapy for a variety of reasons, including:

- hearing impairments,
- cognitive (intellectual; thinking) or other developmental delays,
- weak oral muscles,
- birth defects such as cleft lip or cleft palate,
- autism,
- motor planning problems,
- respiratory problems (breathing disorders),
- swallowing disorders,
- traumatic brain injury.

Therapy should begin as soon as possible. Children enrolled in therapy early in their development (younger than three years) tend to have better outcomes than children who begin therapy later.

This does not mean that older children can't make progress in therapy; they may progress at a slower rate because they often have learned patterns that need to be modified or changed.

Finding Care for Your Child

It's important to make sure that the speech-language therapist is certified by ASHA. That certification means the specialist has at least a master's degree in the field, has passed a national examination, and has successfully completed a supervised clinical fellowship.

Sometimes speech assistants (who have typically earned a two-year associate's or four-year bachelor's degree) may assist with speech-language services under the supervision of ASHA-certified SLP. Your child's SLP should be licensed in their state, and have experience working with children, and your child's specific disorder.

You may also find a specialist by asking your child's doctor or teacher for a referral or by checking your local telephone directory. The state associations for speech-language pathology and audiology also maintain listings of licensed and certified therapists.

Helping Your Child

Speech-language experts agree that parental involvement is crucial to the success of a child's progress in speech or language therapy.

Parents are an extremely important part of their child's therapy program. Parents help determine whether their child's experience in speech-language therapy is a success. Children who complete the program most quickly and with the most lasting results are those whose parents have been involved. It is very important that parents help their child use the stimulation activities that their speech-language pathologist suggests at home to ensure continued progress and carry-over of newly learned skills.

Ask your child's therapist for suggestions on how you can help your child, such as performing speech-language exercises with him at home. The process of overcoming a speech or language disorder may take some time and effort, so it's important that all family members be patient and understanding with the child.

Chapter 40

Building Blocks of Reading Instruction

The characteristics of well-designed reading programs include both instructional content and instructional design. The following are elements that should be included in the content of any basal reading program:

- phonemic awareness instruction
- systematic, explicit phonics instruction
- fluency instruction
- vocabulary instruction
- text comprehension instruction

Instructional design elements that should be present in a well-designed reading program include:

- explicit instructional strategies,
- coordinated instructional sequences,
- ample practice opportunities, and
- aligned student assessments.

If some students are not progressing well in a program, teachers should consider whether the above characteristics are present in the

---

Excerpted from "Questions about Reading Instruction," National Institute for Literacy, February 2007.

instructional reading program they are currently implementing. In addition, some students may need to be administered diagnostic reading assessments to identify areas of specific reading strengths and weaknesses in order to design appropriate interventions for those students.

Phonemic Awareness

In kindergarten, children need to develop phonemic awareness by hearing, identifying, and manipulating the individual sounds, or phonemes, within spoken words. Among the activities that might be practiced to help children acquire phonemic awareness are:

- phoneme isolation (What is the first or last sound in sat?);

- phoneme identity (Which sound is the same in man, mitt, and mess?);

- phoneme categorization (Which word doesn't belong? fat, fan, tap);

- phoneme blending (What word results when you blend these separately pronounced individual sounds together to make a word? /p/ /i/ /t/);

- phoneme segmentation (What are the separate sounds in this word? Show me by tapping or counting each sound as you pronounce the word, or set out a token as you say each sound—ant—/a/ /n/ /t/—three sounds).

Once children acquire letter knowledge, then they can be taught to perform these activities by pointing to or manipulating letters along with the sounds. The most important types of phonemic awareness for children to acquire are blending and segmentation because they provide the foundation for acquiring decoding and spelling skills.

By the end of kindergarten, many children are able to blend and segment phonemes using letters, signaling readiness for phonics in grade one.

Research has indicated that in kindergarten, phonemic awareness can be acquired from instruction usually lasting a total of 20 hours or less, though some individual children might need more instruction to be able to segment words accurately. More than that does not appear to enhance the benefits. It is important to assess students individually to verify that instruction has been successful for all students. More instruction may be required for some than for others.

Phonics

Systematic and explicit phonics programs teach children letter-sound relationships directly in a well-defined sequence. Most systematic phonics programs carefully sequence phonics generalizations from least difficult to more difficult, including all major generalizations for consonants, vowels, consonant or vowel blends, and digraphs. It is important to provide instruction in the application of letter-sound knowledge to reading and writing activities along the way as letter-sounds are acquired.

In systematic phonics instruction, the teacher typically models or demonstrates how to blend letter-sounds to pronounce known words and how to segment sounds in known words to write letters representing those sounds. Children then practice blending and segmenting based on the teacher's example. Children generally begin by blending letter-sounds in simple one-syllable words such as *at* and *in*. Later they advance to more complex syllable patterns. They learn to decode letter patterns that occur in several words as units, for example, -ing and -ock. Also, they learn to apply their knowledge of known words to decode unknown words, for example, reading screen by analogy to green. Students also practice their knowledge of letter-sound relationships by reading text that includes those letter-sound relationships that have been taught systematically and explicitly. In addition, students learn to spell the words they have learned to decode by using these words as part of stories they write.

What is the difference between explicit phonics and embedded phonics?

Explicit phonics approaches teach letter-sound correspondences in a well-defined sequence, providing reading practice with the correspondences that students are learning during instruction. Examples of explicit phonics approaches include blending individual letters and sounds to decode words and blending larger subunits or words such as onsets and rimes (for example: j-ump, st-art) to decode words.

In contrast, in embedded phonics, the teacher teaches letter-sound correspondences as students need them during reading activities. Additionally, students may initially learn to read and write a small number of sight words by word level drill as well as by analyzing letter-sound correspondences in those words. Examples of embedded phonics approaches include literature-based and some basal reading programs that emphasize sight word reading rather than phonetic decoding. Embedded phonics programs may or may not be systematic and explicit.

It is important to examine carefully the approaches used in reading programs to determine whether the materials and strategies represent a systematic and explicit approach to phonics instruction, while providing opportunities for students to practice using their phonics and other word recognition skills when reading text and grade-appropriate children's literature.

Do all children need to be taught phonics? Why or why not?

All children need to acquire knowledge of the alphabetic system to become skilled readers. The most direct way for teachers to accomplish this is by providing explicit, systematic phonics instruction as one part of a comprehensive early reading program. Systematic and explicit phonics instruction is effective for all students in kindergarten and grade one, regardless of socioeconomic status or the ease with which children learn to read.

The amount of explicit phonics instruction appropriate for individual students depends on the student's needs and abilities. Some students learn phonics generalizations easily and move quickly to practicing phonics and other word recognition skills as they read text and grade-appropriate literature. Children who are struggling to learn to read, or who may be at risk for reading difficulties in later years, need more intensive systematic and explicit phonics instruction. Repeated exposure to phonics generalizations and practice applying this knowledge in reading and writing tasks may be necessary to enhance the likelihood that these students will learn to read.

Fluency

Fluency is the ability to read a text accurately, quickly, and with proper expression and comprehension. Students who are able to read orally with speed, accuracy, and expression, but who do not simultaneously understand what they read, are not fluent. Educators value assessments of rate and accuracy because they help determine a child's level of automaticity, or the "fast, effortless word recognition that comes with a great deal of reading practice."

One effective indicator of reading fluency is to have a student read a passage from grade level material aloud for one minute. A score is given representing the number of words the student read correctly. This procedure is valid and reliable and is a good way to monitor student progress over time in reading grade level material. The scores can be easily graphed to illustrate progress and there are published norms for grades 1–3.

Another tool often used to assess both oral reading accuracy and comprehension is the informal reading inventory. A child is typically asked to read aloud a passage at grade level and the teacher records errors. Then the child is asked to orally answer comprehension questions about the passage. Several published informal reading inventories are currently available.

A third tool that can be used to evaluate fluency includes a measure of expression. In the National Assessment of Educational Progress (NAEP), a four point scale was used. When a child's oral reading was word by word, one point was given; when reading showed comprehension with appropriate pauses at meaningful phrases and clauses, four points were awarded.

What is guided oral reading?

Guided repeated oral reading is an instructional strategy that can help students improve a variety of reading skills, including fluency. There are a number of effective procedures that can be used in providing guided oral reading. In general, a teacher, parent, or peer reads a passage aloud, modeling fluent reading. Then students reread the text quietly, on their own, sometimes several times. The text should be at the student's independent reading level. Next, the students read aloud and then reread the same passage. Usually, reading the same text four times is sufficient.

Some examples of more specific techniques that involve rereading with feedback include these:

- An adult or peer reads with the student by modeling fluent reading and then asking the student to read the same passage aloud with encouragement and feedback by the adult or peer.

- A student listens to a tape of a fluent reader reading text at the student's independent level at a pace of about 80–100 words a minute. The student listens to the tape the first time and then practices reading along with the tape until the student is able to read fluently.

- The student reads with a peer partner. Each partner takes a turn reading to the other. A more fluent reader can be paired with a less fluent reader to model fluent reading. The more fluent reader can provide feedback and encouragement to the less fluent reader. Students of similar reading skills can also be paired, particularly if the teacher has modeled fluent reading and the partner reading involves practice.

349

- Readers' theatre can be a motivating way to improve fluency. Students read scripts and rehearse a play to prepare for a performance. The practice in reading and rereading the scripts provides an excellent opportunity to improve fluency skills.

What does the research say about encouraging students to read on their own as a way to improve reading skills?

The National Reading Panel (NRP) found correlational studies indicating that students who read more are generally better readers. Because these were correlational studies, it isn't clear, however, whether the relationship is causal. For example, in a correlational study, it is possible that good readers tend to read more and poor readers tend to read less. What is not clear from correlational studies is the direction of the relationship. What we would ideally like to demonstrate is that the amount of reading a student does determines if one becomes a good reader or a poor reader. In order to establish the direction of the relationship, we would have to do an experimental study that carefully manipulates the amount of reading that the student will do.

Because none of the reviewed studies was experimental, the NRP was not able to make a statement to that effect that encouraging students to read more on their own actually causes them to become better readers. However, the wealth of support from the correlational studies suggests that reading more leads to growth in reading achievement. More research needs to be done to examine the role of increased reading and its impact on both fluency and comprehension. The NRP therefore suggested that sustained silent reading during class time without time set aside for instruction in the numerous skills associated with reading may not be a productive way to spend valuable class time. It is important to note that the NRP did not discourage teachers and others from encouraging students to read more on their own outside of class time.

What is progress monitoring in fluency?

Monitoring progress in reading fluency involves taking samples of students' reading and recording the correct words read per minute. Teachers look for increases in words read correctly per minute from test to test. This measure is highly reliable, valid, and strongly correlated with reading comprehension. Furthermore, it is highly predictive of performance on high-stakes reading tests.

Vocabulary

Knowledge of word meanings is the most important single factor in reading or listening comprehension. Students must be able to interpret the meanings of most of the words in a text in order to make sense of it.

What are some effective ways to teach vocabulary to children in grades K-3?

Young children learn the meanings of new vocabulary words both indirectly and directly. Children learn vocabulary when they participate in daily conversation, especially with fluent adults; when they listen to others read aloud, especially when the reader draws children's attention to new words or engages them in conversations about books; and when children read a wide range of grade-appropriate fiction and nonfiction.

Direct vocabulary learning occurs when teachers provide explicit instruction on the meaning of specific words and word learning strategies. To help students learn specific new words, teachers often introduce vocabulary that students will encounter when they read a specified text, encourage students to use new words in different contexts, and provide repeated exposure to new words in varying contexts. Word learning strategies include the use of dictionaries or other reference aids.

Comprehension

Teaching Comprehension Skills in Grades K–3

The research on comprehension in the *National Reading Panel Report* was conducted primarily on students in grades four and higher. The research evidence indicates that teaching comprehension skills can improve comprehension for children in grades four and above. *Put Reading First* encourages teachers in the primary grades to incorporate direct instruction in comprehension strategies as well.

The direct and explicit teaching of comprehension strategies helps K–3 students become active readers who are engaged in understanding written text. Teachers provide direct and explicit teaching of comprehension strategies through explanation, demonstration or modeling, guided practice, and opportunities for children to practice using comprehension strategies when reading grade-appropriate children's text.

The National Reading Panel identified six comprehension strategies that have potential value for K–3 reading instructional programs:

1. Comprehension monitoring helps students know what they understand or do not understand when reading text. It also helps them use "fix-up" strategies such as re-reading for a particular purpose or adjusting reading speed as related to text difficulty.

2. Graphic and semantic organizers help students categorize or classify concepts in informational text using maps, webs, graphs, or charts.

3. Answering a variety of questions (including literal, inferential, and critical or application types) during pre-reading, reading, and post-reading provides students with a purpose and focus for reading.

4. Asking different types of questions about text meaning during pre-reading, reading, and post-reading activities improves students' active engagement with text.

5. Recognizing story structure helps students understand how characters, events, and settings contribute to plot.

6. Summarizing main ideas and key details is critical to demonstrating understanding of the author's message.

In combination, these six strategies have been shown to be particularly beneficial when students work cooperatively to construct the meaning of text, as is the case with multiple strategy instruction, or reciprocal teaching. In reciprocal teaching, students combine multiple strategies by predicting and confirming text meaning, asking questions when reading, clarifying vocabulary or concepts that are poorly understood, and summarizing text meaning.

Should all children be good readers by the end of third grade? Is that really the correct benchmark?

Learning to read fluently and with comprehension by the end of grade three marks the difference between the "learning to read" phase of reading development and the "reading to learn" phase that typically begins in grade four. By the end of grade three, students are expected to have developed the automaticity to recognize words quickly on the basis of their orthography or spelling. This ability to identify words rapidly facilitates comprehension of connected text, a critical element of middle school reading when students are expected to use their literacy skills to learn sophisticated content across the curriculum.

What are the best strategies for reading interventions for children in grades K–3 who are not benefiting from the reading program?

When K–3 students are not benefiting from the classroom reading instructional program, early interventions should be implemented to bolster students' opportunities to succeed. Research has documented that early intervention based on screening and diagnostic assessment of skills will enhance students' acquisition of early literacy competencies.

Beginning in kindergarten, early interventions in small groups or, when warranted, one-on-one instruction should focus on the needs of individual students as determined by screening or diagnostic assessments. Early interventions may be provided by certified teachers, reading or teaming specialists, or trained aides or tutors within the classroom, or in pull-out programs, depending upon available resources and the needs of children. Screening assessments can be used to identify students who are not making adequate progress toward achievement of grade-specific early reading competencies associated with phonemic awareness, phonics and other word recognition strategies, fluency, vocabulary development, and comprehension strategies. More detailed diagnostic assessment can help teachers to group students who need similar instruction on particular skills.

Chapter 41

Strategic Instruction Model

Strategy instruction is a powerful student-centered approach to teaching that is backed by years of quality research. In fact, strategic approaches to learning new concepts and skills are often what separate good learners from poor ones. Considering that many students with disabilities struggle with developing strategies for learning and remembering on their own, a parent or teacher skilled in introducing this process can make a world of difference.

Strategy instruction supplies students with the same tools and techniques that efficient learners use to understand and learn new material or skills. With continued guidance and ample opportunities for practice, students learn to integrate new information with what they already know, in a way that makes sense—making it easier for them to recall the information or skill at a later time, even in a different situation or setting.

Not only does an impressive body of research exist with respect to strategy instruction, but that library of knowledge is also extremely broad and has direct and immediate application to practice in almost every area of the educational curriculum.

Even better, this method of instruction is appropriate and effective for students who have disabilities, as well as for those who do not. That's right, all students can benefit from understanding

This chapter includes text from "The Power of Strategy Instruction," *Evidence for Education, Volume 1, Issue 1*, National Dissemination Center for Children with Disabilities (NICHCY), 2006.

the strategies that good learners use. What's more, a skillful teacher can play a critical part in guiding students to use strategies until their use becomes an automatic part of each student's repertoire.

Researchers at the University of Kansas have been deeply involved in researching learning strategies since the 1970s and have done much to define and articulate the benefits of strategy instruction, particularly for students with learning disabilities (LD). This work has resulted in one of the most well-researched models for teaching students to use learning strategies. This model has been known for years as the SIM, which stands for the strategic instruction model. Over the past 25 years, SIM has emerged into a multi-system, comprehensive school-wide approach with coordinated evidence-based teaching and learning components at its core.

The teaching component of SIM is made up of a series of teacher focused content enhancement teaching routines designed so that a teacher can deliver organized content in an engaging and learner friendly manner. One set of routines, for example, walks teachers through the planning of individual lessons, whole units, or even complete courses. Other routines offer practical recommendations for guiding students through an exploration of overarching concepts that may connect to material learned previously.

The learning strategies curriculum of SIM is a series of interconnected, student-centered strategies designed to transform weak or passive learners into students who know how to learn and apply their knowledge and skills actively across various learning environments. The learning strategies curriculum has seven discrete strands and contains more than 30 strategies to improve skills and performance related to the following:

- Reading
- Expressive writing
- Math and problem solving
- Studying and remembering
- Assignments and test taking
- Motivation
- Interacting with others

Taken together, these teaching and learning strategies can greatly improve learning outcomes for students entering the classroom with different learning styles and abilities. When this sort of strategic instruction is coordinated and implemented across teachers and environments—for example, a general education and special education classroom—student successes can be even more pronounced.

More on SIM Research

Content Enhancement Teaching Routine

The *Course Organizer Routine* is designed to help teachers plan courses around core content. The routine is used to introduce central concepts to students at the beginning of a course and is revisited throughout the course to relate newly acquired knowledge to main ideas already learned.

Research findings: Teachers who use this routine spend more time introducing main course themes than do teachers who have not learned the routine.

LD students in classes that used the *Course Organizer Routine* correctly answered an average of eight "big idea" questions by the end of the course, while LD students in the class that did not use the routine answered an average of only four.

Learning Strategies Curriculum

SCORE Skills, (Social Skills for Cooperative Groups), is designed to equip students with a set of skills to work effectively in groups. Students learn to:

Share ideas

Compliment others

Offer help or encouragement

Recommend changes nicely

Exercise self-control

Research findings: Students who learned *SCORE Skills* improved from an average of 25% cooperative skills used in a group setting to 78%. By comparison, a group of students who did not receive training had an average of 25% and 28% for the same time periods.

357

SIM Content Literacy Continuum: A Working Example

Content Mastery

What it looks like for students: All students, regardless of level of literacy development, engage in the process of learning core curricular content.

What it looks like for teachers: Teachers promote content mastery by using content enhancement routines, adjusting the routines appropriately for students of differing literacy levels.

Example: When beginning a history unit on "The American Revolution," the teacher works with students to create a unit organizer highlighting the core content to be covered. Teacher and students refer to the organizer throughout the unit to provide context for newly learned content and to reinforce previously learned material.

Embedded Strategy Instruction

What it looks like for students: Students are introduced to a range of learning strategies designed to develop literacy skills across an entire curriculum.

What it looks like for teachers: Teachers first teach a variety of learning strategies directly to students and then embed further strategy instruction when presenting core content. Teachers continue to prompt and model appropriate strategy use and provide opportunities for individual and group practice throughout the year.

Example: At the start of the school year the teacher explains that being able to paraphrase information about the American Revolution is useful for writing reports, answering questions, and discussing main themes. The teacher then outlines the steps of the paraphrasing strategy and models its use for the class. Classroom activities and homework assignments are designed which require students to use paraphrasing strategies, both verbally and in written form. Targeted feedback is given to tailor and encourage strategy use.

Explicit Strategy Instruction Options

What it looks like for students: Students who struggle with learning and implementing strategies in the regular classroom are presented with more focused and explicit instruction by support personnel.

What it looks like for teachers: Supplemental instruction by trained support personnel can take place in a variety of settings, including: general education classrooms, pull-out resource room sessions, or after-school tutoring programs.

Example: The general education teacher may notice that some students are experiencing difficulty paraphrasing core information about the American Revolution. A resource room teacher can then work separately with this group of students to reintroduce and break down the steps of the paraphrasing strategy. Students may learn to paraphrase sentence by sentence, or paragraph by paragraph, working daily for 15–20 minutes for several weeks or more until they are able to readily apply the skills across different classroom situations.

Self-Regulated Strategy Development (SRSD)

Over the past 25 years, the body of research on writing has grown from investigating technical and grammatical requirements to identifying the types of skills and strategies that good writers use when they write. This research has revealed that skilled writers spend time planning, monitoring, evaluating, revising, and managing the writing process. Poor writers, in contrast, often do not employ any of these skills. Teaching struggling students the very skills and strategies used by expert writers has been the sensible next step and key focus of many expressive writing interventions.

One of the instructional interventions with the strongest and most consistent research base is self-regulated strategy development, or SRSD for short. Pioneered by Steve Graham and Karen Harris at the University of Maryland, SRSD has been used in spelling, reading, and math, but the area receiving the most focused attention has been SRSD in writing. Self-regulated strategy development is a method designed to help students learn and use—and eventually adopt as their own—the strategies used by skilled writers. SRSD is more than simply strategy instruction. It encourages students to monitor, evaluate, and revise their writing—promoting self-regulation skills, increasing content knowledge, and improving motivation.

SRSD instruction is built upon six underlying stages:

1. Develop and activate background knowledge (class).
2. Discuss the strategy, including benefits and expectations (class).
3. Model the strategy (teacher).
4. Memorize the strategy (student).

5. Support the strategy collaboratively (teacher and class).

6. Use the strategy by yourself, independently (student).

In turn, these instructional stages are meshed with four general strategies that students are taught to use on their own (hence, the term self-regulation):

- Goal setting

- Self-instruction (for example, talk-aloud)

- Self-monitoring

- Self-reinforcement

Together, the process of explicit strategy instruction and extensive self-regulation has proven effective for students as early as the second grade, improving not only the quality of student writing, but also their knowledge of the writing process.

Fundamental features of SRSD include:

- explicit and extensive strategy instruction on writing, self-regulation, and content knowledge;

- interactive learning and active collaboration;

- individualized instructional support and feedback tailored to student needs and abilities;

- self-paced learning, with proficiency demonstrations required in order to progress from one stage of instruction to the next; and,

- the continuous introduction of new strategies and novel ways to use previously taught strategies.

Combining Strategy Instruction with Direct Instruction

Because children with disabilities differ widely in their individual strengths, weaknesses, and learning styles, it would make sense that no single instructional model can be recommended for all. Regardless, it may be assumed that certain fundamental teaching principles exist and that effective interventions include components that leverage these principles, adapting them for use with students with diverse learning needs, across different content areas and classroom settings.

The impressive teaching and learning gains realized with strategy instruction suggest that many of these fundamental components are embedded within this approach. It's worth noting, however, that an equally strong evidence base exists for direct instruction, an alternative instructional method that emphasizes fast-paced teacher probes and sequenced drill-repetition-practice routines. Surely within direct instruction, fundamental teaching and learning components can also be found, so how does one choose? The answer is—you don't have to.

Lee Swanson at the University of California, Riverside, has conducted several detailed meta-analyses to determine exactly which underlying instructional principles help students with LD learn best. Together with Maureen Hoskyn, Swanson has found that, in fact, academic performance—particularly in the areas of reading comprehension, vocabulary, and creativity—improved significantly whether students were taught using either strategy instruction or direct instruction. Perhaps more interesting, however, was the finding that outcomes were greatest for instructional approaches that combined aspects of each method.

Swanson has taken this work further by conducting a second level of analysis where he identified the following eight clusters of instructional components shared across interventions utilizing strategic or direct instruction:

- Explicit direct instruction (sequencing and segmentation)
- Explicit strategy instruction
- Monitoring
- Individualized training
- Small interactive group instruction
- Teacher-indirect instruction
- Verbal questioning
- Technology-mediated instruction

Though these clusters of components were found across interventions, not all contributed equally, if at all, to improved student outcomes. Of these clusters, explicit strategy instruction was found to have the most significant impact on student performance and was characterized by the following components:

Explicit practice: Encompasses many activities related to review and practice (for example: repeated practice, weekly reviews, and/or daily feedback).

Strategy cues: Includes think-aloud models, the teacher verbalizing steps or procedures during a lesson, and other reminders to use specific strategies or steps.

Elaboration: Includes explanations about concepts, repetition of information or text, or additional information provided by the teacher.

Writing with POW-er!

Students learning to write through SRSD learn the mnemonics "POW" + "TREE" to help them with the process:

Pick an idea

Organize notes

Write and say more

+

Topic sentence

Reasons—at least three

Explain reasons further

Ending, wrap it up right

A recent meta-analysis of 18 research studies supports the effectiveness of SRSD:

- for students with LD;
- with students who are average or poor writers;
- across different writing genres; and,
- at the elementary and middle school levels.

The SODA Strategy

Children diagnosed with Asperger syndrome have particular difficulty engaging in appropriate play and conversational routines with others. The SODA strategy is a step-by-step strategy designed to lead these children through successful social interactions both inside and outside of the classroom.

Stop: Provides a framework for students to evaluate the setting.

1. What activity is taking place here?

2. Who are the participants?

3. Where should I go to observe?

Observe: Prompts students to be aware of social cues used by others

1. What are the people doing?

2. What are the people saying?

3. What nonverbal cues are they using?

Deliberate: Helps students develop a plan for what to do or say.

1. With whom would I like to talk?

2. What would I like to say?

3. How would I know if others would like to visit with me?

Act: Encourages students to act on the plan and engage success-fully with others.

1. Approach person with whom you'd like to visit.

2. Say, "Hello, how are you?"

3. Look for cues that this person would like to visit longer or would like to end this conversation.

Conclusion

Current educational policy initiatives and legislation, including No Child Left Behind (NCLB) and the Individuals with Disabilities Education Act of 2004 (IDEA), rank among the most ambitious educational mandates in our country's history. Embedded within both of these laws are requirements for high-stakes testing and school accountability that have increased the demands placed upon students and teachers.

For many students with disabilities, these new demands have been accompanied by a shift from basic skills instruction delivered in special education classrooms to an engagement in more challenging content in general education settings. Instructional approaches based on the best available research evidence can only help to meet the new challenges faced by students and teachers alike.

It is clear from the research evidence that approaches that include strategy instruction can play a major role in meeting these challenges.

Strategy instruction has the power to transform passive students into active learners equipped with the tools to promote strategic planning and independent reflection. When strategy instruction is implemented as a coordinated, school-wide system, student outcomes can be even greater, leading to transfer of knowledge, skills, and strategies to other academic and social settings.

Of course, caution should be taken to avoid a focus on teaching strategies at the expense of core content instruction. Quality professional development can help educators strike the proper balance as well as ensure faithful and sustained implementation designed to maximize instructional impact.

Chapter 42

Multisensory Teaching and Sensory Words

Did You Know?

- Research shows that effective teachers make a conscious effort to design instruction that incorporates a broad variety of learning preferences beyond their own (Doolan and Honigsfeld, 2000; Sadler-Smith and Smith, 2004).

- Research shows that varying teaching strategies to address all sensory preferences increases learning, regardless of the individual student's primary preference (Thomas, Cox, and Kojima, 2000).

- Research shows that by using multisensory strategies, teachers can engage and sustain the attention of all students. By employing a variety of strategies, the teacher may address the mixed efficiencies of those students as well as the dominant and secondary preferences of others. Thus, they reinforce strong preferences and strengthen weaker ones (Silver et al., 2000; Haggart, 2003).

- "I had a great feeling of relief when I began to understand that a youngster needs more than just subject matter. Oh, I know mathematics well, and I teach it well. I used to think that that was all I needed to do. Now I teach children, not math." (Everett Shostrom in *Man, the Manipulator*)

The Benefits of Multisensory Teaching and Sensory Words

As a teacher, you know that students learn differently. Some prefer to learn by doing. Others like to watch a demonstration of what they need to do. Some want to listen to what is expected. Most students appreciate a combination of methods: a little bit of doing it, a little bit of seeing it, and a little bit of hearing it. When you teach using a combination of methods that appeal to different learning styles (kinesthetic, tactual, auditory, and visual), you are using multisensory teaching.

Following is an overview of the four major learning styles and their representation in the general population. As you read, you will probably think of past or present students who demonstrate characteristics of each style.

Kinesthetic style: Learning through doing. The kinesthetic learner must do something to learn it. This person is actively involved in learning and loves to flex those large motor muscles. There is a lot of body movement going on when these learners are in the throes of learning. Research in the learning styles area shows that 25 to 35 percent of the general population are kinesthetic learners.

Tactual style: Learning through sensations and feelings. The tactual learner learns through the sense of touch and small motor experiences. Tactual learners are also often very aware of the emotional signals, subtle and blatant, that others send. They may be sensitive to odors in their environment. They often are adept at using their hands, and they benefit from touching things to get to know them better. These are the true hands-on learners. Research indicates that 15 to 25 percent of the general population prefers the tactual modality.

Auditory style: Learning through hearing and speaking. The auditory learner is very focused on speaking and listening. This person enjoys discussions and often needs to say it to learn it. This individual is tuned in to all the sounds in his or her environment and often benefits when trying to concentrate from soft music or white noise in the background. This person frequently needs to say it to herself, or move her lips as though talking to herself, to process the material in the most efficient way. Auditory learners compose about 10 to 15 percent of the general population.

Visual style: Learning through seeing. Visual learners process information best when they see it. They enjoy videos, movies, compact discs read-only memory (CD-ROM), and watching demonstrations. Colors attract the attention of this person. This person must see it to believe it, and see it to learn it. Visualization often comes easily to this individual, and he might also have a good visual-spatial sense. Maps, graphic organizers, and pictures of all kinds are this learner's best friends. In the general population, about 35 to 40 percent of people share this learning preference.

Chances are high that you have students representing each of these four learning styles in varying degrees in your classroom. Ideally, teachers create multisensory activities that appeal to kinesthetic, tactual, auditory, and visual learners. Activities can also become multisensory—appealing to more than one learning style—by adding sensory words to them.

Using Sensory Words to Reach All Students

Sensory words are words that appeal to the senses associated with the four main learning styles: kinesthetic, tactual, auditory, and visual.

- Kinesthetic: jump, kick, run
- Tactual: pat, write, hold
- Auditory: whisper, cheer, growl
- Visual: glance, peek, notice

There are four occasions when you can use sensory words to enhance your teaching.

1. When lack of time limits an opportunity for sensory experiences. When there is no time to create a multisensory experience, and you want students to understand something through their senses, using sensory words can provide a comparable experience for students.

2. When a real sensory experience is not possible. For example, you want to study the ocean but you are living 400 miles away.

3. When you are teaching an interpersonal skill such as "participate," tell what it looks like, sounds like, and feels like when
you are "participating."

4. To build rapport, mirror verbs. Use action-oriented words to
describe non-physical things—if a person is kinesthetic, say,
"Let's slam our ideas together" when suggesting action for a
cerebral activity.

Vary sensory words when you communicate with students. For
example, the rule "Walk in the halls" is kinesthetic. If students continue to run or horse around in the halls, you might change how you
present the rule by varying sensory words. For instance:

- When I see you running in the hall, it looks like a herd of el-
ephants. Please slow down. (visual)

- It sounds like thunder when you run in the hall. Please tread
quietly. (auditory)

- It feels like the building is shaking when you run in the hall.
Please walk gently. (tactual)

- Running in the hall distracts people from learning. Please walk.
(neutral/kinesthetic)

Encourage students to vary sensory words when they communicate with one another and work on projects. Learning to communicate with others, including those whose learning styles are different
from their own, is a life skill that will benefit students during their
education as well as when they enter the work force. As a teacher,
varying sensory words is an essential part of our jobs. You can take
this skill a step further by encouraging your students to practice it
as well.

Put students in groups of three or four and ask them to help create or modify classroom rules. If your students are not versed in learning styles, simply hand out a list of sensory words from which they
can choose. Groups must choose at least one word from each category—kinesthetic (K), tactual (T), auditory (A), and visual (V).

When students respond to one another or to questions you ask
in class, ask them to stretch their responses to include a variety of
KTAV responses. For example, rather than "I hear what you are saying" (auditory), a student could respond, "That feels right to me" (tactual).

For Younger Students

Use a kinesthetic activity where students toss a ball to one another. Each time the ball is caught, the student has to make a kinesthetic, tactual, auditory, or visual statement such as: "I saw that ball coming" then toss it to someone else, who might make a tactual comment such as: "That catch felt great." Students can choose from a list of words you write on the board, or can even use vocabulary words when appropriate.

For Older Students

1. Put students in groups to practice rotating sensory words.

    - Person 1 makes a statement beginning with "fortunately, . . ." using a kinesthetic word.

    - Person 2 makes a statement beginning with "unfortunately, . . ." using a tactual word.

    - Person 3 makes a statement beginning with "fortunately, . . ." using an auditory word.

    - Back to Person 1, this time for a statement beginning with "unfortunately, . . ." and using a visual word.

    - Person 2 makes a statement beginning with "fortunately, . . ." using a neutral word, and so forth.

2. Each person uses the previous statement as a springboard, so that each statement connects with the previous one and the group's statements make a continuing conversation.

3. Have students do four rounds of this activity. An added challenge is to make the responses content-specific. Here is an example for health class:

    - Fortunately, I am up and moving around after my bout with chicken pox. (kinesthetic)

    - Unfortunately, I sense that my older brother is getting it, as he has a fever and a rash. (tactual)

    - Fortunately, I heard him say that he thinks it won't be so bad for him. (auditory)

    - Unfortunately, I picture him being in pretty bad shape, like a human polka dot. (visual)

    - Fortunately, I will be back at school by then. (neutral)

Source: The tips are based on Performance Learning System's graduate course "Teaching Through Learning Channels®."

References

Doolan, L. S., and Honigsfeld, A. (2000). Illuminating the new standards with learning style: Striking a perfect match. *Clearing House*, 73(5), 274–278.

Haggart, W. (2003). *Discipline and learning styles: An educator's guide*. Nevada City, CA: Performance Learning Systems.

Sadler-Smith, E., and Smith, J. P. (2004). Strategies for accommodating individuals' styles and preferences in flexible learning programmes. *British Journal of Educational Technology*, 35(4), 395–412.

Silver, H. F., Strong, R. W., and Perini, M. J. (2000). *So each may learn: Integrating learning styles and multiple intelligences*. Alexandria, VA: Association for Supervision and Curriculum Development.

Thomas, H., Cox, R., and Kojima, T. (2000). *Relating preferred learning style to student achievement*. Paper presented at the Annual Meeting of the Teachers of English to Speakers of Other Languages, Vancouver, BC [Canada]. (ERIC Document Reproduction Service No. 445 513).

Chapter 43

Learning Disabilities and the Arts

LD (Learning Disabilities) and the Arts

The arts are more than a fun, superficial way to keep kids occupied. Art activities can help children with learning disabilities begin to overcome the challenges they face in learning in many different ways. Of course, having a learning disability does not necessarily mean that a person has an exceptional artistic talent. However, music, art, crafts, and dance can give students with learning disabilities a chance to express themselves through different media and gain confidence along the way.

Unlocking Confidence

A feeling of self-worth—the knowledge that you can do something—is a critical part of the learning process. Children with learning disabilities often come to think they are incapable of learning because of their ongoing difficulties in school. A paintbrush; a costume; a drum; or paper, scissors, and glue can be new tools for self-expression that boost confidence while providing opportunities for learning and practice.

Learning through Art

The arts can open the world of learning to students who have trouble with traditional teaching methods. The arts are intellectual disciplines—requiring complex thinking and problem solving—that offer students the opportunity to construct their own understanding of the world.

- Drawing and painting reinforce motor skills and can also be a way of learning shapes, contrasts, boundaries, spatial relationships, size, and other math concepts.

- Music teaches children about rhythm, sound, and pitch. Beats can help children learn rhymes and other features of reading such as phonological awareness. Using repetitive songs to learn academic facts (like the alphabet song or multiplication tables) can make the learning experience easier and more fun.

- Dance provides children with a social way to learn about sequencing, rhythm, and following directions. While developing coordination and motor control, students can also learn counting and directionality, which can enhance reading and writing concepts—such as understanding the difference between similar looking letters (like p/b/d/q) and telling left from right.

- Performing plays is an opportunity for children to immerse themselves in a theme and learn about it in a profound and personal way. Acting out historical or literary figures and events gives students a sense of ownership about what they've learned, allowing them to acquire a deeper appreciation of the subject matter.

- Crafts offer children the opportunity to express themselves in two- and three-dimensional ways. Students can develop vital problem-solving skills without having to rely on areas of expression that may be more challenging.

Arts as a Means of Assessment

- Timed tests and take-home reports are traditional means of academic assessment that can be especially difficult for individuals with learning disabilities. Creative projects offer these students the freedom to show what they know without the constraints of printed text. Offering students art projects or multimedia presentations as a way to demonstrate an understanding of material they've learned can be an excellent alternative.

372

- Because a person has difficulty learning through hearing alone or seeing alone, that does not mean they cannot learn. The arts offer individuals with learning disabilities dynamic ways of learning, and just as importantly, a way to fully discover their own self-worth.

Art Therapy Outcome and Single Subject Studies for Attention Deficit Disorder (ADD), Attention Deficit/Hyperactivity Disorder (AD/HD), and Asperger Syndrome

Study: Kearns, D. (2004). Art therapy with a child experiencing sensory integration difficulty. *Art Therapy: Journal of the American Art Therapy Association*, 21(2), 95–101.

Aim and Method: An increasing number of students diagnosed with difficulties such as attention deficit/hyperactivity disorder and Asperger syndrome are being seen in schools. Sensory integration difficulties may be part of the symptomatology of these disorders. These difficulties may result in difficulties with both classroom behaviors and academic performance. This single-case study investigated the effectiveness of art therapy with a five-year old white male with sensory integration difficulties. Art therapy focused on pre-art activities using three media. The pre/post test measurement tool was the *Formal Elements Art Therapy Scales (FEATS)* (Gantt and Tabone, 1998) to assess a "person picking an apple from a tree." Scales were rated for "changes in various qualities over the course of the research period" including: prominence of color, color fit, implied energy, use of space, integration, realism, details of objects and environment, and developmental level. Teacher ratings based on observation, assessed classroom behavior for improvement. A recording form "had a series of boxes, one for each 30-minute segment of Michael's school day" (p. 97). Ratings were positive or negative. Each of the varied media sessions was compared to control sessions where a non-art experience was offered.

Results: Results indicated an increase in positive behaviors after art sessions as well as postponement of the first incidence of negative behaviors. Art therapy was found to be a useful intervention (Kearns, 2004, p. 95; P. St. John, 8/14/05).

Study: Smitheman-Brown, V., and Church, R. P. (1996). Mandala drawing: Facilitating creative growth in children with ADD or ADHD.

Art Therapy: Journal of the American Art Therapy Association, 13(4), 252–262.

Aim and Method: Using a single-subject, multiple-baseline research design, this study investigates the creative growth and behavioral changes precipitated by the work done in art therapy through employment of the mandala as an active centering device with children (N = 8: four experimental and four control, ages 10–13) who have been diagnosed with attention deficit disorder (ADD) or attention deficit/ hyperactivity disorder (AD/HD), accompanied by a history of impulsivity. During specified intervals of treatment, a drawing was requested. "Draw a person picking an apple from a tree" was rated according to the guidelines of the *Formal Elements Art Therapy Scales (FEATS)* (Gantt and Tabone, 1998). Four scales were used: Number 5, Integration; Number 8, Problem Solving; Number 9, Developmental; and Number 10, Details of Objects and Environment. "Baseline data were gathered from historical and observable patterns of behavior, use of the *Child Behavioral Checklist* (Attenbach, 1979), general artwork produced before the intervention, and the repeated drawing task—produced prior to the introduction of the intervention" (p. 253). "Ongoing behavioral data were charted through direct observation. The [5-minute minimum, mandala-drawing] intervention was considered to begin during the art therapy sessions in which the mandala drawing was first introduced" (p. 253).

Results: Through examination of the drawings by three independent trained raters and objective findings of this scale, it appears that a visual measurement of creative growth was achieved. Preliminary findings indicate that the mandala exercise has the effect of increasing attentional abilities and decreasing impulsive behaviors over time, allowing for better decision making, completion of task, general growth in developmental level, and an interest in personal aesthetics (Smitheman-Brown and Church, 1996, p. 252; P. St. John, 8/14/05).

Chapter 44

Vision Therapy Not Supported by Scientific Evidence

Description of Vision Therapy

Vision therapy, also referred to as visual training or vision training, is a method attempting to correct or improve presumed ocular disorders, visual processing, and perceptual disorders. Vision therapy can be broadly divided into two categories. In the first category, classic orthoptic techniques are used to correct accommodative (focusing) and convergence dysfunctions as well as heterophorias (latent misaligned eyes) and refractive errors (need for glasses) that might be responsible for asthenopic symptoms (eye fatigue and discomfort often aggravated by close work). In the second category, often referred to as behavioral vision therapy, eye movement and hand-eye coordination training techniques are used to improve visual processing skills, learning efficiency, and visual-motor integration. Behavioral vision therapy is based on the premise that differences in children's visual perceptual motor abilities exist and that these perceptual motor abilities influence cognitive and adaptive skills such as reading, writing, and motor activities used in activities of daily living. Behavioral vision therapy has been recommended to improve visual skills and processing in the belief that this will improve learning disabilities, including speech and language disorders, and nonverbal learning disorders. Colored overlays or lenses are sometimes used as part of vision therapy to alter contrast.

Excerpted from "Vision Therapies for Learning Disabilities," © 2007 EyeCare America (www.eyecareamerica.org), a program of the Foundation of the American Academy of Ophthalmology. Reprinted with permission.

Conclusions

To date, there appears to be no consistent scientific evidence that supports behavioral vision therapy, orthoptic vision therapy, or colored overlays and lenses as effective treatments for learning disabilities. It seems intuitive that oculomotor abilities and visual perception play a role in learning skills such as reading and writing. However, several studies in the literature demonstrate that eye movements and visual perception are not critical factors in the reading impairment found in dyslexia, but that brain processing of language plays a greater role. Furthermore, the vast majority of individuals with known ocular motility and eye movement defects appear to read and comprehend normally. Many individuals born with severely misaligned eyes excel in reading and academics.

Regarding the benefits of treatment, no well-performed randomized controlled trials were found in the literature. In this complex field, controlled studies are difficult to conduct, because there are so many variables involved, and possibly confounding factors. There is no standard definition for what techniques comprise vision therapy. Children included in the studies have been diagnosed with learning disabilities using different criteria, or may have been misdiagnosed, or may have additional conditions that may confound the findings. Furthermore, during a course of vision therapy, children are simultaneously receiving continued and even enhanced instruction in a standard or remedial educational setting, as well as undergoing natural maturational changes. Behavioral vision therapy studies that were found in the peer-reviewed literature reported findings that are inconsistent. A team approach utilizing multidisciplinary educational specialists to assess the effectiveness of vision therapy in scientifically valid studies seems indicated.

Description of Vision Therapy

Vision therapy, also referred to as visual training or vision training, is a method attempting to correct or improve ocular, visual processing, and perceptual disorders. The American Optometric Association defines vision therapy as "a sequence of activities individually prescribed and monitored by the doctor to develop efficient visual skills and processing."

Vision therapy is based on the premise that differences in children's visual perceptual motor abilities exist and influence skills such as reading, writing, and motor activities used in activities of daily living. Vision therapy aims to improve a child's motor awareness, motor planning and motor sequencing on the premise that this will improve learning disabilities, including speech and language disorders, and nonverbal learning disorders. In order to understand this premise, it is important to know that vision therapy practitioners identify three interrelated domains of visual function, all of which they believe must be evaluated fully to identify learning-related vision problems.

- Visual pathway integrity, including eye health, visual acuity, and refractive status.

- Visual skills, including accommodation status (eye focusing), binocular vision (eye teaming), and eye movements (eye tracking).

- Visual information processing including identification, discrimination, spatial awareness, and integration with other senses.

Different treatment areas within vision therapy are orthoptic vision therapy, behavioral vision therapy, and the use of colored lenses and overlays. While these three treatment areas are defined, this assessment will discuss the evidence supporting behavioral vision therapy and colored lenses and overlays.

Orthoptic Vision Therapy

Asthenopia (eye fatigue and discomfort often aggravated by close work) is believed by some to be related to reading inefficiency. The aim of the orthoptic aspect of vision therapy is to improve vergence amplitudes (measure of the ability to bring the eyes into alignment) in cases of convergence insufficiency (eye muscle problem causing outward deviation of the eyes when looking at a near object that can cause eye fatigue or double vision) by teaching diplopia (double vision) awareness. Other asthenopic symptoms due to heterophorias (latent misaligned eyes) or accommodative dysfunction (focusing problems) are addressed using a variety of refractive lens powers, prisms, bifocals, and haploscopic (simultaneously presents separate visual targets to each eye) devices. In general, children have normal accommodative and vergence amplitudes. It is important to distinguish the role of the orthoptist in pediatric eye care from these types of orthoptic vision therapy that are being used to treat learning disabilities. An orthoptist is a professional trained in the diagnosis and treatment of strabismus and amblyopia and often works in a pediatric ophthalmology practice.

Behavioral Vision Therapy

Behavioral vision therapy involves eye exercises, eye-hand coordination tasks, and exercises designed to improve the patient's motor memory activity. Vision therapy requires a number of office visits depending upon the severity of the problem diagnosed by the vision therapy provider. The typical length of the program ranges from several weeks to several months and usually includes activities to perform at home.

Colored Lenses and Overlays

Vision therapy may include the use of colored overlays or filters, and glasses for mild refractive errors with or without prisms. Colored overlay filters are said to reduce pattern glare, which is a hypersensitivity to repetitive patterns, including lines of print on a page.

Definition of the Problem

It is important to recognize that children often have visual complaints from normal visual phenomena. Wright and Boger review many normal, common physiologic visual experiences such as blurred or double vision. A child's description of these experiences can be misinterpreted by the patient, parent, or practitioner as abnormal, and lead them to believe that the complaints are the basis of a reported learning or reading problem. Experiences that children complain of include blurring or "swimming together" of print while reading due to normal relaxation of accommodation or convergence, and from physiologic diplopia. It is important to note that pathologic conditions such as high refractive errors, heterotropias (misaligned eyes), and true convergence insufficiency can cause these complaints and these conditions should be diagnosed and treated. Children with abnormalities identified at routine vision screening examinations as described in national standards should be referred for comprehensive eye examination.

U.S. Food and Drug Administration (FDA) Status

There are no legal or FDA controls or restraints on orthoptic or behavioral vision therapy.

Chapter 45

Assistive Technology (AT) at School or Work for Individuals with Learning Disabilities

Assistive Technology (AT) for Individuals with Learning Disabilities

General Facts about Assistive Technology

Individuals with learning disabilities often have difficulty with tasks that others take for granted—like reading, listening, organizing information, or writing—and may benefit from the use of assistive technology (AT) in order to increase their daily independence.

Appropriate assistive technology for students and adults with learning disabilities can include but is not limited to:

- computers with adaptive software;

- books on tape, or electronic format;

- speller and grammar checkers;

- specialized four-track tape recorders;

- audio players;

- computer screen readers;

This chapter includes text from "Assistive Technology (AT) for Individuals with Learning Disabilities," © 2004 Learning Disabilities Association of America (www.ldanatl.org). Reprinted with permission. And, "A Process for Choosing AT for Employees with Disabilities," by Beth Loy, Ph.D., and Linda Carter Batiste, J.D., Job Accommodation Network (JAN), January 2007.

- talking word processors and calculators;
- electronic data organizers.

Assistive technology may be considered to be one of the following:

- **High-tech:** Usually costs more, requires training, and equipment and software such as voice recognition or word prediction software.
- **Low-tech:** Usually costs less than high-tech and requires only limited training and inexpensive equipment such as a talking watch, pencil grippers, highlighting marker tape, and ear plugs to reduce distraction.

Assistive technology can be used to accommodate and/or modify specific tasks, or be incorporated into performing tasks. Assistive technology providers (for example, rehabilitation engineers, certified assistive technology professionals) evaluate formally, and in some cases informally, the functional limitation of the disability to match the appropriate assistive technology.

Definitions

With this in mind, the re-authorized Assistive Technology Act (Tech Act) of 1998 defines an assistive technology device as any item, piece of equipment, product, or system, whether acquired commercially, modified, or customized, that is used to increase, maintain, or improve functional capabilities of individuals with disabilities (Authority: 29 U.S.C. 3002).

As defined in the Individuals with Disabilities Education Act of 1997 (IDEA 97) the term assistive technology device means "any item, piece of equipment, or product system, whether acquired commercially off the shelf, modified, or customized, that is used to increase, maintain, or improve the functional capabilities of a child with a disability." 34 CFR 300.5 (Authority: 20 U.S. C. 1401 (1)). The term assistive technology service means "any service that directly assists a child with a disability in the selection, acquisition, or use of an assistive technology device." 34 CFR 300.6 (Authority: 20 U.S.C. 1401 (2)).

Facts about Assistive Technology and the Individualized Education Program (IEP)

1. Assistive technology needs must be considered along with the child's other educational needs.

2. Needs for technology must be identified on an individual basis.

3. Identification of technology needs must involve family members and a multidisciplinary team.

4. Parents or IEP members can ask for additional evaluations or an independent evaluation to determine assistive technology needs.

5. When an evaluation is being conducted, consider fine-motor skills, communication, and alternatives to traditional learning approaches.

6. Lack of availability of equipment or cost alone cannot be used as an excuse for denying an assistive technology service.

7. If included in the IEP, assistive technology services and devices must be provided at no cost to the family and, if so indicated, devices must be allowed to go home with the student.

8. Parents always have the right to appeal if assistive technology services are denied.

The need for assistive technology must be considered like other needs, on a case-by-case basis. Assessments can also be requested through the IEP process. Individualized education programs that include assistive technology should be written so that students have access to these accommodations not only for in-class work, but also for projects and all types of tests, including high-stakes assessment. To support the need for assistive technology, parents and professionals should document precisely how the student benefits educationally. For instance, documentation could include information such as: "Mary usually takes one hour to do eight long-division math problems. With a voice output (talking) calculator, she can do the same number of problems in 20 minutes."

Facts about Assistive Technology and Employment

Individuals and employers can get help identifying appropriate assistive technology and/or accommodations in the workplace by contacting the Job Accommodations Network (JAN) at 800-526-7234, or at http://janweb.icdi.wvu.edu.

JAN consultants can provide comprehensive, up-to-date information about accommodations, devices, and strategies. Calls to JAN are confidential. Information is provided about job accommodations, the Americans with Disabilities Act, and the employability of individuals with disabilities.

In addition, some companies have taken the lead in providing accessibility services. For example, Microsoft Corporation has developed a website that features products and resources for assistive technology. For more information, visit http://www.microsoft.com/enable/default.aspx.

Nationwide Technical Assistive Projects

With the passage of the Assistive Technology Act of 1998 (Tech Act), the National Institute on Disability and Rehabilitation Research (NIDRR) is responsible for its implementation. The Tech Act provides grants to states to help bring about systems change to increase the availability of, access to, and funding for assistive technology. NIDRR also helps states provide legal advocacy to individuals with disabilities concerning assistive technology issues. The most effective way to learn about your local Tech Act project is to go to the Rehabilitation Engineering and Assistive Technology Society of North America (RESNA) website (http://www.resna.org) which will offer contact information for state Technical Assistive Projects.

A Process for Choosing AT for Employees with Disabilities

The following steps are helpful when choosing AT to meet the specific accommodation needs of an employee with a disability:

Step 1: Define the Situation

The first step in choosing AT to accommodate an individual with a disability is to define the situation. An effective way to do this is to determine what job functions need to be accommodated by evaluating the individual's work site, work station, and work activities. Answering the following questions will assist with defining the situation:

- What are the individual's functional limitations? A functional limitation involves difficulty in performing one or more specific work activities (for example: difficulty communicating during meetings, using a telephone, reading print material, lifting boxes, and using a keyboard).

- What is the extent and type of impairment? Determining whether a condition is progressive or stable may not always be a factor to consider. However, knowing how the individual's condition will improve or worsen over time can be important when choosing AT. For example: an employee with progressive vision loss may benefit from screen magnification now, but may need screen reading software in the future as his condition worsens. In some cases, it may make more sense to go ahead and purchase the screen reading software now.

- What job tasks are difficult to perform as a result of the impairment? This may be a good time to study the individual's job description to determine the essential and marginal functions of the position (for example: distinguishing color, entering data, lifting materials, and tolerating stress).

Step 2: Explore Available AT Options

Once the situation has been defined, the next step is to explore available AT options. A good starting point is consulting with the individual who needs the accommodation. Often the individual knows what AT is available. Also, talking with the individual can help determine whether the individual is proficient in using a certain type of AT, which can save research and training time. Another way to explore available AT options is to contact Job Accommodation Network (JAN) directly to speak with an AT specialist or access the JAN Searchable Online Accommodation Resource (SOAR), which lets users explore various accommodation options for people with disabilities in work settings. SOAR is available at: http://www.jan.wvu.edu/soar.

Other resources that can help employers explore available AT options include the following agencies:

- State vocational rehabilitation (VR) agencies provide services to ensure gainful employment for people with disabilities. In addition to job placement, services may include, but are not limited to counseling, vocational evaluation, assessment, on-the-job training, rehabilitation technology services, and possible assistance with funding accommodations. For a list of state VR agencies, go to: http://www.jan.wvu.edu/cgi-win/TypeQuery.exe?902.

- State AT projects provide technical assistance on AT, consultation, product demonstrations, equipment borrowing, and low-interest loans for individuals with disabilities. For a list of state AT projects, go to: http://www.jan.wvu.edu/cgi-win/TypeQuery.exe?735.

- The Rehabilitation Engineering and Assistive Technology Society of North America (RESNA) provides information on assistive technology practitioners (ATP) or rehabilitation engineering technologists (RET). To access a directory of ATP and RET from RESNA, go to: http://www.resna.org.

- Disability specific organizations can also be helpful resources. For a listing of organizations by specific disability, go to: http://www.jan.wvu.edu/links/disspec.htm.

A final option for exploring available AT is to consult with the computer technician or information technology team at the individual's workplace. Compatibility and feasibility issues should be addressed and it may be possible for an IT representative to download trial versions and test free demos of AT.

Step 3: Choose AT

Once steps one and two are completed, an informed choice can be made about the AT. When choosing AT, consider the following:

- Is there technical support available?
- Is there a money back guarantee and warranty?
- Is there an option to upgrade with newer versions?
- Is the product compatible with other technology used?
- Is training available?
- Does the electronic infrastructure support interoperability with the AT?
- How will the AT be funded?

Tax incentives, vocational rehabilitation services, and local civic organizations may assist with funding AT. For more information on funding options, go to: http://www.jan.wvu.edu/links/Funding/GeneralInfo.html.

Step 4: Implement AT

Once a potential AT solution is chosen, the next step is to implement the AT, which involves purchasing the product or service, providing appropriate training, and ensuring that the individual with the disability can successfully use the AT.

Step 5: Monitor and Upgrade AT

Providing AT as an accommodation is an ongoing process between an employee and his or her employer. It is important to keep the lines of communication open, to monitor the effectiveness of the accommodation to ensure that the AT is meeting the needs of the employee and employer, and to upgrade the AT as needed. Some questions to consider include:

- If training was provided, was it effective?
- Is the AT being used properly?
- Is the AT being maintained?
- Should other accommodations besides AT be considered?

Take into account any changes in the individual's functional limitations or job duties that would alter current accommodation needs and the effectiveness of the AT. When changes occur, an employer may need to communicate with employees who use AT in the workplace.

Chapter 46

Principles of Effective Instruction for Adults with Learning Disabilities

There are six general principles of instruction that should be used when developing instructional methods and materials for adults with learning disabilities:

1. Provide direct instruction.
2. Prevent overloading.
3. Provide systematic, sequential instruction.
4. Teach to mastery.
5. Prevent forgetting through practice.
6. Provide feedback.

1. Provide Direct Instruction

People with learning disabilities are not good incidental learners. They need direct instruction that addresses the literacy, math, and daily living problems they experience. Adults who are reading at low levels need help to improve their basic reading skills. Basic reading skills include sight word knowledge (the ability to read words quickly by sight) and decoding (the ability to figure out unfamiliar words using the sound and syllable structure of words). It is vital that adults with learning disabilities be provided with direct instruction in these basic skills.

2. Prevent Overloading

Adults with learning disabilities can be easily overloaded with new information. Overloading can affect a person's ability to learn new information and can disrupt previously learned information. Appropriately designed instruction helps to circumvent the problems of overloading and to compensate for the poor attention skills that many adults have.

Instruction that is designed to prevent overloading limits the amount of new information taught at one time. We need to think about how much new information is being presented. There is no rule of thumb for determining the amount of new information any given individual can absorb. Observations during teaching help to determine an appropriate amount for a particular person. It is easy to tell when too much new information is being presented. People start to make mistakes while they are learning and may even make mistakes on things we thought they had mastered.

3. Provide Sequential Instruction

Just as with children, instruction for adults should not be haphazard. Don't wait for teachable moments when a person needs a specific skill or piece of information. Rather, make all moments teachable and sequence instruction so that people learn new things in a sensible way that provides a good basis for moving on to more sophisticated skills.

We need to present learning disabled adults with instruction that is carefully sequenced to prevent gaps in their knowledge, to provide foundations for future learning, and to compensate for difficulties in integrating separate skills and in generalizing or abstracting information.

Prevent overloading in basic decoding instruction—look for programs that:

- teach only one short vowel sound at a time;
- introduce consonants a few at a time since they are usually easier to learn;

388

- do not introduce new short vowels until mastery is attained;
- introduce rules for long vowels one at a time.

4. Teach to Mastery

Adults with learning disabilities may forget new words or sounds they have been taught. This occurs in part because the words or sounds were not really mastered and information that is not mastered is readily forgotten. Each new skill that is taught should be practiced to a point of automatic mastery. An automatic response is one that the person does not have to stop and think about.

Look for programs that provide a good sequence for decoding instruction such as the following progression:

- Letter names
- Consonant sounds
- Short vowels
- Consonant combinations (blends and digraphs)
- Long vowels (silent e, vowel digraphs)
- R-controlled vowels and vowel diphthongs
- Exceptions and more difficult sounds (for example, soft g and c)

Insuring that each new skill is learned to a point of automatic mastery helps compensate for problems in memory, attention, and discrimination. Keep in mind, though, that even when new concepts and new learning are mastered and well understood, they can—and will—be lost over time if they are not practiced and used. For example, most of us cannot remember the foreign language we learned in high school with the same degree of proficiency we displayed at that time if we have not used the language since graduation.

5. Prevent Forgetting through Practice and Repetition

"Use it or lose it." This saying applies to most things in life, but it is of particular importance for individuals with learning disabilities. Two strategies need to be used to help learning disabled adults remember what they learn. First, provide a great deal of practice and repetition. Although some people moan at the thought of repetition, it is vital that learning disabled adults get as much practice as possible. Practice and repetition don't have to be boring. It gives adults enormous enjoyment to read things they have mastered. And it is a teaching challenge to locate or prepare materials that allow for successful practice and eventual mastery.

6. Provide Informative Feedback

Once we understand that learning disabled adults are not good discovery learners or incidental learners we can begin to understand their need for informative feedback. We can't be reluctant to tell someone that they have read something incorrectly. Adults do not want to be patronized or told that anything they do is just fine. They want to communicate with other adults as adults. But, we can't just tell adults they are wrong and to please try again. We need to give them opportunities to correct their errors or to supply correct responses and give them the opportunity to practice the correct responses.

Given their emotional sensitivity, it is important to provide feedback to learning disabled adults in a positive and constructive way.

Table 46.1. Feedback for Learning Disabled Adults

Avoid these:	Try this feedback instead:
That's not right.	Try it this way.
That's wrong.	Make this change and it will be right.
You've made a mistake.	Here is another way of doing it.
That's not the right way.	My turn—I'll show you.
You have five words wrong.	You have 15 words correct.
We covered that already.	Let's go over that again.
Try to remember.	Let's go over that again.

Part Six

Legal and Financial Information for Individuals with Learning Disabilities

Chapter 47

What Parents of Students with Disabilities Need to Know about the No Child Left Behind Act (NCLB) and the Individuals with Disabilities Education Act (IDEA)

Overview

The No Child Left Behind Act (NCLB) and the Individuals with Disabilities Education Act (IDEA) are two of the nation's most important federal laws relating to the education of children. While NCLB seeks to improve the education of all children—with an emphasis on children from low-income families—IDEA focuses on the individual child and seeks to ensure specialized services for children with disabilities so that they may benefit from education.

Lately, these two laws have taken on new importance to parents of students with disabilities. NCLB provisions apply to all students, including those whose disabilities require special education. So it's important that parents understand the requirements of NCLB. IDEA, in its latest update by Congress, has been more closely aligned with NCLB, making it equally important that parents become familiar with the ways the two laws have been positioned to work together to improve academic achievement of students with disabilities.

The No Child Left Behind Act (NCLB)

The No Child Left Behind Act (NCLB) is the latest version of the Elementary and Secondary Education Act (ESEA), the nation's major federal law related to education in grades pre-kindergarten through high school. Congress first passed the ESEA in 1965 as part of the nation's war on poverty. The centerpiece of the ESEA, Title I, was designed to improve achievement among the nation's poor and disadvantaged students.

When NCLB was signed into law in 2002, it ushered in some of the most sweeping changes the American educational system has seen in decades. New requirements introduced in NCLB were intended to increase the quality and effectiveness not only of the Title I program, but of the entire elementary and secondary education system—raising the achievement of all students, particularly those with the lowest achievement levels. NCLB is built on four basic principles:

- Accountability for results
- An emphasis on doing what works based on scientific research
- Expanded parental involvement and options
- Expanded local control and flexibility

Building on the standards-based reform efforts put into place under the previous version of ESEA, NCLB seeks to:

- raise the academic achievement of all students; and
- close the achievement gap between groups of students that historically perform poorly and their higher performing peers.

The purpose of this title is to ensure that all children have a fair, equal, and significant opportunity to obtain a high-quality education and reach, at a minimum, proficiency on challenging state academic achievement standards and state academic assessments. (No Child Left Behind Act of 2001)

Title I programs serve 16.5 million school children. Currently all states accept Title I funds. Almost all school districts and 55 percent of all public schools accept funds through a Title I grant. Federal funding for Title I programs was almost $13 billion in 2006.

What All States Must Do

NCLB requires all states that accept Title I funds to bring all students to a proficient level in reading and math by 2014. To achieve that goal, every state is required to do the following:

- Develop challenging academic standards that are the same for every student.

- Develop annual academic assessments for all students.

- Ensure that there is a highly qualified teacher in every classroom.

- Define the amount of academic progress that school districts and schools must achieve each year in order to reach the proficiency goal by 2014.

- Ensure that schools and school districts test at least 95 percent of all students.

- Determine a minimum size for required subgroups of students to be included in yearly progress calculations, based on technical considerations.

- Ensure the availability of reasonable adaptations and accommodations for students with disabilities.

- Produce an annual statewide Report Card of performance and make the report available to the public.

Annual statewide assessments (or tests) of student progress are the centerpiece of the accountability principle of NCLB. Data from these assessments, combined with other important indicators, are used to determine if schools and school districts achieve adequate yearly progress (AYP).

NCLB: The Bottom Line

All provisions contained in NCLB are designed to hold schools, school districts, and states accountable for student achievement. By requiring that all students in the required grades participate in assessments of reading/language arts and math, schools are graded on how well students are learning the knowledge and skills defined by the content standards. By requiring that the performance of certain groups of students (subgroups) is reported, schools' grades are based on how well these particular groups of students are learning—not just the total school population. This approach holds schools accountable for the learning of all students.

Nothing in NCLB requires or even encourages states to attach high-stakes consequences to student achievement on large-scale assessments. Policies to make high-stakes decisions based on a student's performance on a state or district-wide assessment (such as receiving a standard diploma or being promoted to the next grade) are made at the state or local level, generally by state legislatures, state boards of education, or local school boards.

The Individuals with Disabilities Education Act

The Individuals with Disabilities Education Act (IDEA) is the federal law dealing with the education of children with disabilities. Congress first passed IDEA in 1975, recognizing the need to provide a federal law to help ensure that local schools would serve the educational needs of students with disabilities. The law originally passed was titled the Education for All Handicapped Children Act. That first special education law has undergone several updates over the past 30 years. In 1990, the law got a new name—the Individuals with Disabilities Education Act, or IDEA. The most recent version of IDEA was passed by Congress in 2004. It can be referred to as either IDEA 2004 or IDEA.

In updating IDEA in 2004, Congress found that the education of students with disabilities has been impeded by "low expectations and an insufficient focus on applying replicable research on proven methods of teaching and learning...." Significant changes to IDEA as well as a close alignment to NCLB are designed to provide students with disabilities access to high expectations and to the general education curriculum in the regular classroom, to the maximum extent possible, in order to "meet developmental goals and, to the extent possible, the challenging expectations that have been established for all children...."

The purposes of this title are to ensure that all children with disabilities have available to them a free appropriate public education that emphasizes special education and related services designed to meet their unique needs and prepare them for further education, employment and independent living. (Individuals with Disabilities Education Improvement Act of 2004)

IDEA serves 6.1 million school age children and almost one million children ages birth to five. Federal funding for IDEA was $10.6 billion in 2006. These funds are distributed to all states to assist with the cost of providing special education services.

What All States Must Do

IDEA requires all states that accept IDEA funds to provide a free appropriate public education to all children with disabilities in the state. To achieve that goal, every state is required to do the following:

- Establish a goal of providing full educational opportunity to all children with disabilities and a timetable for accomplishing that goal.

- Identify, locate, and evaluate all children with disabilities residing in the state who are in need of special education and related services.

- Ensure that all special education teachers are highly qualified.

- Evaluate every child suspected of having a disability in accordance with the requirements of IDEA.

- Annually develop an individualized education program (IEP) for each child with a disability.

- Provide education services in the least restrictive environment— removing children from the regular education environment only when the nature or severity of their disability makes it necessary to do so.

- Provide all procedural safeguards required by IDEA to children with disabilities and their parents.

- Establish goals for the performance of children with disabilities that are the same as the state's definition of adequate yearly progress (AYP) and are consistent with any other goals and standards for children established by the state.

- Include all children with disabilities in all general state and districtwide assessment programs, including those assessments required by NCLB—students must be given appropriate accommodations and alternate assessments as indicated in their IEP.

The special education provided to children with disabilities must be specially designed instruction to meet the unique needs resulting from the child's disability and must enable the child to be involved and make progress in the general education curriculum.

IDEA: The Bottom Line

Requirements of IDEA are designed to ensure that all schools, school districts, and states provide a free appropriate public education to children with disabilities. IDEA focuses on the individual child—requiring the development of an individualized education program (IEP) outlining the specially designed instruction necessary to allow the child to participate and progress in the same curriculum as all children.

However, nothing in IDEA holds schools accountable for the progress and performance of children with disabilities. While IDEA allows parents to challenge the adequacy of special education services, the law does not contain any measures of total school performance for IDEA-eligible students, as is required by NCLB.

NCLB and IDEA: Better Together

Together, NCLB and IDEA provisions and requirements combine to provide both individualized instruction and school accountability for students with disabilities. The progress and performance of students with disabilities is now a shared responsibility of general and special education teachers. Enhanced accountability for students with disabilities has elevated them in the consciousness of school, school district, and state level administrators. Never before have the nation's federal education laws been aligned to provide such powerful opportunities for children with disabilities.

To understand this powerful connection, let's look more closely at four key ways that NCLB and IDEA work together to improve the academic performance of students with disabilities.

Academic Content and Achievement Standards

NCLB requires all states to have challenging academic content standards—what students need to know—and academic achievement standards—how well students need to know the content standards. More importantly, NCLB requires that these content and achievement standards are the same for all students, including students with disabilities. It is this requirement that establishes high expectations for all students regardless of the history of their performance.

IDEA requires all states to establish performance goals and indicators to promote the progress of students with disabilities. Every student must have an individualized education program (IEP) that outlines the special education services—specially designed instruction—and related services that will be needed for the student to access and progress in the general education curriculum. In the case of reading/language arts, and math, the general education curriculum is based on the challenging academic content standards each state has established as required by NCLB. While the IEP is a statement of what the student needs, it is not a performance document and does not guarantee educational progress.

NCLB's requirement for challenging academic content standards and achievement standards for all students must be aligned with IDEA's requirement to carefully plan the specially designed instruction each student with a disability needs to participate in the general curriculum and make progress toward proficiency. This alignment ensures that students with disabilities have the extra support they need to achieve the same high standards as other students.

To Do

The individualized education programs (IEP) of students with disabilities should be connected to the state's academic content standards. This IEP linkage—sometimes called standards-based IEP—ensures that students with disabilities are working toward the same state grade-level content and skills as their grade-level peers. The location where students with disabilities receive their specially designed instruction should ensure access to the general curriculum. Access to the general education curriculum means that students with disabilities are actively engaged in learning the content and skills that define the general education curriculum. It is not enough to simply be placed in the general education classroom—students must be actively engaged in learning the content and skills that define the curriculum.

At the same time, each student's IEP must define how the student will participate in any state and districtwide assessments, including the state assessments required by NCLB.

Annual Assessments

NCLB requires every state to implement annual assessments in reading/language arts and math in grades 3–8 and at least once in grades 10–12. Science assessments are also required beginning in 2008. However, schools are not held accountable for student performance on science assessments. The assessments must be aligned with the challenging state academic content standards and based on academic achievement standards that have been set by the state.

Results of this testing must be reported for the overall school and must also be disaggregated, or broken out, by specific groups of students that historically underachieve. These groups are known as subgroups. A student's performance data are included in every applicable subgroup. The performance of subgroups is only reported if the number of students in the subgroup meets or exceeds the minimum set by the state. The minimum size of each subgroup varies greatly among states.

IDEA requires students with disabilities to participate in all state assessments. If a state has a more comprehensive assessment program than required by NCLB, IDEA requires that students with disabilities participate in those assessments as well.

The required subgroups that must be reported are:

- students from major racial/ethnic groups;
- economically disadvantaged students;
- students with limited English proficiency; and
- students with disabilities (eligible for services under IDEA)— such students must have an IEP in place annually.

The results of the testing, along with other indicators such as attendance and graduation rates, are used to determine if schools are providing substantial and continuous improvement in the academic achievement of its students and to determine if schools are making AYP.

NCLB expects that the vast majority of students with disabilities will participate in the same assessment as all other students. Some may need accommodations such as extra breaks, reading the math test, or a Braille edition. However, the academic content being tested and the achievement standard that is expected does not differ from that of all other students.

There are several options available to students with disabilities to participate in the regular assessments—the same assessments that all students take.

Accommodations for Students with Disabilities

States must provide appropriate accommodations that are needed by students with disabilities to fully participate in state and districtwide assessments. Accommodations level the playing field so that the test measures what a student knows and can do and not the effect of the child's disability.

IDEA requires every state to establish guidelines for accommodations to make sure that students use only accommodations that produce a score that is valid for school accountability purposes. For example, if the reading assessment is supposed to measure how well a student can decode text, then reading the test aloud to the student as an accommodation would result in an invalid score on the test because the accommodation would interfere with the skill being measured. If, however, the skill is comprehension of text, reading the test aloud might be a permissible accommodation.

Accommodations used in state and districtwide assessments should mirror those used in day-to-day classroom instruction and classroom tests, to the extent possible. An accommodation should never be introduced for the first time in a state assessment. The student's IEP team must make decisions about the accommodations needed on state assessments. These accommodations must be clearly listed in the student's IEP.

Accommodations are generally grouped into the following categories:

- Presentation (repeat directions, read aloud, use of larger bubbles on answer sheets)

- Response (mark answers in book, use reference aids, point, use of computer)

- Timing or scheduling (extended time, frequent breaks)

- Setting (study carrel, special lighting, separate room)

Alternate Assessment on Grade-Level Achievement Standards

An alternate assessment based on grade-level achievement standards (with or without accommodations) assesses the same content as a regular grade-level assessment and holds the student to the same expectations based on the same definition of proficiency. However, unlike the regular assessment, this option provides different ways for students to show what they know. Results from such an assessment are treated in the same manner as results from regular assessments. There is no limit to the numbers of students who can be assessed in this manner. This option, however, is not available in all states.

Alternate Assessment on Alternate Achievement Standards

NCLB recognizes that some students may have significant cognitive disabilities that prevent them from attaining grade-level achievement standards, even with the very best instruction. For such students, NCLB allows an alternate assessment based on alternate achievement standards—in other words, an assessment that measures student progress on state grade-level content standards but at reduced breadth, depth, or complexity, and judged against a different definition of proficiency from the regular assessment. Instruction for these students should be linked to the same challenging academic content standards that apply to their same age peers. This linkage ensures that students with the most significant cognitive disabilities are given access to academic skills and concepts—something that has been missing from much of their instructional program until now.

As with all other assessment options, the decision that a student will participate in an alternate assessment based on alternate achievement standards is made by the IEP team—including the parents. NCLB places a limitation on the scores of students assessed using this option that can be used in a school district's AYP calculation. This limitation is based on research about students with significant cognitive disabilities—including the numbers of such students within the general population—and is designed to ensure that only those students who truly need this type of assessment are assigned to participate in this manner. Out-of-level testing is considered an alternate assessment based on alternate achievement standards, and the scores of students assessed in this manner are subject to the same limitation. Rigorous standard-setting criteria and other considerations must be met before out-of-level testing can be used as an alternate assessment based on alternate achievement standards.

Out-of-Level Testing

Out-of-level testing generally refers to the practice of giving a student a test intended for students at a lower grade level. Out-of-level testing is often associated with lower expectations for students with disabilities, tracking such students into lower-level curricula with limited opportunities. It may also limit student opportunities for advancing to the next grade or graduating with a regular high school diploma. According to the National Center on Educational Outcomes, research does not support the use of out-of-level test scores from state assessments when measuring student proficiency on standards for the grade level in which a student is enrolled.

To Do

IEP teams must make careful decisions about how a student will participate in state and districtwide assessments. A student's participation at the most challenging level will ensure that every student is being provided with full access to the general curriculum, appropriate accommodations, and high expectations.

IEP teams must also make careful decisions about the accommodations a student needs in order to participate in regular assessments. State guidelines on accommodations should be reviewed and selected accommodations should result in a valid score on the test. Accommodation decisions should not be made based on a student's disability or placement or on the school's ability to administer the accommodation.

Each state is required to establish clear guidelines for IEP teams to use when deciding if a student should be assessed using an alternate assessment based on alternate achievement standards. These guidelines should provide parameters and direction to ensure that students are not assessed based on their placement, their disability category, or their racial or economic background.

An assessment should not be selected because the student has not been exposed to the material on the test, because the student's placement has restricted access to the general curriculum, or the student's teacher isn't qualified to teach the academic content being tested. A decision should not be made based on whether the assessment option will help a school's AYP calculations.

Understanding the implications of each assessment option is a critical component of making a wise decision. Some assessment options may eventually mean that the student will not be able to earn a regular diploma because of a state's requirements for awarding diplomas. While NCLB doesn't require or even encourage that the results of assessments required by NCLB should be used to make decisions regarding a student's promotion or graduation, many states have policies in effect that link a student's performance on state assessments with grade promotion or graduation with a standard diploma. Also, in many states, the same high school assessment is used to make graduation decisions and to satisfy the NCLB requirement for an assessment in reading/language arts and math once between grades 10 and 12.

School Accountability

NCLB's school accountability system is based on three components—annual measurable objectives (AMO), adequate yearly progress (AYP), and report cards. Much of what makes up AMO and AYP is set by individual states—just as the specifics of the academic content standards and academic achievement standards.

Annual measurable objectives: In order to reach NCLB's goal of all students achieving at the level of proficiency or better by the year 2013–2014, each state must set annual targets that ultimately lead to the 100% goal. These targets—called annual measurable objectives—represent the percentage of students who must perform at the proficient level each year. Some states have AMO that increase every year, some have AMO that increase every three years, and some have AMO that expect slow growth in the early years then very quick growth in the years approaching 2014.

Adequate yearly progress: This is the term used to describe the achievement of the AMO. The results of student assessments, both overall and by subgroups, plus two other components, contribute to AYP—student participation and one other measure, generally attendance rates in elementary schools and graduation rates in high schools.

Report cards: Every year, every school must issue a report card to the public that details the school's performance in each AYP element for the total school and for each subgroup of students. For schools that directly receive Title I funding, the AYP performance is also used to make determinations about offering learning alternatives to students—such as opportunities to change schools or receive supplemental instruction such as after school tutoring.

In addition to the school report cards issued to the public, parents receive a report about the individual performance of their child on the state assessments required by NCLB. These individual reports should be used by schools and teachers to plan instructional changes that will improve the student's performance. Data from the statewide assessments should be supplemented with classroom data to ensure you have a full picture of how your child is doing.

To Do

School report cards should be used to learn how the school is performing—both in terms of overall student achievement and the achievement of students with disabilities. The NCLB requirement that schools separate out the performance of several important subgroups of students— including students with disabilities—is essential to learning what lies beneath the total school performance. Too often the total school performance indicates adequate, even outstanding, performance while certain groups of students within the school population are in fact doing very poorly. NCLB's requirement to report the performance of students with disabilities is critical to improving achievement for these students.

Highly Qualified Teachers

NCLB recognizes that student performance is directly linked to effective teaching. In order to improve teacher quality, NCLB introduced requirements for every teacher of core academic subjects. These requirements are intended to elevate the quality of the nation's teaching force and that quality is expected to have a positive impact on the achievement of all students.

Following this same principle, IDEA also now sets qualification requirements for all special education teachers. Additionally, for the first time, special education teachers who teach core academic subjects to students with disabilities—without the support or collaboration of a general education teacher—must be highly qualified in both the academic subject(s) and special education. This requirement is intended to provide students with disabilities who receive instruction outside of the general education classroom the same access to teachers who are qualified in academic content as all other students. Core academic subjects include the following:

- English
- Reading/language arts
- Mathematics
- Science
- Foreign languages

- Civics/government
- Economics
- Arts
- History
- Geography

Special education is not a core academic subject.

While most students with disabilities spend much of their instructional time in general education classrooms (see Table 47.1), those who receive instruction in academic subjects from special education teachers deserve the same opportunity to receive that instruction from teachers who are qualified.

To Do

The new requirements for teacher qualifications are central to improving students' performance. While special education teachers possess a unique set of skills, such as understanding of curriculum accommodations and adaptations as well as knowledge about disabilities themselves, teaching core academic skills such as reading and math require additional training. Now, NCLB and IDEA teacher quality requirements combine to ensure that students with disabilities get quality instruction.

Parents should inquire about the qualifications of their student's teachers—both general education and special education teachers. If a student is receiving instruction in academics such as reading and

Table 47.1. Where Students with Disabilities Spend Their School Day

Location	Percent of Students
In a regular education classroom more than 80% of the day	48%
In a regular education classroom at least 40% of the day	29%
Outside a regular education classroom more than 60% of the day	23%

Source: 26th Annual Report to Congress on the Implementation of the Individuals with Disabilities Education Act 2004.

math from a special education teacher, inquire about the teacher's qualifications to teach the academic content.

Frequently Asked Questions

Why shouldn't IEP teams be able to exempt a student from taking the assessments required by NCLB?

The full participation requirement of NCLB is a key part of the school accountability system. Only by requiring that schools include all students—including those with disabilities—in the assessments will the performance and progress of all students be of equal importance to schools. As U.S. Department of Education Secretary Spellings has said, "What gets measured gets done." Too often in the past, students with disabilities were excluded from assessments and accountability systems, and the consequence was that they did not receive the academic attention and resources they deserved.

My child's school told me that my child will not receive a standard diploma unless he can pass the test required by NCLB.

NCLB is strictly about school accountability. Furthermore, the federal government does not set requirements for grade promotion or graduation. Such requirements and policies are set at the state level. While some states may use the same tests to satisfy NCLB's testing requirements and make decisions about students as required by state or local policies, parents should not confuse the requirements of NCLB with those of their individual state or local school district.

Why can't adequate yearly progress for students with disabilities be determined by the attainment of their IEP goals?

There are several reasons why IEP goals are not appropriate for school accountability purposes. In general, IEP goals are individualized for each student and may cover a range of needs beyond reading/language arts and mathematics, such as behavior and social skills. They are not necessarily aligned with state standards, and they are not designed to ensure consistent judgments about schools—a fundamental requirement for AYP determinations. The IEP is used to provide parents with information about their child's progress and for making individualized decisions about the special education and related services a student needs to succeed. Assessments used for school accountability purposes must be aligned to state content and achievement standards.

Why are some accommodations not allowed on state assessments? Shouldn't my child be given any accommodation that will help him?

Some accommodations invalidate the test by compromising the skill that is being tested. Only by truly measuring the skill can the results of the test be meaningful and valid. These scores can then be used to make school AYP determinations and improvements to the instruction of individual students. Students with invalid scores must be counted as non-participants in AYP determinations.

I hear that many schools fail to make AYP only because of students with disabilities. Isn't it unfair to expect students in special education to achieve the same level of proficiency as other students?

There is no clear evidence that schools are failing to make AYP only because of the performance of students with disabilities. The picture of AYP attainment is very cloudy in many states, due to complex state accountability formulas. Most students in special education can and should be expected to reach the same level of proficiency in reading and math as all other students—especially when provided with the appropriate level of specialized, individualized instruction, related services and accommodations. This additional support—provided to them because of their disability—is what allows them to achieve the same as other students. For the small number of special education students who may not be able to participate in the general assessments required by NCLB there are options that states have available to them. These alternates provide ample flexibility for schools and school districts. Given this flexibility, it is critical that the performance of special education students be a component of AYP achievement. Without such accountability for this and other subgroups of students, schools may not provide the necessary level of attention to the instruction of these students.

Will the requirement to include the assessment results of students with disabilities lead to schools attempting to exclude these students?

The assessment options allowed by NCLB provide adequate alternate assessments for students with disabilities who need an alternate achievement standard to demonstrate their grade-level content knowledge and skills in reading/language arts and math. In addition, the limitations placed on the alternate assessment option do not apply at the school level, only at the district and state level. So, individual schools should not have any incentives to exclude students with disabilities.

Chapter 48

Preschool Services under IDEA

We don't usually think of specific learning disabilities in connection with children below school age. When we think about children age birth to six, we think first of their learning abilities in the achievement of developmental milestones—walking, running, climbing, talking in sentences, acquiring vocabulary concepts, learning to read, and learning to play alone and with others. While the preschool years are a time of triumphs for most children and families, approximately 8% of all young children are identified as having disabilities that may prevent their reaching these important milestones as expected. It was with these children and their families in mind that Congress created the Part C Infant/Toddler Program and the Preschool Special Education Program in 1986 when it reauthorized the Individuals with Disabilities Education Act (IDEA). Some children with diagnosed conditions such as Down syndrome or cerebral palsy identified at birth or shortly thereafter receive services through the Part C Infant/Toddler Program. They may make the transition to the preschool special education program at age three. Other children do not raise concerns until after the third birthday and, if eligible, may be enrolled in what is commonly referred to as the Section 619 Preschool Program.

I'm not sure my preschool child is developing normally. What should I do?

You and/or others who know your child may have questions or concerns about his or her development. Your pediatrician, well-child clinic staff, or preschool teacher can help to answer your questions and suggest next steps. It may be that no next steps are necessary as your child is developing within the normal range. However, if there is concern, you can contact your local school system's director of special education programs for a diagnostic screening at no cost to you through the IDEA process called Child Find. This screening will help you confirm whether or not a disability or delay exists. (Local public school systems are required to conduct Child Find to locate and identify children and students from birth–21.) The superintendent of schools' office can tell you how to reach this individual. Your local school system may also have a staff member whose job is exclusively to coordinate preschool special education referrals.

No two children grow and develop at the same pace or in the same way. Some children who are not identified at birth as having a disability may have more subtle issues that can cause parents and/or professionals to suspect that there is a problem around the ages of three–five. They may have speech and language delays or disorders, put shoes or mittens on the wrong feet or hands, have difficulty remembering directions, be uninterested in playing early learning games or listening to stories, or seem generally mildly uncoordinated. If this is your child, you may be saying "Something's going on. I don't know what it is." On one hand, preschool special education may be needed to ensure that your young child will make progress in later school years. On the other hand, emphasis on failures and problems and prescriptive teaching can damage a child's self image. National Center for Learning Disabilities (NCLD) offers a parent-friendly checklist (http://www.ncld.org/images/stories/downloads/parent_center/ldchecklist.pdf) that may help you determine whether your observations and feelings may be valid. If you decide to seek preschool screening that may lead to special education services for your child at home or at school, IDEA offers two eligibility categories that may reflect what is happening with your child. You can download the "Next Steps" document at http://www.getreadytoread.org/transition_nextsteps.

What is a developmental delay? What is a specific learning disability?

Developmental delay means that a young child has a delay or disorder in sensory, physical, mental, or social/emotional development or has multiple delays in comparison to his or her peers, as documented by diagnostic testing. IDEA allows states to use this eligibility category up to age nine and to establish their own criteria such as developmental inventories and/or informed clinical opinion (IDEA Section 1402). Young children who may later be identified as learning disabled are frequently included in this category.

Specific learning disability (SLD) means that a child has a disorder in one or more of the basic psychological processes involved in understanding or in using language, spoken or written. These difficulties may manifest themselves in the imperfect ability to listen, think, speak, read, write, spell, or do mathematical calculations. The term includes such conditions as perceptual disabilities, brain injury, minimal brain dysfunction, dyslexia, and developmental aphasia. It does not include mental retardation, cultural difference, or environmental disadvantage (IDEA Section 1402 (30)). In making the decision to identify a young child as learning disabled, professionals have to rule out other factors such as speech/language delays, "late blooming," environmental factors, and emotional issues. The IDEA Amendments of 2004 did away with the absolute requirement for a severe discrepancy between age and achievement to be needed in the determination of an SLD, although severe discrepancy is still in use by some states.

The decision can now also be based on criteria established by each state based on a child's response to scientific research-based interventions (Response to Intervention, (RTI)) and on a pattern of strengths and weaknesses in performance in light of age, grade level standards, or intellectual development (IDEA 2004 Final Regulations Update, http://www.ncld.org).

In 2005–2006, 260,692 children age 3–5 were identified as having developmental delays. During the same period 12,065 children age 3–5 were identified with specific learning disabilities. (Source: http://www.ideadata.org)

What is the federal special education program for children age 3–5?

Section 619 of Part B of IDEA, defines the preschool program which guarantees a free appropriate public education (FAPE) to children with disabilities age three through five. Under this program, preschool children who have disabilities are entitled to special education and related services in the least restrictive environment (LRE). Young children, who have been identified as having any of the conditions named in Part B of IDEA including developmental delays, are eligible to receive services under Section 619 of IDEA.

In each state department of education, there is a staff member, the preschool grant coordinator, who is responsible for administering the state's Section 619 preschool grant moneys for developing, maintaining and providing information about the program in the state. The "shorthand" title for these individuals is "619 Coordinator." The National Early Childhood Technical Assistance Center provides contact information for the 619 coordinators at http://www .NECTAC.org. In addition to contacting your local director of special education or early childhood special education coordinator, you may want to speak with your state's 619 coordinator. He or she can provide you with helpful information about your rights, about local programs and services, and in some cases be present at meetings to assist with the process.

Doesn't universal public education begin at age 5–6?

Yes. However, across the country, many children are enrolled in some type of preschool program. In implementing IDEA Section 619, the states have made it possible for 500,000 children with disabilities to receive their special education preschool services either totally in a general preschool school, child care, or Head Start setting or in a combination of these settings with special education (http:// www.ideadata.org). As much as possible, preschool children with disabilities need to spend time in early childhood settings in order to learn the "give and take" of play, to hear normal spoken language, and to learn pre-reading and other cognitive learning skills presented in the regular preschool curriculum. Preschool-age children with disabilities are first and foremost children and need to be with their same age peers. Each child's team must take the individual child's needs into account when deciding on the best educational environment. Sometimes children will learn best in settings other than the general preschool classroom. NCLD's *IDEA Parent Guide* provides information about the continuum of placements that moves from the mainstream to self-contained settings.

- In the fall of 2005, 704,087 children age 3–5 were being served through Section 619 or approximately 8% of this age group in the general U.S. population. (Source: http://www.ideadata.org)

- $380 million dollars was awarded to the states and territories to help with the cost of the program in 2005–2006.

The Recognition and Response website, http://www.recognitionand
response.org, offers information and resources to help early educators
address the needs of young children (3–5 year-olds) who show signs
that they may not be learning in an expected manner, even before they
begin kindergarten.

How do the public schools provide general education classroom learning environments for young children with disabilities?

Public schools in 23 states work with Head Start, public and private childcare, and preschool providers to offer integrated learning
environments for young children, including those with disabilities. This
collaboration may be supported by written interagency agreements or
memorandums of understanding at the state and/or local levels. In
some cases, the schools look within their own programs to offer settings such as a vocational education lab preschool setting or a "reverse
mainstream" classroom. Examples of these types of programs can be
found in the District of Columbia, Kansas, Louisiana, Maine, New York,
and Pennsylvania (National Association for the Education of Young
Children, http://www.naeyc.org). In these settings, preschool special
education staff work side by side with early childhood classroom teachers to provide services for all children within the classroom setting.

Who decides if my child is eligible for preschool special education?

A team, which includes you the parent, and professionals specializing in evaluating the needs of young children, will assess and review test results, reports, and all other pertinent information. This
team must carefully consider all information about the child's development and medical history before making a decision. As you can
imagine, eligibility decisions for young children are complicated and
depend on consideration of environmental, language, and socioeconomic factors in addition to any testing results. For more information
about team membership and eligibility determination, see the *IDEA
Parents' Guide* at http://www.ld.org/ideaguide.

What happens after my child is found eligible for pre-school special education?

Once eligibility is determined, the same team, including parents, develops an individualized education plan (IEP). The IEP is a "blueprint"

413

for teaching the child and is based on the information about the child gained from the screening and diagnostic testing. It includes goals and services for the child, and is implemented by preschool classroom teachers with the help of special educators and related service professionals. In some states, home-based services are provided for young children who do not require additional preschool services.

The team that develops the IEP determines what educationally related services are needed. These may include speech therapy, occupational therapy, and physical therapy, to name a few. Preschool-specific services may include social activities with typically developing young children in the community. The IEP will include goals in all areas identified during assessment and evaluation as needing attention. Typically, these include cognitive, speech and language, gross and fine motor, and social and emotional development.

Where would my child receive preschool special education services?

Your child may already be attending preschool. Your local public school system may agree to have your child continue in that setting and pay for the portion of the time that the IEP is implemented in that setting. Or, your child may receive specialized services at home by a specialist (for example, speech language or occupational therapy). If your child needs some services that can only be implemented in a special setting, the school system must pay for the child's transportation to and from that setting. If your child is not enrolled in a preschool, childcare, or Head Start program, the school system must work with you in determining the right setting for your child. Although there is no universal pre-kindergarten program in this country, many states have public pre-kindergarten programs for specific age groups and populations.

What if I disagree with my child's education team about eligibility or any part of the IEP and services?

If test results or other information lead you or members of your child's team to disagree about your child's disability or desired learning environment, or on the way the process has been implemented, you can do several things.

- Refuse to sign the IEP.
- Request an independent educational evaluation.

- Request an informal due process hearing (maybe named a different term, for example, administrative hearing) to share your concerns with a district representative.

- File a formal due process request to present your case to an officer appointed by the state department of education.

- File a formal complaint if you think that the procedural safeguards have not been followed.

- Request that any disputes be mediated by a trained professional.

A successful mediation will result in an agreement that reflects the consensus of all parties. A formal complaint will be investigated by someone appointed by your state department of education, who will review the information and make a report of findings and recommend a solution. A due process hearing is the most formal of these steps. It is led by a hearing officer who hears the arguments of both sides, which are usually presented by attorneys. The hearing officer makes a decision based on the facts presented.

Any of the steps in dispute resolution might seem challenging to parents of young children, especially to those who speak a language other than English. For this reason, IDEA supports a network of Parent Training and Information Centers. Each state has one or more of these centers. NCLD's *IDEA Guide* (http://www.ld.org/ideaguide) provides a full explanation of the options listed as well as additional resources.

What is the Part C option? Is my preschool child eligible for enrollment in my state's Part C program?

Part C of IDEA regulates the process by which infants and toddlers (from birth to age three) receive services. The 2004 amendments to the IDEA created an option for children identified before age three and enrolled in the Part C program to continue in that program up to age six. If a child was not enrolled in the Part C program prior to December 2004, this option is not open. The purpose of the option is to allow flexibility, if wanted, for states to make Part C services available to children from age three until eligible to enter kindergarten or elementary school. This allows for a smoother transition for children who have received services from a very young age while promoting school readiness, early literacy, language, and numeracy skills in the services offered. For children who are newly identified at age three through pre-kindergarten, services must be provided under Part B

415

Section 619 of IDEA. The final regulations for Part C including this option were published in the fall of 2007.

Where can I learn more about learning disabilities and young children, the law, and my child's and my rights?

Many information resources are available to you if you are the parent of a young child who may have a learning disability.

- *IDEA Parent Guide:* NCLD offers an *IDEA Parent Guide* at http://www.ncld.org as well as a parent center and guidance on early literacy and early childhood education at http://www.getreadytoread.org.

- **The U.S. Department of Education:** The U.S. Department of Education, Office of Special Education Programs has created a website, http://www.ed.gov, that contains IDEA 2004 resources.

- **The National Early Childhood Technical Assistance Center (NECTAC):** NECTAC (http://www.nectac.org) includes information on the Section 619 Preschool Program and state contacts' mailing addresses.

- **Parent Training and Information Centers:** In every state there is at least one parent center. To locate the parent center or centers in your state you can contact the National Technical Assistance Center at its nationwide toll-free number 888-248-0822, or locate a center near you at http://www.taalliance.org. Parent centers serve families of children and young adults from birth to age 22 with all disabilities. Their purpose is to help families obtain appropriate education results for all children.

In Conclusion

The IDEA Preschool Program (Section 619) supports education services for young children with disabilities who are identified after their third birthday. It offers early learning experiences in language, reading and writing skills, play, and other social emotional areas. Preschool special education is available through your public school system.

Activities and studies being conducted in different states and by the U.S. Department of Education are starting to provide information that show that the program does help children to succeed in their later school years. You can look at evaluation activities in the different states at the Early Childhood Outcomes Center website to learn how states are working to become accountable for children's learning (http://www.fpg.unc.edu/~eco/index.cfm).

Becoming informed about the Section 619 program, whether or not you choose to pursue enrollment for your child, can help you with present and future decisions about your child's school years.

—Luzanne Pierce

About the Author: Luzanne Pierce, MAT, is a former Section 619 Coordinator for the state of New Hampshire. From 1992 to 2003 she directed the NECTAC (National Early Childhood Technical Assistance Center) sub-contract at NASDSE (National Association of State Directors of Special Education). She is the co-author of early childhood documents on autism, preschool inclusion, transitions, and other topics for NECTAC and NASDSE and a contributor to the 20th Annual Report to Congress on the IDEA implementation. The discovery of her daughter's learning disability led her to become a preschool special education teacher.

Chapter 49

IDEA Regulations for Children Enrolled in Private Schools

The reauthorized Individuals with Disabilities Education Act (IDEA) was signed into law on December 3, 2004, by President George W. Bush. The provisions of the Act became effective on July 1, 2005, with the exception of some of the elements pertaining to the definition of a "highly qualified teacher" that took effect upon the signing of the Act. The final regulations were published on August 14, 2006. This information was prepared by the Office of Special Education and Rehabilitative Services (OSERS) in the U.S. Department of Education. It addresses significant changes from preexisting regulations to the final regulatory requirements regarding children enrolled by their parents in private schools.

IDEA Regulations

1. Define parentally placed private school children with disabilities: Parentally placed private school children with disabilities means children with disabilities enrolled by their parents in private, including religious, schools or facilities that meet the definition of elementary school or secondary school, other than children with disabilities covered under 34 CFR 300.145-300.147.

2. Clarify treatment of children with disabilities, aged three through five: Children aged three through five are considered to be

Excerpted from "IDEA Regulations: Children Enrolled by Their Parents in Private Schools," U.S. Department of Education, November 2006.

parentally placed private school children with disabilities enrolled by their parents in private, including religious, elementary schools, if they are enrolled in a private school that meets the definition of elementary school in 34 CFR 300.13.

3. Explain the manner in which services are provided to children enrolled in private schools: Assigns responsibility for equitable participation to the local educational agency (LEA) where the private school is located. [Under prior law, this was the responsibility of the LEA of the parent's residence.] To the extent consistent with the number and location of children with disabilities who are enrolled by their parents in private, including religious, elementary schools and secondary schools located in the school district served by the LEA, provision is made for the participation of those children in the program assisted or carried out under Part B of the Act by providing them with special education and related services, including direct services determined in accordance with 34 CFR 300.137, unless the secretary has arranged for services to those children under the by-pass provisions in 34 CFR 300.190 through 300.198.

Child Find

4. Requires Child Find for children in private schools: Each LEA must locate, identify, and evaluate all children with disabilities who are enrolled by their parents in private, including religious, elementary schools and secondary schools located in the school district served by the LEA, in accordance with 34 CFR 300.131(b) through 300.131(e), 300.111 and 300.201.

In carrying out the requirements of this section, the LEA, or, if applicable, the state educational agency (SEA), must undertake activities similar to the activities undertaken for the agency's public school children.

The Child Find process must be completed in a time period comparable to that for students attending public schools in the LEA consistent with 34 CFR 300.301. Such Child Find process shall be completed in a time period comparable to that for other students attending public schools in the LEA.

Each LEA in which private, including religious, elementary schools and secondary schools are located must, in carrying out the Child Find requirements in this section, include parentally placed private school children who reside in a state other than the state in which the private schools that they attend are located.

The cost of carrying out Child Find, including individual evaluations, may not be considered in determining whether an LEA has met its obligations under 34 CFR 300.133 (expenditures).

5. Requires that Child Find ensure equitable participation: The Child Find process must be designed to ensure the equitable participation of parentally placed private school children; and an accurate count of those children.

6. Requires maintenance of records on number of children evaluated and number found eligible as part of Child Find and the number of children served: Each LEA must maintain in its records, and provide to the SEA, the following information related to parentally placed private school children covered under 34 CFR 300.130 through 300.144:

- the number of children evaluated;
- the number of children determined to be children with disabilities; and
- the number of children served.

7. Clarifies that no parentally placed child with a disability has an individual right to services: No parentally placed private school child with a disability has an individual right to receive some or all of the special education and related services that the child would receive if enrolled in a public school.

8. Contains requirements for services plans: In accordance with 34 CFR 300.132(a) and 300.137 through 300.139, a services plan must be developed and implemented for each private school child with a disability who has been designated by the LEA in which the private school is located to receive special education and related services under 34 CFR Part 300. The LEA must initiate and conduct meetings to develop, review, and revise a services plan for a child designated to receive services. The LEA must ensure that a representative of the religious or other private school attends each meeting. The LEA must use other methods to ensure participation by the religious or other private school, including individual or conference telephone calls, if the representative cannot attend. The services plan must describe the specific special education and related services that the LEA will provide to the child in light of the services that the LEA has determined through the consultation process that it will make available to its population of parentally placed private school children with disabilities. The services plan must, to the extent appropriate:

- meet the requirements of 34 CFR 300.320, or for a child ages three through five, meet the requirements of 34 CFR 300.323(b) with respect to the services provided; and

- be developed, reviewed, and revised consistent with 34 CFR 300.321 through 300.324.

9. Contains consultation requirements: Consultation must be timely and meaningful. To ensure that this occurs, an LEA, or, if appropriate, an SEA, must consult with private school representatives and representatives of parents of parentally placed private school children with disabilities during the design and development of special education and related services for parentally placed children regarding the following:

- The Child Find process, including: how parentally placed private school children suspected of having a disability can participate equitably; and how parents, teachers, and private school officials will be informed of the process.

- The determination of the proportionate share of federal funds available to serve parentally placed private school children with disabilities under 34 CFR 300.133(b), including the determination of how the proportionate share of those funds was calculated.

- The consultation process among the LEA, private school officials, and representatives of parents of parentally placed private school children with disabilities, including how the process will operate throughout the school year to ensure that parentally placed children with disabilities identified through the Child Find process can meaningfully participate in special education and related services.

- How, where, and by whom special education and related services will be provided for parentally placed private school children with disabilities, including a discussion of: the types of services, including direct services and alternate service delivery mechanisms; how special education and related services will be apportioned if funds are insufficient to serve all parentally placed private school children; and how and when those decisions will be made.

- If the LEA disagrees with the views of the private school officials on the provision of services or the types of services (whether provided directly or through a contract), how the LEA will provide to the private school officials a written explanation of the reasons why the LEA chose not to provide services directly or through a contract.

10. Requires annual count of number of parentally placed private school children with disabilities: Each LEA must:

- after timely and meaningful consultation with representatives of parentally placed private school children with disabilities (consistent with 34 CFR 300.134), determine the number of parentally placed private school children with disabilities attending private schools located in the LEA; and,

- ensure that the count is conducted on any date between October 1 and December 1, inclusive, of each year.

The count must be used to determine the amount that the LEA must spend on providing special education and related services to parentally placed private school children with disabilities in the next subsequent fiscal year.

Funding Requirements

11. Requires each LEA to use funds for services for parentally placed private school children with disabilities according to a formula: Each LEA must spend an amount to meet its obligations to parentally placed private school children with disabilities that is equal to a proportionate amount of federal funds made available under the Act. Each LEA must expend the following on providing special education and related services (including direct services) to parentally placed private school children with disabilities:

- For children aged 3–21, an amount that is the same proportion of the LEA's total subgrant under section 611(f) of the Act as the number of private school children with disabilities aged 3–21 who are enrolled by their parents in private, including religious, elementary schools and secondary schools located in the school district served by the LEA, is to the total number of children with disabilities in its jurisdiction aged 3–21.

- For children aged three through five, an amount that is the same proportion of the LEA's total subgrant under section 619(g) of the Act as the number of parentally placed private school children with disabilities aged three through five who are enrolled by their parents in a private, including religious, elementary school located in the school district served by the LEA, is to the total number of children with disabilities in its jurisdiction aged three through five.

12. Provides that state and local funds may supplement and not supplant proportionate amount of federal funds: State and local funds may supplement and in no case supplant the proportionate amount of federal funds required to be expended for parentally placed private school children with disabilities under Part 300.

13. Makes provision for carry-over of unexpended funds: If an LEA has not expended for equitable services all of the funds described in 34 CFR 300.133(a)(1) and (a)(2) by the end of the fiscal year for which Congress appropriated the funds, the LEA must obligate the remaining funds for special education and related services (including direct services) to parentally placed private school children with disabilities during a carry-over period of one additional year.

14. Contains requirements regarding how services to this population are provided: The provision of services pursuant to 34 CFR 300.138 and 300.139 through 300.143 must be provided by employees of a public agency or through contract by the public agency with an individual, association, agency, organization, or other entity.

Special education and related services provided to parentally placed private school children with disabilities, including materials and equipment, must be secular, neutral, and non-ideological.

15. Explains that IDEA does not prohibit on-premises services: Services to parentally placed private school children with disabilities may be provided on the premises of private, including religious, schools, to the extent consistent with law.

16. Contains requirements regarding when transportation must be provided: If necessary for the child to benefit from or participate in the services provided under Part 300, a parentally placed private school child with a disability must be provided transportation from the child's school or the child's home to a site other than the private school and from the service site to the private school, or to the child's home, depending on the timing of the services. LEAs are not required to provide transportation from the child's home to the private school.

17. Contains requirements for control of property, equipment, and supplies: A public agency must control and administer the funds used to provide special education and related services under 34 CFR 300.137 through 300.139, and hold title to and administer materials, equipment, and property purchased with those funds for the uses and purposes provided in the Act.

The public agency may place equipment and supplies in a private school for the period of time needed for the Part B program. The public agency must ensure that the equipment and supplies placed in a private school are used only for Part B purposes and can be removed from the private school without remodeling the private school facility.

The public agency must remove equipment and supplies from a private school if the equipment and supplies are no longer needed for Part B purposes or removal is necessary to avoid unauthorized use of the equipment and supplies for other than Part B purposes.

No funds under Part B of the Act may be used for repairs, minor remodeling, or construction of private school facilities.

Complaint Process Applicable to Consultation

18. Requires written affirmation and provides a right to complain: When timely and meaningful consultation as required by 34 CFR 300.134 has occurred, the LEA must obtain a written affirmation signed by the representatives of participating private schools. If such representatives do not provide such affirmation within a reasonable period of time, the LEA shall forward the documentation of the consultation process to the SEA.

A private school official has the right to submit a complaint to the SEA that the LEA did not engage in consultation that was meaningful and timely or did not give due consideration to the views of the private school official.

If the private school official wishes to submit a complaint, the official must provide to the SEA the basis of the noncompliance by the LEA with the applicable private school provisions in 34 CFR 300.132 through 300.135 and 300.137 through 300.144 and the LEA must forward the appropriate documentation to the SEA.

If the private school official is dissatisfied with the decision of the SEA, the official may submit a complaint to the secretary by providing the information on noncompliance described in 34 CFR 300.136(b)(1) of this section and the SEA must forward the appropriate documentation to the secretary.

Other Provisions

19. Defines personnel standards for parentally placed private school children with disabilities: The services provided to parentally placed private school children with disabilities must be provided by personnel meeting the same standards as personnel providing services in the public schools, except that private elementary school and secondary school teachers who are providing equitable services to parentally placed private school children with disabilities do not have to meet the highly qualified special education teacher requirements of 34 CFR 300.18.

20. Establishes criteria for due process hearing requests: The procedures in 34 CFR 300.504 through 300.519 apply to due process complaints that an LEA has failed to meet the Child Find requirements in 34 CFR 300.131, including the requirements in 34 CFR 300.300 through 300.311. Any due process complaint regarding the Child Find requirements for parentally placed private school children must be filed with the LEA in which the private school is located.

21. Establishes criteria for state complaints: Any complaint that an SEA or LEA has failed to meet the requirements in 34 CFR 300.132 through 300.135 and 300.137 through 300.144 must be filed in accordance with the procedures described in 34 CFR 300.151 through 300.153. A complaint filed by a private school official under 34 CFR 300.136(a) must be filed with the SEA in accordance with the procedures in 34 CFR 300.136(b).

22. Establishes requirements for parental consent: If a child is enrolled, or is going to enroll in a private school that is not located in the LEA of the parent's residence, parental consent must be obtained before any personally identifiable information about the child is released between officials in the LEA where the private school is located and officials in the LEA of the parent's residence.

If a parent of a child who is home schooled or placed in a private school by the parents at their own expense does not provide consent for the initial evaluation or the reevaluation, or the parent fails to respond to a request to provide consent, the public agency may not use the consent override procedures described in 34 CFR 300.300(a)(3) and (c)(1) and the public agency is not required to consider the child as eligible for services under 34 CFR 300.132 through 300.144.

Chapter 50

Alternate Assessments and Modified Academic Achievement Standards for Students with Learning Disabilities

Measuring the Achievement of Students with Disabilities

The U.S. Department of Education has released final regulations under the No Child Left Behind Act (NCLB) and the Individuals with Disabilities Education Act (IDEA) providing additional flexibility to states to more appropriately measure the achievement of certain students with disabilities. These regulations allow states to develop modified academic achievement standards that are challenging for eligible students and measure a student's mastery of grade-level content, but are less difficult than grade-level achievement standards. The new regulations are part of an ongoing effort to ensure that all students, including those with disabilities, fully participate in a state's accountability system and are assessed in an appropriate and accurate manner.

Modified achievement standards are intended for a small group of students whose disability has prevented them from achieving grade-level proficiency and who likely will not reach grade-level achievement in the same timeframe as other students. Currently, these students must take either the grade-level assessment, which

This chapter includes: "Measuring the Achievement of Students with Disabilities," U.S. Department of Education, April 2007; and, "Alternate Assessments for Students with Disabilities: Frequently Asked Questions," is reprinted with permission from the National Center on Educational Outcomes, College of Education and Development at the University of Minnesota. © 2007 Regents of the University of Minnesota.

is often too difficult, or an alternate assessment for students with the most significant cognitive disabilities, which is too easy. Neither of these options provides an accurate assessment of what these students know and can do. Alternate assessments based on modified academic achievement standards will provide a more appropriate measure of these students' achievement of grade-level content, and give teachers and parents information that can be used to better inform instruction.

For this group of students, states may develop alternate assessments based on modified academic achievement standards. States may count the proficient and advanced scores on those assessments when measuring adequate yearly progress (AYP) under NCLB, as long as the number of those scores does not exceed 2.0 percent of all students assessed.

A student's individualized education program (IEP) team, which includes the student's parents, will determine whether the student will be assessed based on modified academic achievement standards.

- States must develop guidelines for IEP teams to ensure that they are appropriately identifying students to be assessed based on modified academic achievement standards.

- The regulations include several safeguards to ensure that students are not inappropriately assessed based on modified academic achievement standards, including not choosing such an assessment solely because of a particular disability; considering the student's performance on multiple items of objective evidence over time; and evaluating annually whether it is appropriate to continue using such assessments.

IEP goals that are based on grade-level content standards must be included in the IEP of students who are assessed based on modified academic achievement standards. This will help ensure that these students receive instruction in grade-level content so that they can make progress toward meeting grade-level achievement. IEP goals that are based on grade-level content standards focus the teacher, student, and parents on grade-level content and on providing the educational supports and services that a student needs to reach those standards.

With the addition of the final regulations on modified academic achievement standards under NCLB, students with disabilities may be assessed in the following ways (unless otherwise noted, the proficient and advanced scores for all students being appropriately assessed may be counted towards AYP):

- General state assessment

- General state assessment with appropriate accommodations

- Alternate assessment based on grade-level academic achievement standards

- Alternate assessment based on modified academic achievement standards (up to two percent of all proficient and advanced scores may count towards AYP)

- Alternate assessment based on alternate academic achievement standards (up to one percent of all proficient and advanced scores may count towards AYP)

As part of a new special education partnership to help states implement the new regulations, the U.S. Department of Education (DOE) is providing funding to develop assessments—$21.1 million is available to help states develop assessments based on modified academic achievement standards. Competitive funds will be available as follows:

- $7.6 million under the Title I Enhanced Assessment Grants program that states can use to develop these new assessments.

- $13.5 million under the IDEA General Supervision Enhancement Grants program.

States also may use funds from Title I, Title VI State Assessment Grants, and the IDEA to develop these new assessments.

The special education partnership is also providing technical assistance to states including the following:

- Non-regulatory guidance has been released simultaneously with the new regulations to provide further details and information and is accessible on the department's website.

- Monthly teleconferences to provide ongoing assistance to states that wish to implement this regulation. Title I staff will also be available to provide ongoing technical assistance and additional guidance.

The DOE also recognizes the need to provide this information to parents of students with disabilities. The Office of Special Education Programs (OSEP) is undertaking outreach efforts with parent groups to ensure that information about this new flexibility is communicated to parents.

Frequently Asked Questions about Alternate Assessments for Students with Disabilities

Why provide alternate assessments?

To ensure educational accountability: Alternate assessments are necessary in order to achieve educational accountability for all students. Students who are excluded from the state assessment and reporting of results are not considered when decisions are made about how to improve programs, and they may be denied educational opportunities available to other students.

Requirements of federal legislation: The Individuals with Disabilities Education Act of 1997 (IDEA) first identified alternate assessments as an option for some students. The No Child Left Behind Act of 2001 (NCLB) specifies that each state, district, and school must be held accountable for the achievement of all students. Alternate assessments are intended to provide the missing piece that makes it possible to include all students with disabilities in state and district assessments.

Who should participate in alternate assessments?

In general, alternate assessment participants are those students with disabilities who are unable to participate in regular assessments even with accommodations. Some of these students may have significant cognitive disabilities and can be assessed using alternate formats aligned to the grade-level content, but based on alternate achievement standards that define proficiency differently from the general assessment. Other students may require alternate assessments aligned to grade-level content that is based on grade-level achievement standards, or the same definition of proficiency as the general assessment.

New regulations in April 2007 added an additional option. According to the DOE: "Modified achievement standards are intended for a small group of students whose disability has prevented them from achieving grade-level proficiency and who likely will not reach grade-level achievement in the same timeframe as other students. Currently, these students must take either the grade-level assessment, which is often too difficult, or an alternate assessment for students with the most significant cognitive disabilities, which is too easy. Neither of these options provides an accurate assessment of what these students know and can do. Alternate assessments based on modified academic achievement standards will provide a more appropriate measure of these students' achievement of grade-level content, and give teachers and parents information that can be used to better inform instruction."

What are some sample guidelines?

Guidelines might include, for example: A student with a significant cognitive disability

- who requires substantial modifications, adaptations, or supports to meaningfully access the grade-level content;

- who requires intensive individualized instruction in order to acquire and generalize knowledge; and,

- who is unable to demonstrate achievement of academic content standards on a paper and pencil test, even with accommodations.

Who should participate in alternate assessments on grade-level achievement standards?

Guidelines might include, for example: A student with a disability

- who requires accommodations that are not available on the general assessment to demonstrate skill and knowledge on the grade-level content and grade-level achievement standards; and,

- who demonstrates achievement in different formats or contexts than are provided by the general assessment.

What should be included in an alternate assessment?

All assessments for NCLB accountability purposes should measure student achievement on the grade-level content. How these assessments reflect the depth and breadth of the grade-level content depends on whether the alternate assessment is based on grade-level achievement standards or alternate achievement standards. For alternate assessments based on grade-level achievement standards, the depth and breadth of assessed content should be the same as on the general assessment in order to draw accurate inferences of student proficiency.

Alternate assessments based on alternate achievement standards must also assess student achievement on the grade-level content. In states with checklists and performance tasks, stakeholders typically have prioritized content to be covered for students with significant cognitive disabilities. States that use portfolio or body of evidence approaches may permit IEP teams to select a limited number of grade-level content standards and benchmarks to assess; or the state may require specific content standards or benchmarks for each tested grade. In portfolio or body-of-evidence states that require specific content coverage, stakeholders have generally prioritized specific content for that purpose.

Many states that had earlier identified one set of prioritized content standards across all grade levels for their alternate assessment students now require grade-level content alignment. This reflects NCLB regulations and guidance requirements that all assessments must be aligned to the grade-level definitions of content for the enrolled grade of the student being assessed.

What do alternate assessments look like?

States use a variety of approaches in the design of alternate assessments. Definitions of the most common types of alternate assessment approaches follow.

Definitions (based on Roeber, 2002; available at http://education .umn.edu/NCEO/OnlinePubs/Synthesis42.html)

- **Portfolio:** Student portfolios are a purposeful and systematic collection of student work that is evaluated and measured against predetermined scoring criteria.

- **Performance assessment:** These assessments are direct measures of a skill, usually in a one-on-one assessment. These can range from highly structured one-on-one assessments similar to traditional pencil and paper test, to a more flexible approach that can be adjusted based on student needs.

- **Checklist:** This method relies on teachers to remember whether students are able to carry out certain activities. Scores reported are usually based on the number of skills that the student was able to successfully perform.

How should alternate assessments be incorporated into the accountability system?

States typically report the assessment results from their assessment programs by achievement levels, also known as proficiency or performance levels. Terms such as novice, basic, proficient, meeting the standard, advanced, or exceeding the standard may be used to describe the achievement level of each student. Achievement standards include labels for the various achievement levels, descriptions of competencies associated with each achievement level, and assessment scores (cut scores) that differentiate among the achievement levels. Achievement standards must be defined using a rigorous process and must be aligned with academic content standards.

The December 9, 2003 NCLB Regulations permit states to develop alternate assessments based on grade-level achievement standards, and alternate assessments for students with the most significant cognitive disabilities based on alternate achievement standards. The process of setting achievement standards (describing various levels of proficiency and identifying cut-scores) is required for both options. Achievement standards for alternate assessments based on grade-level achievement standards must be equivalent to those on the general assessment. Setting alternate achievement standards based on grade-level content standards is a challenging but rewarding process, and requires the active participation of test company partners, measurement experts, curriculum and special education state leadership, as well as educators, parents, and higher education standard-setting panelists.

According to the December 9, 2003 NCLB Regulations, once achievement standards have been set, all scores determined to be proficient are included as proficient in accountability indices whether they are on alternate achievement standards or on grade-level achievement standards, provided that the number of proficient and advanced scores based on the alternate achievement standards does not exceed 1.0 percent of all students in the grades tested at the state or LEA level, unless a special exception has been granted.

435

Chapter 51

Summary of Performance Fosters Postsecondary Supports for Students with Learning Disabilities

Summary of Performance Facts

The summary of performance (SOP) is a new requirement in evaluation procedures as contained in IDEA 2004. (§300.305.(3)(e). The language is as follows: "For a child whose eligibility under special education terminates due to graduation with a regular diploma or due to exceeding the age of eligibility, the local education agency shall provide the child with a summary of the child's academic achievement and functional performance, which shall include recommendations on how to assist the child in meeting the child's postsecondary goals."

What Is a Summary of Performance?

The word summary provides a clue to what the intent of the law may be. While the SOP is very closely tied to the information contained in the individualized education program (IEP), it should be a separate document which condenses and organizes the key information that should follow the student. It is a summary of existing data and of performance in academic and functional areas. The SOP must also include recommendations on how to assist the student in meeting the

This chapter includes: "Summary of Performance Fact Sheet," © North Dakota Department of Public Instruction. Reprinted with permission. And, "Summary of Performance Completion Guidelines," reprinted with permission from the Colorado Department of Education Exceptional Student Leadership Unit (http://www.cde.state.co.us/cdesped).

student's measurable postsecondary goals. This SOP is in lieu of an exit evaluation.

Goal of the SOP: To foster access to postsecondary supports for students with disabilities.

SOP is most useful when linked with the IEP process: The student should have the opportunity to actively participate in the development of this document. The individual that develops the SOP should typically be the IEP case manager for the student. The final draft of the SOP should be presented to the IEP team for its review, revision, and formal approval.

An SOP that includes a review: A student's previous disability documentation and current data on the functional impact of the student's disability will significantly assist the student in gaining access to, and participating in, further education and employment.

An SOP may need additional information: Data to document the disability and describe current limitations and accommodations needed in secondary school is needed, and if not provided, the SOP will need to be supplemented by additional information.

The summary document is required upon the student's graduation with a regular diploma or upon aging out from special education services: As a best practice, however, educators should choose to prepare an SOP earlier for students who are transferring to another school, meeting with the disability coordinator at a college, applying for vocational rehabilitative services, or similar transitions. The intent of the SOP is to provide crucial information to those people who may assist the student in the future, therefore providing that information when it is most timely makes sense. If an early SOP is prepared for a student, it is recommended that an electronic copy be saved. Therefore, if the student's contact information changes, or if there are substantial performance changes prior to graduation or ageing out, the appropriate section(s) of the electronic copy can be updated fairly easily.

The IDEA 2004 also mandates: State education agencies are to collect data on the number of students who were on an IEP in secondary school, that have been employed or attended postsecondary education or training within one year after exiting the secondary school system. Students with disabilities will be contacted one year after graduation, aging out, or dropping out of school. Since the summary of performance will be one of the last things done with students before they leave special education, it is an opportune time to inform the student and parents about any upcoming follow-up interviews and at the same time obtain current contact information for the parent(s) and student.

Summary of Performance Completion Guidelines

The Law

One new transition requirement contained in Individuals with Disabilities Education Improvement Act of 2004 (IDEIA 2004) impacts special education students who are finishing their high school or secondary education. Specifically, §300.304 of IDEIA 2004 requires the following evaluation procedures:

(B)   In case of a reevaluation of a child, whether the child continues to have such a disability, and the educational needs of the child.

(e)   Evaluations before change in placement.
   (1)   Except as provided in paragraph (e)(2) of this section, a public agency must evaluate a child with a disability in accordance with §§300.304 through 300.311 before determining that the child is no longer a child with a disability.
   (2)   The evaluation described in paragraph (e) (1) of this section is not required before the termination of a child's eligibility under this part due to graduation from secondary school with a regular diploma, or due to exceeding the age eligibility for FAPE under state law.
   (3)   For a child whose eligibility terminates under circumstances described in paragraph (e)(2) of this section, a public agency must provide the child with *a summary of the child's academic achievement and functional performance, which shall include recommendations on how to assist the child in meeting the child's post high school goals.*

Analysis

The word summary provides a clue to the intent of the new requirement. Special education professionals accumulate a wealth of information regarding their students, including: life goals, preferences and interests, functional and academic strengths and needs, needed accommodations, strategies for success, and so forth. In the past, much of this information simply ended up in a dead file, and even when file documents were copied for future service providers, they were not always in a useful and up-to-date format for the next provider. IDEIA 2004 requires that in lieu of an exit evaluation, a summary of performance be prepared during the student's exit year. A well-written summary of performance may make the reader feel like they know the student.

The summary of performance (SOP) is discussed as part of evaluation procedures. While the SOP is very closely tied to information contained in the IEP, it should be a separate document, which condenses and organizes the key information that should follow the student.

For the first time, IDEIA 2004 also mandates that follow-up contacts be made with special education students one year after graduation, age-out, or dropping out of school. Since the summary of performance is one of the last things done with students before they leave special education, it should contain the up-to-date post high school goals that will be addressed (measured) during the follow-up contacts.

A summary of performance should contain the following information.

1. Student Information

This section contains student contact and demographic information that may be helpful to future service providers. A school contact person is also listed. Complete and up-to-date information is crucial to the follow-up process. When completing the forms, be sure to address every line, print clearly or type and ensure data is current and correct. When indicating primary and secondary disability, please use the following terminology exactly and include the appropriate numerical code with the disability.

- significant limited intellectual capacity
- physical disability
- emotional disability
- speech Language
- perceptual/communication
- deaf-blind
- hearing disability
- multiple disabilities
- visual disability

- preschooler with a disability
- infant with a disability
- autism
- traumatic brain injury

2. *Measurable Post High School Goals*

IDEIA 2004 requires that special education students aged 16 and above have measurable post high school goals (based upon age appropriate transition assessments) related to:

- training,
- education,
- employment, and
- independent living skills (where appropriate).

Under IDEIA 2004, measurable post high school goals are required in three and possibly four areas. These goals are the vision statements for the student. To encourage the consideration of further education for students with disabilities, Congress has mandated that long-term goals in the areas of post high school training and education be part of the transition planning process. Measurable post high school goals for independent living are now included where appropriate. Again, the measurable post high school goals are to be based on age-appropriate transition assessment.

To help make the post high school goals measurable, consider incorporating descriptors like the following—identified in the *Enderle-Severson Transition Rating Scales–Appendix A, 3rd Edition*—when writing the student's goals:

- Employment—paid (competitive, supported, sheltered), unpaid, non-employment

- Education—four-year college or university, technical school, two-year college, military

- Training—specific vocational or career field, independent living skill training, vocational training program, apprenticeship, military, Job Corps

- Independent living skills—adult living, daily living, independent living, financial, transportation

3. Summary of Performance

Student's strengths and needs should be written in an objective manner. Assessment language (average, below average, above average) rather than value words (good, nice, significant, brilliant, slow) should be used to establish these areas. It is of utmost importance that the actual levels of performance be documented clearly and without an overly positive bias. Eligibility for most adult agency services is dependent upon a need, a deficit, and a disability. This need is the key to attaining the essential services necessary for success in post-secondary settings. Over complimentary language can falsely hinder a student's ability to gain access to certain essential services. It is important then that present levels of performance are honest, objective, clear, and concise.

IDEIA 2004 separates the old "present levels of performance" concept into:

- **Academic achievement and cognitive performance:** This should include reading, math, writing, and other related academic skills as well as general ability, problem solving skills, attention, and organization. What are the student's present levels? Include: strengths, needs, necessary accommodations, modifications, assistive technology, and so forth. Remember that the purpose of the document is to help that next service provider to better understand how to help the student. What do you think is the most relevant information to convey?

- **Functional performance:** This could include present levels for social, interpersonal, and behavior skills; independent living skills; self care and personal hygiene; environmental access; motor and mobility skills; self-determination, advocacy, direction, and communication abilities; career, vocational, work tolerance, and work skills.

4. Recommendations to Assist the Student in Achieving Measurable Post High School Goals

This section is unique to the SOP in that it provides specific recommendations to the student, the family, and post high school agencies who may utilize the SOP for information regarding specific and meaningful steps the student, family, and provider might or should do as the student exits public education. This may include specific

442

activities, agency linkages, recommended supports for the student, and contact information for further connection with post high school agencies and service providers, and should include what steps or activities still need to take place after the student leaves school to help the student to achieve the measurable post high school goals.

5. Student Input

Asking the student about what supports and services have helped him or her to be successful in high school, and about what services or supports will be needed in the future, can be very enlightening.

Chapter 52

Rights and Responsibilities of Students with Disabilities Preparing for Postsecondary Education

More and more high school students with disabilities are planning to continue their education in postsecondary schools, including vocational and career schools, two- and four- year colleges, and universities. As a student with a disability, you need to be well informed about your rights and responsibilities as well as the responsibilities postsecondary schools have toward you. Being well informed will help ensure you have a full opportunity to enjoy the benefits of the postsecondary education experience without confusion or delay.

The information in this chapter provided by the Office for Civil Rights (OCR) in the U. S. Department of Education, explains the rights and responsibilities of students with disabilities who are preparing to attend postsecondary schools. This chapter also explains the obligations of a postsecondary school to provide academic adjustments, including auxiliary aids and services, to ensure the school does not discriminate on the basis of disability.

OCR enforces Section 504 of the Rehabilitation Act of 1973 (Section 504) and Title II of the Americans with Disabilities Act of 1990 (Title II), which prohibit discrimination on the basis of disability. Practically every school district and postsecondary school in the United States is subject to one or both of these laws, which have similar requirements. Although both school districts and postsecondary schools must comply with these same laws, the responsibilities of postsecondary schools are

---

"Students with Disabilities Preparing for Postsecondary Education: Know Your Rights and Responsibilities," U.S. Department of Education, March 2007.

significantly different from those of school districts. Moreover, you will have responsibilities as a postsecondary student that you do not have as a high school student. OCR strongly encourages you to know your responsibilities and those of postsecondary schools under Section 504 and Title II. Doing so will improve your opportunity to succeed as you enter postsecondary education.

As a student with a disability leaving high school and entering postsecondary education, will I see differences in my rights and how they are addressed?

Yes. Section 504 and Title II protect elementary, secondary, and postsecondary students from discrimination. Nevertheless, several of the requirements that apply through high school are different from the requirements that apply beyond high school. For instance, Section 504 requires a school district to provide a free appropriate public education (FAPE) to each child with a disability in the district's jurisdiction. Whatever the disability, a school district must identify an individual's education needs and provide any regular or special education and related aids and services necessary to meet those needs as well as it is meeting the needs of students without disabilities.

Unlike your high school, your postsecondary school is not required to provide FAPE. Rather, your postsecondary school is required to provide appropriate academic adjustments as necessary to ensure that it does not discriminate on the basis of disability. In addition, if a postsecondary school provides housing to non-disabled students, it must provide comparable, convenient, and accessible housing to students with disabilities at the same cost.

May a postsecondary school deny my admission because I have a disability?

No. If you meet the essential requirements for admission, a postsecondary school may not deny your admission simply because you have a disability.

Do I have to inform a postsecondary school that I have a disability?

No. However, if you want the school to provide an academic adjustment, you must identify yourself as having a disability. Likewise, you should let the school know about your disability if you want to ensure that you are assigned to accessible facilities. In any event, your disclosure of a disability is always voluntary.

What academic adjustments must a postsecondary school provide?

The appropriate academic adjustment must be determined based on your disability and individual needs. Academic adjustments may include auxiliary aids and modifications to academic requirements as are necessary to ensure equal educational opportunity. Examples of such adjustments are: arranging for priority registration; reducing a course load; substituting one course for another; and providing note takers, recording devices, sign language interpreters, extended time for testing, and if telephones are provided in dorm rooms, a teletypewriter (TTY) in your dorm room, and equipping school computers with screen-reading and voice recognition or other adaptive software or hardware.

In providing an academic adjustment, your postsecondary school is not required to lower or effect substantial modifications to essential requirements. For example, although your school may be required to provide extended testing time, it is not required to change the substantive content of the test. In addition, your postsecondary school does not have to make modifications that would fundamentally alter the nature of a service, program, or activity, or that would result in undue financial or administrative burdens. Finally, your postsecondary school does not have to provide personal attendants, individually prescribed devices, readers for personal use or study, or other devices or services of a personal nature, such as tutoring and typing.

If I want an academic adjustment, what must I do?

You must inform the school that you have a disability and need an academic adjustment. Unlike your school district, your postsecondary school is not required to identify you as having a disability or to assess your needs.

Your postsecondary school may require you to follow reasonable procedures to request an academic adjustment. You are responsible for knowing and following these procedures. Postsecondary schools usually include, in their publications providing general information, information on the procedures and contacts for requesting an academic adjustment. Such publications include recruitment materials, catalogs, and student handbooks, and are often available on school websites. Many schools also have staff whose purpose is to assist students with disabilities. If you are unable to locate the procedures, ask a school official, such as an admissions officer or counselor.

When should I request an academic adjustment?

Although you may request an academic adjustment from your postsecondary school at any time, you should request it as early as possible. Some academic adjustments may take more time to provide than others. You should follow your school's procedures to ensure that your school has enough time to review your request and provide an appropriate academic adjustment.

Do I have to prove that I have a disability to obtain an academic adjustment?

Generally, yes. Your school will probably require you to provide documentation that shows you have a current disability and need an academic adjustment.

What documentation should I provide?

Schools may set reasonable standards for documentation. Some schools require more documentation than others. They may require you to provide documentation prepared by an appropriate professional, such as a medical doctor, psychologist, or other qualified diagnostician. The required documentation may include one or more of the following: a diagnosis of your current disability, the date of the diagnosis, how the diagnosis was reached, the credentials of the professional, how your disability affects a major life activity, and how the disability affects your academic performance. The documentation should provide enough information for you and your school to decide what is an appropriate academic adjustment.

Although an individualized education program (IEP) or Section 504 plan, if you have one, may help identify services that have been effective for you, it generally is not sufficient documentation. This is because postsecondary education presents different demands than high school education, and what you need to meet these new demands may be different. Also, in some cases, the nature of a disability may change.

If the documentation that you have does not meet the postsecondary school's requirements, a school official should tell you in a timely manner what additional documentation you need to provide. You may need a new evaluation in order to provide the required documentation.

Who has to pay for a new evaluation?

Neither your high school nor your postsecondary school is required to conduct or pay for a new evaluation to document your disability and need for an academic adjustment. This may mean that you have to pay or find funding to pay an appropriate professional for an evaluation. If you are eligible for services through your state vocational rehabilitation agency, you may qualify for an evaluation at no cost to you. You may locate your state vocational rehabilitation agency through the Job Accommodation Network's website at http://www.jan.wvu.edu/cgi-win/TypeQuery.exe?902.

Once the school has received the necessary documentation from me, what should I expect?

The school will review your request in light of the essential requirements for the relevant program to help determine an appropriate academic adjustment. It is important to remember that the school is not required to lower or waive essential requirements. If you have requested a specific academic adjustment, the school may offer that academic adjustment or an alternative one if the alternative would also be effective. The school may also conduct its own evaluation of your disability and needs at its own expense.

You should expect your school to work with you in an interactive process to identify an appropriate academic adjustment. Unlike the experience you may have had in high school, however, do not expect your postsecondary school to invite your parents to participate in the process or to develop an IEP for you.

What if the academic adjustment we identified is not working?

Let the school know as soon as you become aware that the results are not what you expected. It may be too late to correct the problem if you wait until the course or activity is completed. You and your school should work together to resolve the problem.

May a postsecondary school charge me for providing an academic adjustment?

No. Furthermore, it may not charge students with disabilities more for participating in its programs or activities than it charges students who do not have disabilities.

What can I do if I believe the school is discriminating against me?

Practically every postsecondary school must have a person—frequently called the Section 504 coordinator, Americans with Disabilities (ADA) coordinator, or disability services coordinator—who coordinates the school's compliance with Section 504 or Title II or both laws. You may contact this person for information about how to address your concerns.

The school must also have grievance procedures. These procedures are not the same as the due process procedures with which you may be familiar from high school. However, the postsecondary school's grievance procedures must include steps to ensure that you may raise your concerns fully and fairly and must provide for the prompt and equitable resolution of complaints.

School publications, such as student handbooks and catalogs, usually describe the steps you must take to start the grievance process. Often, schools have both formal and informal processes. If you decide to use a grievance process, you should be prepared to present all the reasons that support your request.

If you are dissatisfied with the outcome from using the school's grievance procedures or you wish to pursue an alternative to using the grievance procedures, you may file a complaint against the school with the Office for Civil Rights (OCR) or in a court.

Students with disabilities who know their rights and responsibilities are much better equipped to succeed in postsecondary school. We encourage you to work with the staff at your school because they, too, want you to succeed. Seek the support of family, friends, and fellow students, including those with disabilities. Know your talents and capitalize on them, and believe in yourself as you embrace new challenges in your education.

For More Information

U.S. Department of Education
Office for Civil Rights
400 Maryland Ave. S.W.
Washington, DC 20202-1100
Toll-Free: 800-421-3481
Toll-Free TDD: 877-521-2172
Fax: 202-245-6840
Website: http://www.ed.gov/ocr
E-mail: ocr@ed.gov

Chapter 53

American Disabilities Act and Individuals with Learning Disabilities

Civil Rights for You

Almost three decades after the passage of the Civil Rights Act of 1964, a federal law was passed giving people with disabilities the same rights as minorities and women. This law, the Americans with Disabilities Act (ADA) of 1990, gives people with disabilities the right to compete fairly for jobs. ADA also gives people with disabilities the right to shop where they please, stay in whatever hotel they choose, and patronize any establishment open to the public; the right to use public transportation; and many other rights. Because finding and keeping a job is the topic of this chapter, this section will focus on the employment provisions of the law (Title 1).

Before the ADA became law, it was legal for most employers to look a person with a disability in the eye and say, "You have dyslexia. I will not hire you." Today, employers (with 15 or more employees) cannot do that.

The goal of the law is simple. It is to eliminate discrimination against people with disabilities. But figuring out what it all means is complicated. The interpretation of the law changes when cases are decided in court. New regulations come out, clarifying the intent of

"The Americans with Disabilities Act," reprinted with permission from Learning a Living: Guide to Planing Your Career and Finding a Job for People with Learning Disabilities, Attention Deficit Disorder, and Dyslexia, by Dale S. Brown, (Woodbine House, 2000), pp. 227–238. Available at LD OnLine at http://www.ldonline.org/article/5999. © 2000 Dale S. Brown. Contact information was verified in August 2008.

the law. That means that the law may have changed by the time you read this chapter. In addition, the law has many exceptions, and listing them all would be boring and confusing, as many of them probably do not apply to you. This author's goal is therefore to explain the truth about the law as it applies to most readers of this book.

If you decide to use the Americans with Disabilities Act to obtain your rights, research the latest changes in the law using your public library and the organizations at the end of the chapter. Study the latest court cases. In addition, it may be helpful to consult an attorney.

Most likely, you will not be involved in a lawsuit or complaint. Learning about your rights, however, can give you confidence and bargaining power. That is the purpose of this chapter.

Who Is Covered?

In an adversarial situation, proving that you are covered by the Americans with Disabilities Act is the first, and sometimes hardest, step to obtaining your rights. Because of the widespread belief that learning disabilities, attention deficit disorder, and dyslexia are not severe, it is possible that an employer will try to claim that you do not have a disability. In addition, if you are able to mitigate the effects of your disability—such as by medication or even by accommodating yourself—you may not be covered. This section explains the standards that determine whether you are considered to have a disability under ADA.

You are covered by the ADA if you are discriminated against for a reason related to disability. Under this provision, you are protected from discrimination if:

- You are perceived as having a disability. Maybe your employer thinks you have a disability, but you don't. Or, you have special education records that say you have a disability. But you don't think your old diagnosis has any bearing on the jobs you are investigating. A prospective employer, however, just found out about that history and now says she won't hire you. This is legally questionable under the ADA.

- You are related to, or associated with, a person who has a disability. Suppose someone won't hire you because they think it's too time-consuming for you to take care of your child with a disability. That is illegal under the law.

- You have a bona fide disability, as discussed in the next paragraph.

Your learning disability, attention deficit disorder, dyslexia, or other condition substantially limits a major life activity. Let's look at what this means. Major life activities include caring for yourself, performing manual tasks, walking, seeing, hearing, speaking, breathing, learning, working, thinking, concentrating, and interacting with other people.

Speaking, working, thinking, concentrating, and interacting with other people are the major life activities that are usually affected for people with learning disabilities, attention deficit disorder, and dyslexia.

In order to be considered "substantially limited" in working, you must be unable to perform many jobs, not just one position. So, if your disability affects your ability to drive, read, write, take phone messages, or work in an "open space environment" it will probably affect your ability to do more than one job. On the other hand, if your disability makes it impossible to use a software system that only your employer uses, it could be argued that you are only limited in doing that particular job.

Myths about The Americans with Disabilities Act

The Americans with Disabilities Act does not do the following:

- Give you the right to a job because you have a disability. You must be qualified and compete. And you may be rejected from jobs just like anyone else.

- Give you extra points in getting a job. The ADA is not an affirmative action statute. That is, it is not intended to make up for past discrimination by requiring the employers hire a certain number of people with disabilities or giving them incentives to do so.

- Fund training, scholarships, or reasonable accommodations. The United States government receives funds to enforce the law and to provide information to organizations so they can comply. However, employers have to pay for accommodations themselves. If they cannot pay, then you become responsible.

- Allow any special privileges on the job. Although sometimes reasonable accommodation might look like special privileges to other people, you have the same responsibilities and challenges as your fellow employees.

The term "substantially limited" protects employers against people whose minor limitations could be misused as a disability. For example, if you take a long time to learn to spell complicated medical terms, it would not constitute a disability. Many people without dyslexia have that problem. Or, you would not be able to claim you had an auditory perceptual problem because you had trouble taking notes regarding unfamiliar technical information. To be protected under ADA, you also must be qualified for the job.

You Are Qualified for the Job

The Americans with Disabilities Act only covers people who can do the job. So, a blind person who wanted to drive a bus would not be protected. The fact is that very few people apply for positions which their disabilities prevent them from doing. On the other hand, the law is balanced to assure that employers are not forced to hire people who are not qualified.

You must meet any job-related requirements. If you don't have a medical doctor license, you can't become a doctor. If a job requires three years experience working in a stockroom, you must have three years experience working in a stockroom.

Even though attention deficit disorders, dyslexia, and learning disabilities give people tremendous difficulties in earning degrees, passing standardized tests, and gaining credentials, it is legal for the employer to demand them. The employer must, however, demand the same degrees, test scores, and credentials of every applicant. That is why education is so important and why using informal ways of looking for jobs is often a good move for people with learning disabilities. Unless we have a hand in determining the qualifications for the job, we often can be legally removed from consideration.

In ADA lingo, you are qualified if you are "able to perform the essential functions of the job with or without reasonable accommodation."

You Can Do the Essential Functions of the Job

"Essential functions" refers to those activities that are intrinsic to the job. What must a person do to perform the core responsibilities of a job? For example, landing and taking off a plane are essential functions of a pilot's job.

Essential functions are determined individually for each job. For example, reading would be an essential function for an abstractor, where the job is to read and summarize articles. But it might not be an essential function for a retail clerk, even if that clerk must read instructions occasionally. Many employers have written job descriptions that state the essential functions.

Essential functions that sometimes are challenging for people with attention deficit disorder, dyslexia, and learning disabilities are:

- reading;
- writing;
- mathematical calculations;
- attending work regularly each day;
- coming in at a specific time;
- driving a vehicle;
- getting along with your boss, team leader, supervisor, or team.

The exact definition from the law reads: "The term 'qualified individual with a disability' means an individual with a disability, who, with or without reasonable accommodation, can perform the essential functions of the employment position..." (Title 1, Section 101, (8)).

So, you are still considered qualified if reasonable accommodation is required to meet these functions. As it applies to employers, making "reasonable accommodation" usually means removing obstacles from the job, the workplace, or the terms and condition of employment that would otherwise prevent an otherwise qualified person with a disability from doing the job. For example, computers and calculators are accommodations that can help many people who have learning disabilities or dyslexia with routine arithmetic and proofreading functions. And the use of flextime and telecommuting can be accommodations for people who have trouble coming in at a specific time to a specific place. (They can also be options open to all employees.)

A Fair Competition for Each Job

The Americans with Disabilities Act sets the rules to create a level playing field for job applicants and employers. This section explains the most important of those rules.

Protections When You Apply for the Job

Employers may not discriminate by using a test or application process that is particularly challenging for people with disabilities. The exception is if they are testing your ability to do an "essential job function." For example, the employer could include a speed-reading test if most of the time is spent reading quickly and you cannot perform the job unless you can quickly understand written materials.

Pre-employment examinations (tests given when you apply) must measure the skill that is being tested, not your disability. The test must evaluate your ability to do the tasks required by the job. It must "relate to business necessity." So, a math test could be given to applicants for a stockroom job, if you would be measuring, counting, and calculating at work. For an editorial assistant position, a proofreading test would be acceptable. This test probably would not be legal for a position as a server in a restaurant.

The employer must provide reasonable accommodation in pre-employment examinations. So, if you have difficulty reading, the employer must allow you to be evaluated in another way, perhaps by having someone read it to you. People with attention deficit disorder may ask to take tests in a private room. Extended time is another frequent accommodation. In fact, most of classroom accommodations can be considered for pre-employment tests. Employers may, however, ask for proof of your disability, before determining whether they should make the accommodation.

What happens if you start the test hoping that your learning disability will not affect your ability to complete it? Then you find out that it does? You should stop taking the test, talk to the proctor, and arrange to take the test with reasonable accommodation at a different time. Unfortunately, pre-employment testing has become a legal way of forcing disclosure of invisible disabilities.

Employers may test applicants for illegal drugs. Some legal drugs used for attention deficit disorder, such as Ritalin and Dexedrine can be picked up by drug tests, although it does not usually happen. Talk to your doctor. Consider disclosing that you have a prescription for these drugs prior to the drug test.

Protections during the Interview

Employers may not ask whether you have a disability or ask questions about your disability during an interview, unless you bring it up yourself. Then they can ask follow-up questions.

But employers may ask if you can do the activities that the job requires. They can even require you to show how you would do it. Here are some questions that they can legally ask you:

- "We need people who are reliable. Is there any reason why you might unexpectedly be absent from work?"

- "This job is stressful for many people, and we need people who are good at handling it. You will work for three people. They will not always coordinate their work (though we try to get them to talk to each other). They may be quite intense about your meeting their personal deadlines. How will you handle this?"

- "There are constant interruptions in this job. Can you start a task, be interrupted, and then go back to the work?"

- "Here is an example of the type of document you will be responsible for reading and evaluating. You'll be required to handle six of these a day. Does that sound reasonable? Have you done this type of intense reading in the past?"

- "Since we make phone calls for various corporations and the people we call ask questions, you will have to learn specific facts at the beginning of each week. Frankly, some of them are pretty dull. Then you'll have to use them accurately to respond to our customers. Can you give me some examples of your good memory?"

Employers may give you a medical examination after they make a job offer, providing that all applicants for the job must take the examination. The employer can withdraw the offer if the examination shows that even if you are accommodated, you cannot do any one of the essential functions. For example, if the tests showed that you were too farsighted to use a tape measure and you wanted to work in a fabric shop where measuring and cutting fabric was an essential part of the job, the employer could withdraw the offer.

In addition, the employer does not have to hire you if you are a "direct threat" to yourself or others. They must prove this and cannot rely on speculation or prejudice. So, they cannot say, "You have ADD, and I hear that people with ADD are impulsive. We can't have that on this job." On the other hand, it would be helpful for you to be prepared with an explanation of how you handle pressure if you disclose your attention deficit disorder.

Protections after You Are Offered the Job

After a job offer is made and before you begin work may be a good time to disclose your disability and start bargaining for reasonable accommodation. At this point, you may also be negotiating other aspects of the job, such as salary and hours. If the employer then withdraws the job offer, it gives a strong appearance of discrimination—particularly if you have a written job offer. You have not yet begun to work or shown whether you can do the job, with or without accommodation.

Still, employers can discriminate at this stage in ways that are hard to prove in court. Examples include the following:

- Sudden budget cuts are claimed. The job is re-announced months later under another title.

- The employer suddenly offers an unreasonably low salary—and will not budge.

- The employer insists that the accommodation is an undue hardship.

- For some reason, the written job offer never arrives—the start date is mysteriously delayed and delayed.

Deciding what to do in these instances is complicated. On the one hand, if you think you can prove discrimination, it might be worthwhile to contact a lawyer. On the other hand, you may want to keep looking, on the grounds that you don't want to work for a company where you would feel unwelcome. In addition, suing a company takes away time that could be spent finding work.

Protections on the Job

Once you are hired, employers may not discriminate against you on the job. They may not:

- put all people with disabilities in the same job category;

- discriminate against you if you are being considered for a promotion;

- fire you because of your disability;

- refuse to give you training if it is offered to people with similar jobs.

Reasonable Accommodation

Employers must make reasonable accommodation to the "known" disability of the applicant or employee. But, to be covered, you must make your disability known. You must tell them. Many people with learning disabilities, attention deficit disorder, and dyslexia find this difficult. Once the disability is disclosed, discrimination may begin. On the other hand, you can't get accommodation if you don't disclose. (This dilemma has been discussed throughout the book, *Learning a*

458

Living: Guide to Planning Your Career and Finding a Job for People with Learning Disabilities, Attention Deficit Disorder, and Dyslexia, and is debated even further in Chapter 14 of that book).

Once you disclose, your employer can request medical documentation and evaluate it to determine whether your request is appropriate. You and your health care provider must prove that you have a disability that substantially limits a major life activity. The employer can require medical documentation, and not accept a letter from a learning disability specialist. And you must also prove you need the requested accommodation to do the job.

The law mentions these possible accommodations:

- job restructuring—asking co-workers to do some non-essential job functions that are difficult for an employee with disabilities
- part-time or modified work schedules
- reassignment to a vacant position
- equipment and devices that help overcome the disability
- adjustment or modifications to examinations
- adjustment or modification of training materials
- adjustment or modification of policies
- the provision of qualified readers or interpreters

What If You Are Not Covered by ADA?

Your Employer Claims Undue Hardship

The employer does not have to make a reasonable accommodation if it will cause an "undue hardship." This protects employers from having to make an accommodation that is extremely expensive, difficult to implement, or disruptive. Generally, this provision applies to small businesses. The law says that factors to be considered in determining "undue hardship" include how big the employer is and how much money they have available. Examples of accommodations that might be considered an undue hardship include:

- an employee asking for over an hour a day of time from the supervisor to structure her work;
- a secretary asking to be relieved of taking phone messages due to an auditory perceptual problem when she is the only secretary serving the division.

Accommodating Yourself

If you offer to pay for an accommodation, your employer cannot say "no" unless it is disruptive. So, if you want to use colored overlays, a pencil to keep your place, or other eccentric-looking accommodations, you cannot be told that company policy does not allow these self-accommodations. Likewise, the employer cannot prevent you from installing your own spell check or grammar check software on your computer, as long as it doesn't damage the computer network. But you might not be able to dictate your reports into a tape recorder instead of writing them if you cannot find a place to do it without disturbing your office mates.

The employer must prove that an accommodation would cause "undue hardship." Nevertheless, it is helpful to research several accommodations so your employer has options. The Job Accommodation Network, a service of the President's Committee on Employment of People with Disabilities, can tell you about various accommodations and describe various options. Their number is 800-526-7234.

Your Employer Is Too Small or You Are an Independent Contractor

Unfortunately, not all jobs are covered by the Americans with Disabilities Act. You are not covered if your employer has fewer than fifteen employees. Nor are you covered if you are working as an independent contractor.

Fortunately, many small businesses gladly provide accommodations. Ask with a positive attitude. Explain that accommodation would make you more productive—and able to do a better job as an employee.

In addition, consider paying for your own accommodation. You may also be able to trade jobs with co-workers or find ways around your disability. The major difference that you face is that you do not have a right to accommodation. Employers can legally fire you if they wish to discriminate against you for having a disability. In addition, disclosing your disability gives you no legal advantages.

Filing a Complaint

Although the ADA gives you many important rights related to employment, discrimination is very difficult to prove. To date, over nine out of ten cases under the ADA have been won by employers.

If you do decide to file a complaint regarding employment, your first step is to contact the nearest field office of the Equal Employment

Opportunity Commission (EEOC). Look in your phonebook under U.S. Government or call 800-669-4000. The agency may be able to resolve your dispute. If not, your next option is to bring a lawsuit against the employer and let a judge decide whether you have been discriminated against. If you win the lawsuit, the ADA requires that your attorney's fees be reimbursed; if you lose, you will have to pay the costs yourself.

Although it is possible to win an ADA dispute, it is usually easier to avoid one. For most people with learning disabilities, attention deficit disorder, or dyslexia, the smoothest road to a job is to do your research, conduct excellent interviews, and find an employer who wants a worker with your personality and qualifications. And, if you have to sue to get the job, do you really want to work there?

For More Information about the Americans with Disabilities Act

If you are thinking about filing a discrimination complaint under the ADA or would just like additional information about your rights, there are many sources of free information. Your public library is likely to have the latest information about the Americans with Disabilities Act. The government sent 95 ADA publications and a videotape about the ADA to 15,000 libraries across the country. Here are some other sources, which have been adapted from publications of the Disability Rights Section of the U.S. Department of Justice:

U.S. Equal Employment Opportunity Commission
1801 L Street, N.W.
Washington, DC 20007
Toll-Free: 800-669-4000
Toll-Free TTY: 800-669-6820
Phone: 202-663-4900
TTY: 202-663-4494
Website: http://www.eeoc.gov

The EEOC offers technical assistance on the ADA provisions applying to employment and also provides information on how to file ADA complaints.

U.S. Department of Justice
950 Pennsylvania Avenue, N.W.
Civil Rights Division

Disability Rights Section–NYA
Washington, DC 20530
ADA Hotline: 800-466-4232
Fax: 202-307-1198
Website: http://www.usdoj.gov/crt/drssec.htm; or, http://www.ada.gov

This hotline is funded by the Department of Justice to provide technical assistance on the Americans with Disabilities Act. Call the hotline to ask questions or order publications about the ADA.

President's Committee on Employment of People with Disabilities

1331 F Street, N.W.
Washington, DC 20004
Phone: 202-376-6200
Fax: 202-376-6250
Website: http://www.pcepd.gov

The President's Committee answers employment questions and funds the Job Accommodation Network.

Job Accommodation Network (JAN)

West Virginia University
P.O. Box 6080
Morgantown, WV 26506-6080
Toll-Free: 800-526-7234
Toll-Free TTY: 877-781-9403
Fax: 304-293-5407
Website: http://www.jan.wvu.edu
E-mail: jan@jan.wvu.edu

The network has a database of thousands of accommodations. Telephone consultants can provide personalized advice on accommodating employees with disabilities.

Center for Learning Disabilities and the Law

P.O. Box 368
Cabin John, MD 20818

The CLDL is a non-profit organization that provides some counseling, but cannot return all calls. They are the only national organization that specializes in learning disabilities and the law.

Be patient when you call these organizations. Some of the 800 numbers receive so many calls that you may have to hold or wait to have your call returned. And be ready with specific questions to ask. Do not try to tell your entire story on the telephone. Thank everyone who does a good job helping you.

Conclusion

The Americans with Disabilities Act can protect you against job discrimination from all except the smallest employers. Knowing your rights should give you confidence as you search for a job. Once you are offered a job, knowing your rights should also help you negotiate the accommodations you need.

Chapter 54

Special Needs Trusts Can Help Students with Disabilities

Mrs. Client has an adult son, Freddie, who resides in her home. Freddie was born with a developmental disability.[1] Freddie's grandmother wishes to give him a generous bequest in her will. Mrs. Client hopes to set up a trust so that Freddie can some day enjoy his grandmother's money, without jeopardizing his state or federal benefits.

A special needs trust[2] is crucial to Freddie's future. More than likely, he will someday have to face life without his parents' financial help. Without a trust, he will have to survive solely on his supplemental security income (SSI) benefits, which are well below the poverty level.[3] But if he receives an inheritance outright, he will lose his SSI and Medicaid.

Medicaid covers much more than a few doctor bills for Freddie. For example, it pays for his case manager at community mental health. It covers a behavioral therapist to help him relate appropriately with others, and it makes him eligible for a host of local community services. Medicaid may even pay for his dentist, who specializes in providing care for persons with special needs.[4]

There would be no point giving Freddie a testamentary bequest if it meant the loss of all his benefits. Then, Freddie would have to use any inheritance to pay for the things Medicaid now covers. The money would be wasted without a special needs trust; grandmother might as well bequeath it to the State of Michigan.[5]

"Prepare for the Future with a Special Needs Trust," by Martha A. Churchill and Patricia E. Kefalas Dudek. © National Fragile X Foundation (www.fragilex.org). Reprinted with permission.

If Freddie is lucky enough to have a trust, though, his trustee could send him to summer camp, buy him a plane ticket to Albuquerque to visit his favorite aunt, or pay the retainer for an attorney in case of a legal emergency. (Some persons with special needs are interrogated by the police, and confess to crimes that they did not commit, due to their high suggestibility.)

Trust money can be used for uninsured medical or dental treatments. It can pay for private rehabilitation, schooling, and recreation. It can cover ball games, camping trips, roller blades, pizza parties, vitamins, or even a travel companion. The money can assist him in reaching his maximum potential and quality of life, and then eventually pay for his funeral. These are all "extras" he cannot afford on poverty level SSI income and Medicaid, alone.

The hallmark of this trust is that the trustee has full discretion to spend the money however he or she sees fit.[6] Then a governmental agency will not be able to claim that Freddie has any legal right to the trust funds. In doing this, his creditors also should be excluded.

If the money to be placed in a special needs trust originates with the beneficiary (a "self-settled" trust), special language is required for the residuary clause. This is necessary if the beneficiary received a settlement from a lawsuit, an inheritance, or has saved up his own earnings from a part-time job.[7] Trust language required in that situation is further explained later in this chapter.

The attorney should also understand Social Security and Medicaid benefits when working with Mrs. Client. By way of illustration, Freddie is 35 years old, and receives SSI due to his mental disability. When his father retires, dies, or becomes disabled, Freddie will qualify for benefits under SSDI, or Social Security Disability Income, based on his father's earnings.[8]

Freddie currently qualifies for SSI because he does not have liquid assets in excess of $2,000. Neither parent has retired, died, or become disabled. The federal government would allow him to own certain property, such as a car or home,[9] without losing his SSI. Freddie needs flexibility, and the trust can provide that by buying or selling a home for his benefit without affecting his Social Security benefits.[10]

Some day, when Freddie starts receiving SSDI instead of SSI, his assets will no longer affect his right to receive the cash benefits. However, he will still have to keep his bank account, and other liquid assets, below $2,000 to qualify for Medicaid and other services through the public mental health system.

The solution is to make sure Freddie spends the money received from SSI or SSDI on food, clothing, and shelter. If he needs something special or expensive, such as an electronic video game, the trust can buy it for him. The trust should not spend money on his food, clothing, or shelter (his basic needs), since that will be considered "income" for SSI or Medicaid purposes.[11] The trust should be titled the "Irrevocable Special Needs Trust for and on behalf of Freddie (last name)." and include discretionary language such as the following:

> "Under no circumstance shall Freddie have the power or authority to demand any distribution from the Trustee who is under no obligation, implied or otherwise, to make any distribution to Freddie. Further, the Trustee may withhold distributions to Freddie if, in its sole discretion, they would not be consistent with intentions as expressed in this Agreement. The Trustee shall use its best efforts to avoid distributions which may cause disqualification for any entitlement to which Freddie is or may be eligible" or,
>
> "Trustee has full discretion to spend the trust income or principal, or not to spend it, as he or she sees fit. Beneficiary shall have no legal right to the trust assets, even in case of emergency. Any attempt by Beneficiary to assign his or her interest in the trust shall be null and void."

In addition, the trustee needs direction, not to spend trust funds on food, clothing, or shelter, which would cause problems with Freddie's SSI eligibility:

> "To the extent that Freddie is eligible for any public benefits to provide for his basic support and maintenance, during the term of this Trust, Grantor directs that distributions from this Trust Agreement shall be used solely for supplementing those benefits which are available to him. In as much as possible, the Trustee is to administer this Trust so that Freddie's eligibility for public governmental assistance programs is not endangered."

Not making a distribution for food, clothing, and shelter is especially important for SSI purposes, but Medicaid is not as strict. Either government program could consider it "income" if third parties are providing food, clothing, or shelter to a person with a disability. The rules are a bit elaborate; SSI allows Freddie and his family to plant a garden and eat their own tomatoes, without calling it "income,"[12] but if Freddie wins a cash prize for the biggest tomato at the town fair, that would be income.[13]

If the trust buys a house, it should rent it to Freddie. The rent should be low enough so that he can afford to buy his own food and clothing. Another option available to Freddie is a housing subsidy from the local community mental health agency. In sum, he should spend nearly all of his monthly Social Security check on necessities, and let the trust buy the extras that enrich his life.

A wonderful byproduct of the special needs trust, is that it can serve as a Medicaid planning tool for the disabled person's parent or grandparent. Suppose Freddie's grandmother needs long-term care in a nursing facility. Pursuant to 42 U.S.C. § 1396p(c)(2)(B), she can transfer money to a disability trust without penalty for Medicaid eligibility purposes, so long as the beneficiary is under age 65. If Freddie's grandmother needs to qualify for Medicaid, she can do so through the special needs trust without exhausting her life savings. Plus, she will have the satisfaction of assisting Freddie by funding the Irrevocable Special Needs Trust for and on behalf of Freddie.

Choosing a Trustee

A key issue for the estate-planning client is the selection of an appropriate trustee. Most often, the trust will be funded when the parents die. Should the trustee be a close relative, such as a sibling? An agency which serves persons with disabilities, such as a local Arc (formerly know as the Association for Retarded Citizens)? A financial institution? An attorney?

In a few cases, the lucky parents will identify a close family member who is highly responsible and who cares deeply about the person's welfare. If so, that solves the problem of choosing a trustee. There should be some thought given to a successor trustee should the first choice be unable to act.

A bank or other financial institution can serve as trustee. However, financial institutions take a percentage off the top each year for administrative expenses and generally will not accept trusts with less than half a million dollars.[14] Further, a bank will not know when Freddie needs special vocational services or a new fishing pole. Obviously, someone who knows and loves Freddie will have to participate in the trustee's decisions, either as an advisor or as co-trustee, even if a financial institution is appointed trustee.

It is a good policy to have a financial advisor involved in making investment decisions for the trust, but that can be done without making it the trustee. If the trust will not support a bank as trustee, due to the high administrative overhead, consider a pooled accounts trust.[15] The parent or other caregiver could have a hand in how the trust money is spent, but without the hassle.

Tax returns, investment decisions, and intricate rules about what is considered "income," would all be taken care of by the pooled trust administrator. Upon the parent's death, the pooled accounts trust would continue its work, and any money remaining after the beneficiary's death would be used to help other persons with disabilities in the pool.

Another possibility is a small stand-alone trust administered by a committee, to include a financial planner[16] and one or two family members.[17] Several close relatives, working as a team, could likely keep each other on the straight and narrow. The financial member would choose sensible investments at a minimum fee. In case one of the team members dies, the others will be familiar with the beneficiary's needs and desires. They will be ready to step in without waiting to become acquainted with the beneficiary's unique personal characteristics. The remaining trustees could even select a replacement to join their trustee team. It may be beneficial to include a provision which allows a person to be appointed to break a "tie" should one arise.

How do the parents recognize a caring family member? Surprisingly, one of the chief characteristics of a suitable trustee is the person's willingness to speak out against the parents and argue with them about what is in Freddie's best interests. Suppose they have a niece, Janet, who sometimes makes suggestions about where Freddie ought to live, or how Freddie could make more friends. That type of interference is a sure sign that Janet genuinely cares about Freddie, to the point she is willing to speak up for him. As a trustee, she would be an ideal advocate, and she ought to have a say in the administration of his trust.

Certain non-relatives could be considered as candidates for the job of trustee, co-trustee, or advisor to the bank—the family pastor or rabbi, a special education teacher, or anyone else who works professionally with persons with disabilities.

In recruiting someone like Janet to serve as successor trustee, do not scare her away by suggesting that she will have to be his surrogate parent. Her job will be much more limited. She will not have to cook Freddie's dinner, but she may buy a microwave for his kitchen if he needs one.

Finding a trustee is not easy for most families. Anyone with a good heart, and who is responsible with money, has the basic qualifications. Once the new trustee is controlling the trust funds for the welfare of the beneficiary, the person with a disability will be light years ahead of his peers without a trust.

Residual Beneficiary

When the beneficiary has died, anything left in the trust should be earmarked. The money could go to the person's siblings, just as if he or she had died intestate. Another consideration, in choosing a residual beneficiary, is the fact that certain agencies do a tremendous job helping persons with a disability. Some parents generously choose to reward such an agency by making it the residual beneficiary.

What if Freddie's cousin Janet serves as trustee, and is also named as one of the residual beneficiaries? This raises a potential conflict of interest. Janet should be spending the money on Freddie, but might theoretically feel disinclined to do so, since saving the money will benefit her (or her lineal descendants) in the end. Freddie's parents can probably avoid questions by confronting this issue openly:[18]

> "In establishing this trust, we, the Grantors, understand that the trustee is also a residual beneficiary. We believe that any technical conflict of interest is greatly outweighed by the benefit of having Janet as trustee, because we know her to be a responsible person who truly cares about Freddie."

Other protections could be built in to the plan as the facts warrant them. For example, requiring an annual accounting to be reviewed by a third party, or local advocacy agency. Some parents write a specific letter of intent to go with the trust.

Footnotes

1. Some people regard the phrase "mentally retarded" as stigmatized, but it is the legally correct term, as defined by Social Security at 20 C.F.R. Part 404, Subpart P, appendix 1, Part A, Sec. 12.05. "Developmental disability" is more politically correct, but its legal meaning includes persons of high intelligence; 42 U.S.C.A. § 6001(8).

2. Also known as a "discretionary trust," a "supplemental needs trust" or an "amenities trust."

3. Current SSI benefits are close to $500 per month, which is for rent, food, and clothing. However, clearly, no single person can live a proper life independently on that income.

4. M.C.L.A. 400.108.

5. M.C.L.A. section 330.1804; M.S.A. § 14.800(804).

6. Miller vs. Dept. of Mental Health, 432 Mich. 426, 442 N.W.2d 617 (1989).

7. In reference to Johannes Trust, 191 Mich. App. 514, 479 N.W.2d 25 (1991).

8. The parent must earn enough to obtain "insured status." Also, Freddie must remain unmarried all his life to qualify for this extra bonus. The benefits paid to Freddie do not affect the amount of Social Security the father receives. If the mother earned more than the father, her earnings will be used to calculate Freddie's SSDI benefit.

9. The car should not exceed $4,500 in fair market value. For a complete list of assets excluded from SSI's definition of "property," see 42 U.S.C.A. § 1382b(a).

10. Parents desiring to ensure a permanent home for a disabled son or daughter should avoid trying to buy a home, or donating a large endowment to any one residential institution. By funding a trust, the trustee can make sure the person has suitable living arrangements, depending on circumstances which the parents cannot predict. Another option is the use of a charitable remainder trust.

11. See the ICLE reference work, "Michigan Guardianship and Conservatorship Handbook," especially chapter 12 which explains what constitutes "income." The book is available by calling toll-free 877-299-4350.

12. 42 U.S.C.A. § 1382a(b)(8)

13. 42 U.S.C.A. § 1382a(a)(2)(C). However, the first $240 per year of income does not count. 42 U.S.C.A. 1382a(b)(2)(A).

14. Typical financial institutions charge about 1% per year paid monthly, plus $800. Some will not accept a trust below $500,000; others will go down to "only" $250,000. Some financial institutions prefer young beneficiaries, so the financial institution can build up the trust assets over the person's lifetime. Banks often shy away from trusts which own real estate, for fear of environmental entanglements, despite statutory protections for fiduciary owners of contaminated property, such as 42 USCA 9607(n)(1); MCLA 324.20101(y)(ii); and MCLA 700.801(1).

15. Several non-profit organizations in Michigan have established pooled accounts trusts, some of which are open to anyone in

the state. A sub-account in a pooled accounts trust is economical and easy to set up. Contact Attorney (and co-author of this chapter) Patricia E. Kefalas Dudek at 248-586-9820, for a complete list of pooled accounts trusts.

16. Typically, a stock brokerage or a certified public accountant (CPA) will serve as financial advisor for about 1/2 percent annually, which is less expensive than a financial institution. Another alternative: state that the trust funds must be invested with Merrill Lynch (or A.G. Edwards or Paine Webber), and can only be withdrawn by the trustees acting jointly.

17. Specify that a single trustee from the committee can act alone, when dealing with third parties, and that the trustees are responsible for consulting one another about decisions. Otherwise, they will have to act unanimously on every little decision, which could get cumbersome.

18. Childs vs. Nat 'l Bank of Austin, 658 F.2d 487 (7th Cir. 1981).

Chapter 55

Scholarships for Students with Learning Disabilities

This chapter presents a short list of scholarships for students with learning disabilities. Due to the very large and growing number of students who claim to be learning disabled, such awards are often highly competitive.

Scholarships for Students with Disabilities

Bank of America Abilities Scholarship Program

This program awards scholarships to students with disabilities (including learning disabilities) who have a career interest in finance, business, or computer science, a grade point average (GPA) of at least 3.0 on a 4.0 scale, and who reside in Arizona, California, District of Columbia, Florida, Georgia, Idaho, Illinois, Iowa, Kansas, Maryland, Missouri, Nevada, New Mexico, North Carolina, Oklahoma, Oregon, South Carolina, Tennessee, Texas, Virginia or Washington. For more information:

Bank of America Abilities Scholarship Program
P.O. Box 1465
Taylors, SC 29687
Phone: 864-268-3363
Website: https://www.scholarshipprograms.org/bada/bada_2005_ins.htm
E-mail: allisonlee@bellsouth.net

Anne Ford Scholarship

The Anne Ford Scholarship is a $10,000 scholarship awarded by the National Center for Learning Disabilities to a high school senior with a learning disability who can act as a role model for others who are faced with learning disabilities, and who has the potential of contributing to society in a way that increases opportunities for all people with learning disabilities. The application deadline is December 31. For more information:

Anne Ford Scholarship
National Center for Learning Disabilities, Inc.
381 Park Ave. South, Suite 1401
New York, NY 10016-8806
Phone: 212-545-7510
Fax: 212-545-9665
Website: http://www.ncld.org/content/view/871/456074
E-mail: AFScholarship@ncld.org

Yes I Can! Foundation for Exceptional Children

The Yes I Can! Foundation for Exceptional Children offers the Stanley E. Jackson Scholarships and Sara Conlon Memorial Scholarship. Each scholarship is $500 for first year college students with a disability. U.S. citizenship is required. The application deadline is February 1. For more information:

Foundation for Exceptional Children
1110 N. Glebe Rd., Suite 300
Arlington, VA 22201-5704
Toll-Free: 888-232-7733
Toll-Free TTY: 866-915-5000
Fax: 703-264-9494
Website: http://www.cec.sped.org
E-mail: yesican@cec.sped.org

Learning Disabilities Association of Iowa

The Learning Disabilities Association of Iowa awards three $1,000 scholarships to Iowa high school seniors with learning disabilities. The deadline is in mid-March.

Learning Disabilities Association of Iowa
Website: http://www.lda-ia.org

P. Buckley Moss Society Harbison Scholarship

The Anne and Matt Harbison Scholarship is awarded by the P. Buckley Moss Society to high school seniors with language-related learning disabilities for college education. For more information:

P. Buckley Moss Society
601 Shenandoah Village Dr., Suite 1C
Waynesboro, VA 22980
Phone: 540-943-5678
Website: http://www.mosssociety.org/page.php?id=30

National Society of the DAR/Margaret Howard Hamilton Scholarship

This award is for $1,000 (renewable for four years) for a high school senior who has been accepted to the Ben Caudle Learning Center, University of the Ozarks. For more information:

NSDAR Administration Building
1776 D Street N.W.
Washington, DC 20006-5392
Website: http://www.dar.org/natsociety/edout_scholar.cfm

Recording for the Blind/Learning through Listening

This program provides three scholarships of $3,000 each for high school seniors who are learning disabled. The award is based on academic achievement, leadership, enterprise, and service to others. Financial need is not a factor. For more information:

Recording for the Blind and Dyslexic
20 Rozelle Road
Princeton, NJ 08540
Toll-Free: 866-732-3585
Website: http://www.rfbd.org

Canadian Scholarships for Students with Disabilities

Learning Disabilities Association of Canada (LDAC)

LDAC offers three scholarships for students with disabilities: The Donald Cummings Scholarship, the Carol Thomson Memorial Fund Scholarship, and the Doreen Kronick Scholarship. The application deadline is May 15. For more information:

Learning Disabilities Association of Canada

323 Chapel Street, Suite 200
Ottawa, Ontario, K1N 7Z2
Phone: 613-238-5721
Fax: 613-235-5391
Website: http://www.ldac-taac.ca
E-mail: information@ldac-taac.ca

Learning Disabilities Association of Ottawa-Carleton (LDAO-C)

LDAO-C offers information about several scholarships for Canadian students with disabilities, including the Roy Cooper Scholarship, the Mattinson Endowment Fund Scholarship, and the Imperial Tobacco Canada Scholarship Fund.

LDAO-C

Website: http://ldao-c.ncf.ca/scholarships.html

Association of Universities and Colleges of Canada

Website: http://www.aucc.ca/programs/scholarships/index_e.html

Gloria Landis Memorial Bursary

The Gloria Landis Memorial Bursary is a $1,000 scholarship awarded by the Learning Disabilities Association of Ontario to a mature individual with learning disabilities to pursue a post-secondary or vocational program. Candidates must be at least 25 years old and have been absent from full-time education for at least three years. The application deadline is June 15. For more information:

Learning Disabilities Association of Ontario

360 Bloor St. E., Suite 1004
P.O. Box 39
Toronto, Ontario M4W 3L4
Phone: 416-929-4311
Fax: 416-929-3905

Justin Eves Foundation Scholarship

The Justin Eves Foundation Scholarship provides a $3,000 scholarship for students with a learning disability. For more information, contact:

The Justin Eves Foundation
199 Bay St., Suite 2901
Commerce Court W., P.O. Box 322
Toronto, ON M5L 1G1
Phone: 416-586-0085
Fax: 416-586-0050
Website: http://www.justinevesfoundation.com

Learning Disabilities Association of Saskatchewan
Website: http://www.ldas.org/scholarships.htm

Scholarships for Careers in Disabilities

Pilot International Foundation Scholarships

The Pilot International Foundation offers three scholarships for students who are pursuing careers in disabilities and brain-related disorders. A minimum GPA of 3.25 on a 4.0 scale (4.01 on a 5.0 scale) is required. All applicants must be sponsored by their local Pilot Club. For more information:

Pilot International Foundation
Website: http://www.pilotinternational.org/html/foundation/scholar.shtml
E-mail: pifinfo@pilothq.org

P. Buckley Moss Society Cary Scholarship

The Judith Cary Memorial Scholarship is awarded by the P. Buckley Moss Society for study leading to a bachelor's or master's degree in special education. For more information:

P. Buckley Moss Society
20 Stoneridge Dr., Suite 102
Waynesboro, VA 22980
Phone: 540-943-5678
Fax: 540-949-8408
Website: http://www.mosssociety.org/page.php?id=29
E-mail: society@mosssociety.org

Part Seven

Living with a Learning Disability

Chapter 56

Coping with a
Learning Disability

The following account is written for parents, school administrators, teachers, coaches, and individuals coping with a learning disability (LD). My aim is to present one insider's perspective, which commences with early childhood and transitions through high school into adulthood. This story chronicles my personal struggle, eventual acceptance, and adoption of personal management strategies to cope with my constant companion, a learning disability called dyslexia.

End of the School Year, Second Grade

Sometime during the last week of second grade the teacher, Ms. Baugher, asked me to meet with her in the back of the room. In a gentle, inviting tone she asked if I would like to stay in second grade and help her with the incoming class. In my young mind, I knew I was not qualified to be her teaching assistant. In fact, I was pretty sure I was not qualified to move onto the third grade, and that, I realized, was the bottom line of our conversation. I was going to be held back. But she left me some wiggle room. I declined the offer and returned to my desk. That night my parents were more direct regarding my status for the following year; there was no wiggle room. I liked Ms. Baugher and the notion of spending another year with her was not all that bad. On the other hand, the embarrassment of staying in second grade while my classmates moved on to third would be exquisite. I comforted myself with the notion that I had the summer to get used to the idea.

This was not the first sign that something was interfering with my ability to learn. When I was in first grade, my poor mother would cringe when she saw the teacher standing with me in the carpool line, my plump, white-knuckled fist full of the red-inked casualties that were my handiwork. Somehow I survived first grade. My performance in second grade, however, called for drastic measures. This was okay with my parents, as the school was engaged and working a solution rather than throwing in the towel on their son.

Richard Lavoie, a nationally recognized expert in the special education field, opens a workshop for educators with, "We all know LD means lazy and dumb." This elicits some knowing chuckles from an audience of teachers, but it's like a punch in the stomach to me. "Lazy and dumb" were often used to characterize my academic performance.

First Day of Second Grade, Take 2

In spite of my hopes, summer did not last forever and I reported back to the old second grade room. While experiencing some embarrassment meeting old classmates headed to third grade, things were going okay. After sitting through the introductions, rules of the classroom and so forth, we started our first class—math. The book was the same text used the year before. I turned to the first page with the teacher. I ran my hand down the smooth new page and wondered what had happened to my old book. By now, Ms. Baugher and the rest of the class were six pages ahead while I considered the disposition of used textbooks.

Ms. Baugher determined quickly that repeating second grade was not the answer to my inability to read, write, and learn math in step with the rest of the class. It was 1965 and there was not a clear understanding of what we refer to as a learning disability today. However, I seemed intelligent and normal in every other way, so sometime early in the school year Ms. Baugher referred me to the head of the lower school, Mrs. Smith. For the purposes of the school in those days, Mrs. Smith was the learning specialist. I spent about an hour with Mrs. Smith and was given a number of square-peg-in-round-hole type tasks and a few problem-solving exercises. I remember that I enjoyed talking through and solving hypothetical problems. Mrs. Smith reported back to my parents that she believed my problems could be associated with a disorder she had been reading about recently called dyslexia. She believed that the problem was not serious and that I was capable of being an effective student at the school, with some additional help.

My parents were not thoroughly convinced that I had any disorder and sought an outside opinion. I have a relatively clear memory of my one and only meeting with the psychologist. He told my father that I was an auditory learner, that I possessed high verbal ability, that I was certainly intelligent and certainly dyslexic. However, they were not to worry because dyslexia normally disappears around the onset of puberty. "He'll grow out of it," he assured my father.

Now, no parent is particularly receptive to the notion that their child is anything but normal. My mother continued to insist that she knew deep down that I was intelligent and, therefore, normal. My father, a physician, embraced the words "he'll grow out of it" and saw the solution in tutoring and athletics to refine coordination.

High School, Fall of Freshman Year

Our freshman English instructor was a gentleman named Ambrose Short. He was tall, balding, and reminded me of the British actor, Alistair Sims. Mr. Short was from the old school. An early requirement for his class was to memorize Rudyard Kipling's "If" and Ernest Henley's "Invictus." Mr. Short was a man of expectations, discipline, and standards. He expected the poems to be memorized by a certain date, and failure to do so meant detention. Memorization was not a strong point for me. I had the attention span of a three-year-old in a K-mart and could not focus long enough to sit down and memorize the poems although I had tried.

This was bad. I was on the football team. As a freshman, I was little more than a blocking dummy, but I showed promise. I was having success at something, and I was part of a team. Detention meant missed practice, and missed practice meant I would not play in Saturday's game. Coach Tattersall was also a man of expectations and standards. I reported to Mr. Short after school to serve my detention in despair. Mr. Short looked up from his papers over his bifocals and said, "Mr. Beattie, you will go to football practice as I do not have the time for you right now."

I hi-tailed it down to the locker room and was out on the practice field before anyone knew I was missing. I was in the act of getting in a three-point stance when I spotted Mr. Short making his way across the field toward our group. He was dressed for the cold, fedora hat pulled low against the wind. In horror, I knew Mr. Short was there for me! The coach confirmed the same, "Beattie, go over there and say your poems for Mr. Short."

I stood there with Mr. Short off to the side, helmet off cradled in the crook of my arm. "If you can keep your head when all around you are losing theirs and blaming it on you..." I recited the poems cued by Mr. Short as needed. Eventually satisfied with my progress, Mr. Short told me to come by his room the next day at lunch and recite the poems for record. The poems were internalized and I had no trouble reciting them the next day as he ate a sandwich in his room. Certainly the extra attention from Mr. Short helped. The extra (undesirable) attention afforded me by the older football players for reciting poetry during football practice was a motivator in itself.

When a kid is struggling in class, the knee-jerk reaction is to yank him from sports or other positive things where he is having some success. Mr. Short realized this and somewhere during the school day struck a deal with Coach Tattersall. Together they practiced an intervention that met the standards of Mr. Short's class, the expectations of the varsity football team, and my need to be good at something.

Now there are those who would maintain that the extra time afforded me by Mr. Short was not fair to the other students in his class. Again, I like Richard Lavoie's thoughts on the concept of fairness: "Fairness means that everyone gets what he or she needs." What else did I need? As an auditory learner I could not take notes and listen for one activity cancels out the other. I managed in language arts on my own. I was not particularly setting the world on fire, but I coped. All math required a tutor. Tutors kept me focused and on task. In the end, administrators, teachers, and coaches at Wilmington Friends School ensured that I got what I needed.

Mr. Short died of Hodgkin's disease before the end of my freshman year. He was sick when he trudged out on the practice field that blustery October day. It was five minutes of his time, and I received what I needed.

Transitioning to Adulthood

I struggled through my senior year in high school with the notion that I had grown out of my dyslexia. In fact, my parents and I ensured that any mention of a LD was expunged from my record as we felt it might hurt my prospects for college.

I was accepted into a small liberal arts college where I played football, wrestled, and, if the mood struck me, went to class. I dropped out after three semesters. I came home, worked in construction, and went to night school, eventually working my way into the full-time program at the local university. While I was no longer playing football or wrestling, my life lacked structure and I was eventually dropped from the university. Again, I went back to night school. About this time, Coach Tattersall of Wilmington Friends School called and offered me a job as head wrestling coach. I readily accepted the job and learned to translate the structure and discipline that I demanded of my wrestlers into my own life.

I gritted my teeth and compressed three years of undergraduate work into three semesters. I graduated with a Bachelor of Arts (BA) degree, last in my class, last in my major, but I graduated. As a young adult I surmised that since I had grown out of my dyslexia (if I ever had it at all) obviously my problems were a character issue. My reality was that I was in fact LD—lazy and dumb.

The Uhwarrie National Forest, North Carolina, the Special Forces Qualification Course

Since I had entered the military I had wanted to be in Special Forces, a Green Beret. To be accepted for the training, one had to have been in the Army at least four years, be a qualified paratrooper, and pass a battery of physical and mental tests. Once in the course, it was an arduous six to twelve months' worth of tough, dangerous training before you were awarded the Green Beret.

Things weren't looking good for me in September of 1987. I was in the middle of my re-test for the long-range land navigation final exam. This is a twenty-four hour, 30-kilometer event to test navigation skills, endurance, and ability to work independently in the woods. Failure (you got two chances) meant relief from the course. I was in trouble; I failed at the first attempt. Somewhere in the process of plotting my current position and the position that I was to move to, I reversed a set of numbers within the eight-digit grid coordinate marking a spot on the map. The number reversal put me well out of my way; I could not make up the time lost and failed.

Sympathy was in short supply as I was dropped off in the middle of the woods for my second and final chance. At the first navigation check point, the instructor gave me my new set of coordinates and informed me that I was not moving fast enough to successfully complete the course. I was either minutes away from the final spot that I had (hopefully) correctly plotted, or I was minutes from failure. I was dizzy and my legs were rubber, but I was mad. How had I been so stupid as to reverse the numbers during the first attempt to put myself through so much agony? Muttering to myself I stumbled into the last point with minutes to spare. I passed the course and eventually earned the Green Beret.

The instructors at the Special Forces course did not cut me a break, nor did I expect them to. A dyslexic moment while operating behind enemy lines could get me and others killed or captured. I became acutely aware of my occasional lack of attention to detail in reversing numbers and letters. Under these circumstances I always have another soldier check my work. I know my limitations.

Coping in the Present

I have recently learned that learning disabilities are forever. You don't grow out of it. It appears that dyslexia has, and will continue to be, my constant companion. Automatic teller machines (ATM) present a challenge as I often forget my personal identification number (PIN). Actually, I remember the numbers but not the sequence and the machines are inflexible regarding the sequence thing. Once I've cracked my own code at the ATM, the next problem is what to do with the five hundred dollars I just withdrew when I'd meant to take out fifty.

Recently, I experienced a great deal of anxiety over enrolling in and attending graduate school. This strikes those who know me as odd. As a Special Forces officer, I have routinely operated in hostile areas under dangerous conditions with little trepidation. What's the difference? In a hostile, uncertain environment my training, experience, and confidence mitigate risk and associated fear. In an academic setting, my experience conjures up my demons: frustration, humiliation, shame, and embarrassment.

In spite of it all, some competencies have evolved:

- I am tenacious. I have learned to never give up—never.

- I am goal-oriented. I always have something to work toward.

- I am a problem solver. I have nontraditional problem solving skills which count when time is at a premium or a unique solution is needed.

- I am a motivator. I know what it takes to get myself and others up the hill.

- I am an effective leader. I know my limitations so I delegate tasks and authority to those who can get the job done.

- I have empathy. I have been odd man out, the bottom of the class, the dumb one.

The bottom line and the simple key to success in coping with a LD is to manage it, recognize it, and accept that it exists. I have learned to embrace the lifelong interventions (I get what I need) and most importantly, I do not to let the notion that I have a LD control my life. Yes, dyslexia has been my constant companion, but it is not what I am.

—LTC Taylor Beattie

Mr. Beattie, who has LD, is a Special Forces officer and instructor in the U.S. Army in Fort Leavenworth, Kansas. He has served in the United States and abroad and has earned several awards. He is currently pursuing a master's degree in education.

Chapter 57

Learning Disabilities and the Family: An Emotional Roller Coaster

Let's face it—families and how they work can be very complicated. They reflect the personalities, interests, goals, values, and emotions of each of its members, and as we all know in very personal ways, they are always changing. While certain family members assume specific roles and responsibilities (for example, paying the bills), there are almost always some common beliefs that are shared by everyone, not the least of which is the importance of doing well in school and getting a well-rounded and high quality education. The impact of having a child with learning disabilities (LD) can have an enormous impact upon the delicate balance that keeps family systems purring.

LD Poses Special Challenges

From the moment parents suspect (or become aware of) their child's struggle, the impact of LD quickly becomes a family affair. Consider some of the challenges that families must face when LD enters the conversation.

Parents need to:

- designate (and share) responsibility for establishing and maintaining close contact with school personnel;

- become effective advocates for their child, requesting assessment and intervention services and helping their child to become confident and self-assured in his or her ability to request needed supports;

- focus on individualized education program (IEP) goals and strategies and find ways to support school success at home;

- provide assistance with school work, studying, calendaring, and organizing activities;

- make special efforts to recognize (and celebrate) the strengths and unique qualities of each family member, including the child with LD.

To handle the emotional roller coaster, parents also need to:

- recognize (and overcome) feelings of guilt, sadness, and denial, and develop strong, positive language about what it means to have a child with LD (for example, "my child has a specific learning disability in reading," not "my child is LD");

- address any feelings of resentment that creep up when so much attention is paid to one child in the family;

- include extended family members in identifying challenges that are posed by LD and include them in finding solutions;

- communicate about ways to deal with the ongoing stress of decision-making and agree to devote extra time and attention as needed.

One important key to success for families dealing with LD is to commit to open and honest communication. Phrases like "it doesn't matter" are triggers for underlying problems that deserve attention. Parents may also tend to focus attention on school work all the time and neglect to ask their child about friendships or whether they feel secure and confident in their relationships with teachers.

Another key to success is to appreciate the delicate balance between disclosing LD and your child's feelings about (and rights to) privacy. There is nothing shameful about having learning disabilities, and sharing information about LD is essential to securing the right kinds of services and supports, certainly in pervasive public mythology about learning disabilities. Be prepared to help the listener appreciate what it means to have LD and how to empower your child to be successful.

Coping Strategies: For Better, For Worse

There is no sure way to manage the stress and learn how to cope with the challenges that are faced by individuals with LD and their families. Here are some common ways that people deal with stress—some of which are clearly behaviors that you want to avoid, while others will help you and those around you to become stronger and more effective advocates for your child.

Try not to:

- panic, feel overwhelmed, and helpless;
- look for someone or something to blame;
- worry a lot about what to do now and in the future;
- avoid confronting problems and hope that others will take charge;
- distance yourself from people who know about your child's problem;
- look for a quick fix.

Find ways to:

- get organized, identify critical people, and define the roles they play in helping you and your child;
- seek information and become knowledgeable about LD and strategies for success;
- reach out to school personnel, partner with teachers and others on a regular basis, and be an equal player in implementing strategies for success;
- establish social support networks (for yourself and other family members);
- focus on solving specific problems (versus dealing with everything all at once);
- establish (or join) a network of like-minded parents and professionals who can share experiences, and provide advice and expertise;
- become active in school activities that support students with LD;
- find ways to reduce tension and relieve stress (exercise, hobbies, and so forth);

- seek guidance from professionals;

- plan ahead—anticipate challenges and initiate discussion with your child, other family members, and school personnel before problems arise.

Chapter 58

Parenting a Child with AD/HD

What We Know

Often, when a child is diagnosed with attention deficit/hyperactivity disorder (AD/HD), the first response from his or her concerned parent is, "What can I do about it?" Although life with your child may at times seem challenging, it is important to remember that children with AD/HD can and do succeed. As a parent, you can help create home and school environments that improve your child's chances for success. The earlier you address your child's problems, the more likely you will be able to prevent school and social failure and associated problems such as underachievement and poor self-esteem that may lead to delinquency or drug and alcohol abuse.

Early intervention holds the key to positive outcomes for your child. Here are some ways to get started:

- **Don't waste limited emotional energy on self-blame:** AD/HD is the result of dysfunction in certain areas of the brain and in the majority of cases is inherited. It is not caused by poor

Text in this chapter is from "What We Know: Parenting a Child with AD/HD," © 2004 Children and Adults with Attention-Deficit/Hyperactivity Disorder (CHADD). Reprinted with permission. For more information, write to CHADD at 8181 Professional Place, Suite 150 Landover, MD 20875 or visit the CHADD website at www.chadd.org. Also, included is an excerpt titled "Your Teenager and AD/HD," from "Attention Deficit Hyperactivity Disorder," National Institute of Mental Health (NIMH), 2007.

parenting or a chaotic home environment, although the home environment can make the symptoms of AD/HD worse.

- **Learn all you can about AD/HD:** There is a great deal of information available on the diagnosis and treatment of AD/HD. It is up to you to act as a good consumer and learn to distinguish the accurate information from the inaccurate. But how can you sort out what will be useful and what will not? In general, it is good to be wary about ads claiming to cure AD/HD. Currently, there is no cure for AD/HD, but you can take positive steps to decrease its impact.

- **Make sure your child has a comprehensive assessment:** To complete the diagnostic process, make sure your child has a comprehensive assessment that includes medical, educational, and psychological evaluations and that other disorders that either mimic or commonly occur with AD/HD have been considered and ruled out.

How to Ensure Your Child's Success at School

- **Become an effective case manager:** Keep a record of all information about your child. This includes copies of all evaluations and documents from any meetings concerning your child. You might also include information about AD/HD, a record of your child's prior treatments and placements, and information for the professionals who have worked with your child.

- **Take an active role in forming a team that understands AD/HD and wants to help your child:** Meetings at your child's school should be attended by the principal's designee, as well as a special educator, and a classroom teacher that knows your child. You, however, have the right to request input at these meetings from others that understand AD/HD or your child's special needs. These include your child's physician, the school psychologist, and the nurse or guidance counselor from your child's school. If you have consulted other professionals, such as a psychiatrist, educational advocate, or behavior management specialist, the useful information they have provided should also be made available at these meetings. A thorough understanding of your child's strengths and weaknesses and how AD/HD affects him will help you and members of this team go on to develop an appropriate and effective program that takes into account his or her AD/HD.

- **Learn all you can about AD/HD and your child's educational rights:** The more knowledge you have about your child's rights under the two education laws—the Individuals with Disabilities Education Act (IDEA) and Section 504 of the Rehabilitation Act—the better the chance that you will maximize his or her success. Each state has a parent training and information center that can help you learn more about your child's rights.

- **Become your child's best advocate:** You may have to represent or protect your child's best interest in school situations, both academic and behavioral. Become an active part of the team that determines what services and placements your child receives in an individualized education program (IEP) or Section 504 plan.

How to Make Life at Home Easier

- **Join a support group:** Parents will find additional information, as well as support, by attending local CHADD meetings where available. You can find the nearest chapter to your home on the CHADD chapter locator online at http://www.chadd.org/AM/Template.cfm?Section=Find_Local_CHADD_Chapters&Template=/CustomPages/ChapterLocator/findchap.cfm.

- **Seek professional help:** Ask for help from professionals, particularly if you are feeling depressed, frustrated, and exhausted. Helping yourself feel less stressed will benefit your child as well.

- **Work together to support your child:** It is important that all of the adults that care for your child (parents, grandparents, relatives, and childcare workers) agree on how to approach or handle your child's problem behaviors. Working with a professional, if needed, can help you better understand how to work together to support your child.

- **Learn the tools of successful behavior management:** Parent training will teach you strategies to change behaviors and improve your relationship with your child. Identify parent training classes in your community through your local parent information and resource center or parent training and information center (http://www.taalliance.org).

- **Find out if you have AD/HD:** Since AD/HD is generally inherited, many parents of children with AD/HD often discover that they have AD/HD when their child is diagnosed. Parents with AD/HD may need the same types of evaluation and treatment that they seek for their children in order to function at their best. AD/HD in the parent may make the home more chaotic and affect parenting skills.

Parent training will help you learn the following:

- **Focus on certain behaviors and provide clear, consistent expectations, directions, and limits:** Children with AD/HD need to know exactly what others expect from them. They do not perform well in ambiguous situations that don't specify exactly what is expected and that require they read between the lines. Working with a professional can help you narrow the focus to a few specific behaviors and help you set limits, and consistently follow through.

- **Set up an effective discipline system:** Parents should learn proactive—not reactive—discipline methods that teach and reward appropriate behavior and respond to misbehavior with alternatives such as time out or loss of privileges.

- **Help your child learn from his or her mistakes:** At times, negative consequences will arise naturally out of a child's behavior. However, children with AD/HD have difficulty making the connection between their behaviors and these consequences. Parents can help their child with AD/HD make these connections and learn from his or her mistakes.

How to Boost Your Child's Confidence

- **Tell your child that you love and support him or her unconditionally:** There will be days when you may not believe this yourself. Those will be the days when it is even more important that you acknowledge the difficulties your child faces on a daily basis, and express your love. Let your child know that you will get through the smooth and rough times together.

- **Assist your child with social skills:** Children with AD/HD may be rejected by peers because of hyperactive, impulsive, or aggressive behaviors. Parent training can help you learn how to assist your child in making friends and learning to work cooperatively with others.

- **Identify your child's strengths:** Many children with AD/HD have strengths in certain areas such as art, athletics, computers, or mechanical ability. Build upon these strengths, so that your child will have a sense of pride and accomplishment. Make sure that your child has the opportunity to be successful while pursuing these activities and that his strengths are not undermined by untreated AD/HD. Also, avoid, as much as possible, targeting these activities as contingencies for good behavior or withholding them, as a form of punishment, when your child with AD/HD misbehaves.

- **Set aside a daily special time for your child:** Constant negative feedback can erode a child's self-esteem. A special time, whether it's an outing, playing games, or just time spent in positive interaction, can help fortify your child against assaults to self-worth.

Your Teenager with AD/HD

Your child with AD/HD has successfully navigated the early school years and is beginning his or her journey through middle school and high school. Although your child has been periodically evaluated through the years, this is a good time to have a complete re-evaluation of your child's health.

The teen years are challenging for most children, and for the child with AD/HD these years are doubly hard. All the adolescent problems—peer pressure, the fear of failure in school or socially, low self-esteem— are harder for the AD/HD child to handle. The desire to be independent, to try new and forbidden things—alcohol, drugs, and sexual activity—can lead to unforeseen consequences. The rules that once were, for the most part, followed, are often now flaunted. Parents may not agree with each other on how the teenager's behavior should be handled.

Now, more than ever, rules should be straightforward and easy to understand. Communication between the adolescent and parents can help the teenager to know the reasons for each rule. When a rule is set, it should be clear why the rule is set. Sometimes it helps to have a chart, often posted in the kitchen, which lists all household rules and all rules for outside the home (social and school). Another chart could list household chores with space to check off a chore once it is done.

When rules are broken—and they will be—respond to this inappropriate behavior as calmly and matter-of-factly as possible. Use punishment sparingly. Even with teens, a time-out can work. Impulsivity and hot temper often accompany AD/HD. A short time alone can help.

As the teenager spends more time away from home, there will be demands for a later curfew and the use of the car. Listen to your child's request, give reasons for your opinion, listen to his or her opinion, and negotiate. Communication, negotiation, and compromise will prove helpful.

Your Teenager and the Car

Teenagers, especially boys, begin talking about driving by the time they are 15. In some states, a learner's permit is available at 15 and a driver's license at 16. Statistics show that 16-year-old drivers have more accidents per driving mile than any other age. In the year 2000, 18 percent of those who died in speed-related crashes were youth ages 15 to 19. Sixty-six percent of these youth were not wearing safety belts. Youth with AD/HD, in their first 2–5 years of driving, have nearly four times as many automobile accidents, are more likely to cause bodily injury in accidents, and have three times as many citations for speeding as the young drivers without AD/HD.

Most states, after looking at the statistics for automobile accidents involving teenage drivers, have begun to use a graduated driver licensing system (GDL). This system eases young drivers onto the roads by a slow progression of exposure to more difficult driving experiences. The program, as developed by the National Highway Traffic Safety Administration and the American Association of Motor Vehicle Administrators, consists of three stages: learner's permit, intermediate (provisional) license, and full licensure. Drivers must demonstrate responsible driving behavior at each stage before advancing to the next level. During the learner's permit stage, a licensed adult must be in the car at all times. This period of time will give the learner a chance to practice, practice, and practice. The more your child drives, the more efficient he or she will become. The sense of accomplishment the teenager with AD/HD will feel when the coveted license is finally in his or her hands will make all the time and effort involved worthwhile.

Chapter 59

Social and Emotional Side of Learning Disabilities

How Does It Feel? The Social/Emotional Side of LD

Author's Note: This time last year [2006], my [Dr. Horowitz] *Research Roundup* column was titled "Nonverbal Learning Disabilities (NVLD): A Primer on a Puzzling Population", and I offered some background and perspective on a subtype of learning disabilities (LD) that is typified by significant struggle in the areas of non-academic learning and behavior. Thinking back on this past calendar year and the scores of studies and texts that I've read (okay, maybe skimmed) covering dozens of important topics, I am reminded of how frequently I found myself nodding my head in agreement with Dr. Samuel Kirk's observation of more than 30 years ago that children with LD, in addition to struggles with academic learning, have trouble with "skills needed for social interaction." What are some of the social and emotional variables that pose as barriers to success for students with LD? Read on.

What Are the Social and Emotional Aspects of LD?

Let's take an imaginary walk down the hall with Joseph, a sixth grader, as he makes his way from his first period math class to his second period English class. He's already a few minutes late because he needed extra time to copy the homework assignment from the board. Rushing to his locker (on the far end of the hall) where he will hopefully find the text books he needs for the remainder of his morning classes, he is aware of the chatter and bustling of other students moving about but has not noticed the pervasive agitated mood of the students in the hallway. Apparently Joseph missed the announcement that the cafeteria was closed for repairs and that students would have to eat in their classrooms. Not picking up on any of the all-too-obvious facial expressions and body language, Joseph turns to a group of classmates and asks, "Want to play cards in the cafeteria during lunch?"

- How do you think these students reacted to Joseph's question?
- What was Joseph feeling as this incident unfolded?
- What are the immediate and long-term consequences of Joseph's having a very different and sometimes ineffective social and emotional barometer?

While it is true that some social skills are more easily taught than others, and that over time, established patterns and routines can compensate for difficulties in social and emotional learning and behavior, these types of problems don't just go away. They can have a profound impact upon students (for example: stress, feeling of self-worth) and are linked to all sorts of everyday activities. Social and emotional skills are critical to activities such as personal interactions (meeting and greeting) and talking on the phone or via the internet, and are directly associated with problem-solving, decision-making, self-management, and initiating and maintaining positive social relationships with peers and others.

Some Definitions

It might be helpful to clarify what we mean by the words social and emotional.

Social

This word might be best understood in two different ways:

- Social skills are the specific reactions, responses, techniques, and strategies that a student uses in social situations.
- Social competence is the term used to describe how well (or poorly) a student performs in social situations.

It is the combination of these two things that helps to describe a student's social well-being.

Emotional

While this word is most readily associated with feelings, it is really much more than that. Emotional well-being is associated with what has been called emotional intelligence, which includes the following:

- Knowing one's emotions (how do I feel about this?)
- Managing one's emotions (given how I feel, how should I react?)
- Motivating one's self (regardless of how I feel, I need to...)
- Recognizing others' emotions (I know how you are feeling)
- Making effective use of social skills (the best thing for me to do now is...)

While the building blocks of emotional intelligence are important for all students, they are particularly important for students with LD who may also struggle because of something I will refer to as "goodness of fit." Explained wonderfully in a 2003 book by Barbara Keogh, titled *Temperament in the Classroom: Understanding Individual Differences*, this perspective suggests that social-emotional and learning problems are linked to temperament (or style of behavior), and that temperament, rather than a disability of any sort, might account for how a student behaves in a particular situation. Let's think for a moment about how students do things rather than what they do or why they do them, and pay attention to such things as:

- adaptability,
- reactivity,
- task orientation persistence, and
- flexibility.

What is the connection to LD? What happens when a child's temperament doesn't conform to the expectations of teachers or parents? Could a child's temperament be a risk factor for school achievement in the same way that LD poses barriers to learning? You bet it can.

Some Important Points about the Social-Emotional Side of LD

- There are many students with LD for whom social skills are an area of strength and who are able to negotiate emotional challenges without needing support. Don't assume that every student with LD experiences struggle in this area.

- When compared with non-learning disabled peers, studies have shown that students with LD may be prone to being more poorly accepted by their peers, at greater risk for social alienation from teachers and classmates, less frequently selected to play or join in group activities, and more willing to conform to peer pressure (in adolescence, this is especially troublesome because of the general predisposition to engage in antisocial behaviors). All of these factors clearly have a direct impact on social-emotional well-being.

- Information processing and executive functioning difficulties can make it seem like students with LD are not fitting in and can contribute to strain and frustration in the classroom and even at home and other settings.

- Students with LD often (and appropriately) demand additional time and attention from teachers and others. When these students then ask inappropriate questions, ask the same question that was just answered, respond impulsively rather than waiting their turn, or misread a social cue that results in a disruption (all of which they are prone to do), the outcome can be upsetting for everyone involved.

What Can You Do?

The following is a short list of ways to promote the social and emotional well-being of students with LD.

1. Recognize the child's specific areas of strength (competence) and need, and look for (or create) teachable moments to model and reinforce positive skills.

2. Teach social skills the same way you would academic skills: proceed in small steps, demonstrate and give multiple examples, offer practice and feedback (reinforcement and praise), and systematically find opportunities to generalize (apply) newly learned skills and behaviors to different settings. Some critical skills to address include the following:

   a. Awareness of non-verbal cues (gestures, body language)

   b. Social conversation (initiating greetings, turn-taking, asking for clarification)

    c. Being funny versus acting funny (knowing when to tell a joke and when doing so can be intrusive or offensive, knowing when to clown around and when to stop)

    d. Confidentiality and getting personal (what types of things to share, how to get someone's attention)

    e. Giving and accepting positive feedback (accepting praise without going overboard, offering criticism without being hurtful)

    f. Identifying feelings (yours and others')

    g. Anticipating problems and problem solving before, during and after moments of stress)

3. Find ways to build the student's self-concept, and help them to achieve and sustain a level of appreciation and positive status among their peers. For many students, this is often most easily accomplished by focusing on non-academic activities (for example: art, music, athletics), but may not hold true for students who have very particular areas of weakness. (I am reminded of a phrase used by NCLD's Professional Advisory Board member Dr. Sally Shaywitz, who refers to LD as "an island of weakness in a sea of strengths.")

4. Try to minimize competition and focus instead on cooperative learning. Whether in the home, at a job, or in the classroom, students are quick to compare their work with the performances of others. Rather than asking students to work independently, try to create opportunities for shared learning and joint activities. This is not only a wonderful way to build social and emotional connections, but an approach that has considerable merit in professional literature as a way to enhance student learning.

For More Information

National Center for Learning Disabilities
381 Park Ave. South, Suite 1401
New York, NY 10016
Toll-Free: 888-575-7373
Phone: 212-545-7510
Fax: 212-545-9665
Website: http://www.ld.org

Look here for a directory of useful resources for understanding and accessing information about different aspects of LD, including social and emotional development.

Chapter 60

Building Self-Esteem and Social Competence in Individuals with Learning Disabilities

Self-Esteem

For individuals with and without learning disabilities (LD), self-esteem is a powerful predictor of success. It has been said that positive self-esteem is as important to success in school and on the job as the mastery of individual skills. Learning disabilities, however, often pose formidable hurdles to positive self-esteem, and in turn contribute to a hard-to-break cycle of self-doubt, frustration, and failure.

What is self-esteem?

Self-esteem can be described as how we view ourselves in the context of our surroundings. It is shaped by how well we get along with peers and family members, and by how we judge ourselves in comparison to those around us. Whether at home, school, or the work place, self-esteem also is shaped by how well we understand and respond to ever-changing interpersonal demands. But it is precisely this area—the area of interpersonal relationships—in which individuals with LD may have the greatest difficulty, thus contributing to feelings of inadequacy and low self-esteem.

Not all people with LD have problems with social competence and self-esteem, but many do, and struggling daily with the challenges posed by a learning disability can erode enthusiasm and confidence.

Knowing one's assets and liabilities and feeling good about one's self can be invaluable in negotiating the sometimes tumultuous path to achievement in school, success in the workplace, and acceptance at home and in the community at large.

How does social competence affect self-esteem?

Building social competence is an important step in becoming a self-reliant and confident person. Socially competent people know how to easily move from person to person, or group to group, seemingly relaxed and at ease, regardless of whether they are talking or listening. They also know how to:

- initiate and maintain positive relationships with peers and others;
- interpret social situations, judging how to interact;
- interact without drawing negative attention to themselves;
- sustain attention on the speaker;
- contribute to conversations;
- control their impulses to draw attention to themselves, even in well-intended ways.

Once again, it is these traits that often pose the greatest challenges to individuals with LD.

What are the threats to self-esteem for individuals with LD?

Research has shown that being classified as having specific LD does not, in and of itself, negatively impact self-esteem. However, there are a number of characteristics, frequently observed in people with LD, which contribute to feelings of low self-worth.

Communication style and social awareness:

- May appear to be overly egocentric and disinterested in the opinions of other speakers (when nothing could be father from the truth)
- Has difficulty judging when it is his or her turn to participate in a conversation
- May misinterpret others' feelings
- Is unaware of when his or her behaviors are bothersome or annoying

- May have problems with visual-spatial planning and self-regulation, resulting in difficulties in judgment: they may mis-judge how close to stand to someone during conversation, how to assume and maintain a relaxed posture, or when it might be appropriate to touch

Self knowledge:

- Is unsure how to understand his or her personal strengths and weaknesses, or how to explain them to others
- Has trouble evaluating and reflecting on his or her behavior in social interactions

Language:

- Has limited vocabulary, or has difficulty retrieving the right words for the situation
- Has trouble with topic selection
- Talks around a topic, providing extraneous, less critical information in response to a question
- When asked to expand on something, is more likely to repeat rather than clarify his or her point
- In conversation, is more likely than peers to rely on gestures
- Is unsure when to end a conversation

Self-perceived social status:

- Has difficulty knowing how he or she fits in to a peer group, which often results in hanging back, being passive, or sticking out in a crowd for trying too hard to belong
- Has limited success getting noticed in positive ways within a peer group
- Is perceived as less popular and therefore more frequently rejected or ignored by peers—sometimes resulting in further self-imposed isolation

Self-perceived ability to effect change:

- Believes that outcomes are controlled by external influences (luck, chance, fate) rather than as a result of his or her own efforts

- Assumes a posture of learned helplessness: believes that because he or she struggled with something in the past, there is little they can do to change a negative outcome in the future, so they stop trying and hope for the best

What role do others' expectations play in self-esteem?

Unfortunately, individuals with LD are commonly confronted with low expectations from others. They are frequently, though not intentionally, the target of spoken and unspoken messages of disappointment from peers, parents, supervisors, and so forth. Others' low expectations may influence the expectations individuals with LD have of themselves, thereby serving to erode self-esteem.

What are some strategies for helping individuals with LD build self-esteem and confidence?

In their book, *The Power of Resilience: Achieving Balance, Confidence and Personal Strength in Your Life*, Dr. Robert Brooks and Dr. Sam Goldstein offer parents guideposts to help children and adolescents develop the strength and skills they need to cope successfully with the challenges they face. Here are some key things, adapted from the book, which parents can do to help:

- Be empathetic. See the world through your children's eyes.

- Communicate with respect. Don't interrupt or put them down; answer their questions.

- Give undivided attention. Children feel loved when we spend on-on-one time with them.

- Accept and love children for who they are. This will allow them to feel more secure in reaching out to others and learning how to solve problems.

- Give children a chance to contribute. This communicates your faith in their abilities and gives them a sense of responsibility.

- Treat mistakes as learning experiences. Children whose parents overreact to mistakes tend to avoid taking risks, then end up blaming others for their problems.

- Emphasize their strengths. A sense of accomplishment and pride give children the confidence to persevere when they face challenges.

- Let them solve problems and make decisions. Avoid telling children what to do; encourage them to come up with solutions to problems.

- Discipline to teach. Do not discipline in a way that intimidates or humiliates your child.

The Bottom Line

Throughout one's life, self-esteem and confidence are critical, and often elusive, ingredients for happiness and success. Individuals with LD are especially vulnerable to attacks on their feelings of self-worth; but with help and support, they can build the self-esteem it takes to achieve future success in any arena.

Chapter 61

Bullying among Children and Youth with Disabilities and Special Needs

What is bullying?

Bullying is aggressive behavior that is intentional and that involves an imbalance of power or strength. Often, it is repeated over time. Bullying can take many forms, such as hitting, kicking, or shoving (physical bullying), teasing or name-calling (verbal bullying), intimidation through gestures or social exclusion (nonverbal bullying or emotional bullying), and sending insulting messages by text messaging or e-mail (cyberbullying).

What is known about bullying among children with disabilities and special needs?

There is a small but growing amount of research literature on bullying among children with disabilities and special needs. This research indicates that these children may be at particular risk of being bullied by their peers. For example, research indicates the following:

- Although little research has been conducted on the relation between learning disabilities (LD) and bullying, available information indicates that children with LD are at greater risk of being teased and physically bullied.

This chapter includes text from "Bullying among Children and Youth with Disabilities and Special Needs," Health Resources and Services Administration (HRSA), 2005; and, the heading "Tips to Remember if Your Child Is Being Bullied," contains excerpts from "What to Do If Your Child Is Being Bullied," HRSA, 2004.

- Children with attention deficit/hyperactivity disorder (AD/HD) are more likely than other children to be bullied. They also are somewhat more likely than others to bully their peers.

- Children with medical conditions that affect their appearance (for example: cerebral palsy, muscular dystrophy, and spina bifida) are more likely to be victimized by peers. Frequently, these children report being called names related to their disability.

- Obesity also may place children at higher risk of being bullied. In a study of children aged 11–16, researchers found that overweight and obese girls (aged 11–16) and boys (aged 11–12) were more likely than normal-weight peers to be teased or to be made fun of and to experience relational bullying (to be socially excluded). Overweight and obese girls were also more likely to be physically bullied.

- Children with hemiplegia (paralysis of one side of their body) are more likely than other children their age to be victimized by peers, to be rated as less popular than their peers, and to have fewer friends than other children.

- Children who have diabetes and who are dependent on insulin may be especially vulnerable to peer bullying.

- Children who stutter may be more likely than their peers to be bullied. In one study, 83 percent of adults who had problems with stammering as children said that they had been teased or bullied; 71 percent of those who had been bullied said it happened at least once a week.

How does bullying affect children?

Bullying can have serious consequences. Children and youth who are bullied are more likely than other children to experience the following:

- depression, loneliness, anxiety
- low self-esteem
- headaches, stomachaches, fatigue, poor appetites
- absenteeism and dislike of school
- suicidal thoughts

Can bullying of my child be illegal?

Yes. Bullying behavior may cross the line to become disability harassment, which is illegal under Section 504 of the Rehabilitation Act of 1973 and Title II of the Americans with Disabilities Act of 1990. According to the U.S. Department of Education, disability harassment is "intimidation or abusive behavior toward a student based on disability that creates a hostile environment by interfering with or denying a student's participation in or receipt of benefits, services, or opportunities in the institution's program." This behavior can take different forms including verbal harassment, physical threats, or threatening written statements. When a school finds out that harassment may have occurred, staff must investigate the incident(s) promptly and respond appropriately.

Disability harassment can occur in any location that is connected with school: in classrooms, in the cafeteria, in hallways, on the playground or athletic fields, or on a school bus. It also can occur during school-sponsored events.

What can I do if I think my child is being bullied or is the victim of disability harassment?

- Be supportive of your child and encourage him or her to describe who was involved and how and where the bullying or harassment happened. Be sure to tell your child that it is not his or her fault and that nobody deserves to be bullied or harassed. Do not encourage your child to fight back. This may make the problem much worse.

- Usually children are able to identify when they are being bullied by their peers. Sometimes, however, children with disabilities do not realize they are being targeted. (They may, for example, believe that they have a new friend, when in fact, this "friend" is making fun of them.) Ask your child specific questions about his or her friendships and be alert to possible signs of bullying—even if your child doesn't label the behaviors as bullying.

- Talk with your child's teacher immediately to see whether he or she can help to resolve the problem quickly.

- If the bullying or harassment is severe, or if the teacher doesn't fix the problem quickly, contact the principal and put your concerns in writing. Explain what happened in detail and ask for a prompt response. Keep a written record of all conversations and communications with the school.

- Ask the school district to convene a meeting of the individualized education program (IEP) team or the Section 504 team, a group convened to ensure that the school district is meeting the needs of its students with disabilities. This meeting will allow you to explain what has been happening and will let the team review your child's IEP or 504 plan and make sure that the school is taking steps to stop the harassment. If your child needs counseling or other supportive services because of the harassment, discuss this with the team.

- As the U.S. Department of Education (2000) recognizes, "creating a supportive school climate is the most important step in preventing harassment." Work with the school to help establish a system-wide bullying prevention program that includes support systems for bullied children.

- Sometimes children and youth who are bullied also bully others. Explore whether your child may also be bullying other younger, weaker students at school. If so, his or her IEP may need to be modified to include help to change the aggressive behavior.

- Be persistent. Talk regularly with your child and with school staff to see whether the behavior has stopped.

Tips to Remember If Your Child Is Being Bullied

Children frequently do not tell their parents that they are being bullied because they are embarrassed, ashamed, frightened of the children who are bullying them, or afraid of being seen as a tattler. If your child tells you about being bullied, it has taken a lot of courage to do so. Your child needs your help to stop the bullying.

Focus on Your Child

Be supportive and gather information about the bullying.

- Never tell your child to ignore the bullying. What the child may hear is that you are going to ignore it. If the child were able to simply ignore it, he or she likely would not have told you about it. Often, trying to ignore bullying allows it to become more serious.

- Don't blame the child who is being bullied. Don't assume that your child did something to provoke the bullying. Don't say, "What did you do to aggravate the other child?"

514

- Listen carefully to what your child tells you about the bullying. Ask him or her to describe who was involved and how and where each bullying episode happened.

- Learn as much as you can about the bullying tactics used, and when and where the bullying happened. Can your child name other children or adults who may have witnessed the bullying?

- If you disagree with how your child handled the bullying situation, don't criticize him or her.

- Do not encourage physical retaliation (just hit them back) as a solution. Hitting another student is not likely to end the problem, and it could get your child suspended or expelled or escalate the situation.

- Check your emotions. A parent's protective instincts stir strong emotions. Although it is difficult, a parent is wise to step back and consider the next steps carefully.

Contact Your Child's Teacher or Principal

- Parents are often reluctant to report bullying to school officials, but bullying may not stop without the help of adults.

- Keep your emotions in check. Give factual information about your child's experience of being bullied including who, what, when, where, and how.

- Emphasize that you want to work with the staff at school to find a solution to stop the bullying, for the sake of your child as well as other students.

- Do not contact the parents of the student(s) who bullied your child. This is usually a parent's first response, but sometimes it makes matters worse. School officials should contact the parents of the child or children who did the bullying.

- Expect the bullying to stop. Talk regularly with your child and with school staff to see whether the bullying has stopped. If the bullying persists, contact school authorities again.

Help Your Child Become More Resilient to Bullying

- Help to develop talents or positive attributes of your child. Suggest and facilitate music, athletics, and art activities. Doing so may help your child be more confident among his or her peers.

515

- Encourage your child to make contact with friendly students in his or her class. Your child's teacher may be able to suggest students with whom your child can make friends, spend time, or collaborate on work.

- Help your child meet new friends outside of the school environment. A new environment can provide a fresh start for a child who has been bullied repeatedly.

- Teach your child safety strategies. Teach him or her how to seek help from an adult when feeling threatened by a bully. Talk about whom he or she should go to for help and role-play what he or she should say. Assure your child that reporting bullying is not the same as tattling.

- Ask yourself if your child is being bullied because of a learning difficulty or a lack of social skills? If your child is hyperactive, impulsive, or overly talkative, the child who bullies may be reacting out of annoyance. This doesn't make the bullying right, but it may help to explain why your child is being bullied. If your child easily irritates people, seek help from a counselor so that your child can better learn the informal social rules of his or her peer group.

- Home is where the heart is. Make sure your child has a safe and loving home environment where he or she can take shelter, physically and emotionally. Always maintain open lines of communication with your child.

What If the Bullying or Harassment Does Not Stop?

If your school district, does not take reasonable, appropriate steps to end the bullying or harassment of your child, the district may be violating federal, state, and local laws. For more information about your legal rights, you may want to contact:

U.S. Department of Education Office for Civil Rights
Toll-Free: 800-421-3481
Website: http://www.ed.gov/about/offices/list/ocr/index.html

U.S. Department of Education Office of Special Education Programs
Phone: 202-245-7468
Website: http:////www.ed.gov/about/offices/list/osers/osep/ index.html

Chapter 62

Ten Things You Can Do to Support a Person with Difficult Behaviors

Supporting a person with difficult behaviors begins when we make a commitment to know the person. Sadly, it is often the case that the people who develop an intervention to stop someone from engaging in difficult behaviors do not know the individual in any meaningful sense. Instead, they see the person as someone (or something) that needs to be fixed, or modified. But attacking a person's behavior is usually ineffective and always disrespectful.

Think about someone you know who engages in difficult behaviors. Ask yourself, "What kind of life is this person living?" Consider how you would feel if you lived the person's life. How would you behave?

What follows are ten things you can do to support a person whose behavior is troubling you. It is not a list of "quick fix" strategies for stopping unwanted behavior. It is a list of ideas for uncovering the real things that a person might need so that you can be more supportive.

1. Get to Know the Person

The first step in supporting a person with difficult behaviors almost seems too obvious to state: get to know the person. It is too often the case that people who develop interventions to eliminate unwanted behavior do not know the person in any meaningful sense. They know the person as the sum total of his or her labels, but know little about the person as a "whole" human being.

Make a point of spending time with the person in places that he or she enjoys, during times of the day that he or she chooses. It should be a comfortable place where both of you can feel safe and relaxed (for example: a quiet room, a nice restaurant, a walking trail in a nearby park).

At a time that feels right (you will have to trust your intuition on this one), tell the person about your concerns and ask for permission to help (it's rude not to). If the person has no formal means of communication, ask anyway. Sometimes people understand what is being said, but they have a difficult time letting others know that they understand. The important point, always, is to ask the person for permission to stick your nose into their business, even at the risk of seeming silly in front of people who think the person cannot understand up from down (they're usually wrong).

2. Remember That All Behavior Is Meaningful

Difficult behaviors are messages which can tell us important things about a person and the quality of her life. In the most basic terms: difficult behaviors result from unmet needs. The very presence of a difficult behavior can be a signal that something important that the person needs is missing. Here are some examples of the kinds of the kinds of messages a person may be conveying with his or her behavior:

- *I'm lonely*: Michael's older brother was invited over to a friend's house for a sleep over. Michael is never invited to the homes of children because he goes to a "special" school 35 miles from his neighborhood. Michael has no friends to play with.

- *I'm bored:* Roberta's sister is a doctor at the local hospital. She has her own house and is her parent's pride and joy. Roberta works all day at a sheltered workshop where she packages plastic forks and knives. She lives at home and is tired of packaging. She wants to get a real job. Roberta's case manager says she day dreams too much.

- *I have no power:* John likes to sit down on the sidewalk when the bus arrives to take him to school. His mother becomes very angry and tells him that there will be no dessert when he gets home. John laughs when the bus driver threatens him with time-out.

- *I don't feel safe:* Conrad uses a wheelchair and is not able to defend himself adequately from attacks by another man. Conrad worries that he will be hurt and often cries when left alone. Staff think he has a psychiatric illness.

- *You don't value me:* Gloria has a "severe reputation." People from all over the state have heard stories about her terrible tantrums. No one knows that she is a very caring person who worries about environmental issues. The only part of Gloria people pay attention to is her problem behaviors.

- *I don't know how to tell you what I need:* June does not know how to use words or sign to let other people know what she was thinking. She lives in an institution where she learned that the best way to get people's attention was to bite your arms. It hurts, but it is the only thing that "works."

- *My ears hurt:* Walter hits his ears with his fists. His job coach wants to stop and wrote a behavior plan for "not hitting." Weeks later, at a scheduled doctor's appointment, it was learned that Walter had a low-grade ear infection. Antibiotics cleared up the infection and Walter has stopped hitting his ears.

- *My body does not move like I want it to:* Aaron wanted to order a hamburger at a the restaurant, but his mouth kept saying, "I want pizza." When the waiter brought him pizza, he became so upset he knocked it on the floor. Later, at home, he typed to his mom, "I wanted a hamburger but I couldn't stop saying, 'I want pizza'." Aaron experiences differences from other people in the way his body moves (see Anne Donnellan and Martha Leary's book, *Movement Differences and Diversity in Autism/Mental Retardation: Appreciating and Accommodating Persons with Communication and Behavior Challenges*, available through Autism National Committee Bookstore, 800-378-0386 or http://iodserver.unh.edu/iodbookstore).

Obviously there are many needs that a person may be conveying with his or her behaviors. A single behavior can "mean" many things. The important point is that difficult behaviors do not occur without reason. All behavior, even if it is self-destructive, is "meaning-full."

Ask the person (and/or the person's supporters) what he or she needs to be happy. Find out who he or she counts on in a pinch. How often does he or she see loved ones and friends? What are his or her favorite activities? Where does he or she like to go? Ask the person what leads to unhappiness. Who are the people who the person does not like? How often does he or she see them? What are the person's least favorite activities? Since many people are experiencing physical and/or psychiatric distress, it's also important to know something about the person's physical and emotional health. Does the person have a way to let others know what he or she needs and feels? Is the person experiencing physiological or psychological distress? What kinds of medications is he or she taking? Do they help?

Finally, if you're stumped, ask, "Are there times when the person exhibits this behavior frequently?" and "Are there times when person exhibits this behavior infrequently or not at all?" Answering these two questions can tell you a great deal about the meaning of the person's behavior. With time, you should be able to see a discernible pattern.

For example, you might find that the person engages in the difficult behavior in the morning hours, but rarely in the afternoon. Ask, "What happens in the morning that might cause the person to behave this way?" or, conversely, "What is happening in the afternoon that causes the person not to behave this way?" (Hint: It often has something to do with the things a person is being asked to do, and/or who is asking the person to do it.)

3. Help the Person to Develop a Support Plan

People who exhibit difficult behaviors are usually subjected to a behavior plan at some point in their lives. It is rare that they are asked if they want a plan, let alone invited to the meetings where one is developed. Instead, a plan is developed by strangers (for example, the agency behaviorist who has spent less than two hours "observing" the person).

Think about how difficult it would be to stop a behavior that a stranger thinks you should stop. It can be difficult enough to stop behaviors we choose to stop (for example, smoking or excessive eating).

Instead of a behavior plan to "fix" the person, help the person and the person's supporters to develop a support plan that reflects a real and authentic life. John and Connie Lyle O'Brien suggest the following questions for building a support plan. Note how different these questions are from those we typically ask, such as "How can we reduce this person's problem behaviors?" or "How can we manage this behavior?"

1. How can we help the person to achieve health and well-being?

2. How can we help the person to maintain his or her relationships and make new ones?

3. How can we help the person to increase his or her presence and participation in everyday community life?

4. How can we help the person to have more choices in life?

5. How can we help the person to learn skills that enhance his or her participation in community life?

6. How can we help the person to make a contribution to others? The team can ask, "Is our vision for the person similar to the vision we hold for ourselves and each other? When we think about what the person needs, do we focus on "fixing" deficits, or do we think about supporting the person in achieving a real life?"

4. Develop a Support Plan for the Person's Supporters

Just as it is simplistic to treat a person's behavior without understanding something about the life the person lives, it is simplistic to develop a support plan without considering the needs of the person's supporters.

Many of our school and human service delivery systems are based on the idea that a few people with greater knowledge and power should bestow care and skills to a larger number of people with lesser knowledge and power. "Success" is based on compliance or obedience. A person who engages in difficult behaviors presents a real threat to a caregiver or teacher whose competence is being judged by this "compliance/obedience" yardstick. The caregiver often expends great energy trying to suppress the person's behavior in order to maintain "competence" (in many of our workplaces it is acceptable to share knowledge but not to share power).

Punishment or the fear of punishment (coercion) may be the primary means of "motivating" staff. Many approach each day with a mixture of fear and dread. If they make a mistake, they could be written up, demoted, or fired. If they try something new, it may violate a policy or procedure. The unspoken message is do as you are told or suffer the consequences. Many of our human services environments are toxic with fear.

It is in this context that human services workers are told to be supportive. Workers are trained in positive approaches when the underlying organizational message is "maintain obedience." Under the deadening weight of these systems, even the kindest and most respectful of caregivers may begin to exhibit their own difficult behaviors. They become excessively controlling and resistant to change. They begin to believe that individuals are worthy of their labels and beyond hope. They may even resort to forms of punishment procedures that the average citizen would find repulsive and unacceptable.

Take time with your colleagues to develop support plans for each other. For example, what can you do to increase each other's level of safety and comfort when someone is behaving dangerously? What can you do to have more fun at work? How can you have more control over your schedule and input into decisions? How can managers better support you?

A fundamental question is, "If you stopped responding to the person's difficult behavior the way you do now, who would you be?"

5. Don't Assume Anything

It is easy to make the mistake of underestimating a person's potential because of his or her labels or because he or she has failed to acquire certain skills. This is a tragic mistake.

I have worked in the field for 15 years and am less confident in my ability to predict how much a person understands with every passing day. Recent developments make clear the folly of making predictions about a person's potential on the basis of diagnostic labels or past performance. Hundreds of thousands of people deemed unfit for society have left our institutions and now live in community. One hundred twenty thousand people who were assessed to be unemployable because of the severity of their disability now work and pay taxes thanks to supported employment services.

The very definition of mental retardation itself has changed in recent years. The American Association for Mental Retardation (AAMR) has recently overhauled the definition. Gone are pessimistic predictions that saw little hope for the severely retarded and profoundly retarded. The new definition eliminates such terms altogether and emphasizes the importance of our supports. In short, an individual's potential depends largely upon the adequacy of his or her supports rather than some inherent flaw or defect.

Always remember that people are people first. Labels tell us nothing (in any real sense) about how we can be supportive. We need not forget the person's problem behaviors, but we must understand that people have gifts and capacities that eclipse our labels (or, as Herb Lovett has said, our clinical accusations).

Always remember to speak directly to the person and explain things as clearly as you can, even if the person's labels suggest that he or she cannot understand (at the very least the person will understand the tone of your voice). Never speak about the person as if he or she were not in the room.

6. Relationships Make All the Difference

Loneliness is the most significant disability of our time. Many people with disabilities, young and old, live lives of extraordinary isolation. Some depend entirely upon their families for support. A brother, sister, mom, or dad, are the only source of company. Friends are often absent altogether.

All too often, the only relationships people have are with paid staff. Although staff can offer a great deal, they change jobs frequently or take on new responsibilities. The resulting instability can be devastating to someone who is fundamentally alone.

Remember that there are many people in the community who will benefit from knowing the person. Chances are the person has already made someone's life fuller. Be confident that she or he will make someone's life richer again and again.

Learn more about personal futures planning and other person-centered approaches to planning.

7. Help the Person to Develop a Positive Identity

John Bradshaw writes, "Our identity is the difference about us that makes a difference." Many people with disabilities develop identities as "problem people." They are segregated into "special" programs where they are treated as people who have little to offer. Soon their "treatment" becomes a kind of cage to protect them from themselves and others. The real danger is that if enough people begin to think of the person as a problem, he or she will begin to believe it too.

We all need to be needed: Help the person to find a way to make a contribution. Start when the person is young if you can. Giving is a lifelong endeavor. Things as simple as helping with household chores or helping out at church can teach the person that she can make a contribution.

Pour over the newspaper and find the "Volunteers Needed" section. Talk to the person about joining an organization with you or with a friend (for example: Habitat for Humanity, a local food shelter, an environmental group).

Help the person to learn how to support friends (for example: an invitation to a sleep over, birthday cards, learning to ask "How are you doing?" or "What's new?").

Remember that it is important to overcome the belief that the person has nothing to share. It takes time and determination to help the person and others to see strength and the capacity to give when deficits were all that anyone ever saw before.

8. Instead of Ultimatums, Give Choices

Choice is a powerful alternative to punishment. If the person's behavior challenges you, help him to find more desirable ways to express

523

the needs underlying the behaviors. Instead of ultimatums, give choices. For example: "Bill, I know you're upset. What would help? Would you like to go for a walk, or take a ride? You need a chance to calm down."

Allow the person to make decisions throughout the day. If he or she has trouble making choices, find a way to help. Make sure there are at least three desirable outcomes to choose from. As Norman Kunc has said, "one option = tyranny; two options = a dilemma; three or more options = a real choice."

Don't assume that helping the person to have more choices means letting him or her do whatever he or she wishes. Setting limits is an important and fair part of any relationship. The real question is who is setting the limits and why. If limits are imposed upon the person without their input, and if the limits are part and parcel of a life in which the person is powerless, even your best advice may even be interpreted as one more statement of "do it my way or else." You can expect a general disregard for your advice if the person on the receiving end of the advice is "out of power."

Make a sustained commitment to the person and to fairness in the relationship. If the person has been on the outside of power for too long, you may need to bend more often than not for awhile. The goal is to teach the person that giving is a two-way street.

9. Help the Person to Have More Fun

Fun is a powerful antidote to problem behaviors. People with significant disabilities often live in ghettos of reward. Indeed, it is often this poverty of reward, not a lack of skills, which keeps people separate from other community members. Many must endure reward schedules for good behavior. The very few things that they enjoy are used contingently to reinforce compliance—talk about spoiling a good thing.

Count the number of things the person enjoys, the number of places he or she likes to go. Compare this to the number of things other people enjoy, the number of places other people go. Ask yourself, "Is the person having fun? Is he or she experiencing enough joy? Is this an interesting life with things to look forward to?"

Help the person to add to his or her list of interesting (and really fun) things to do. Spend time in regular community places where people hang out. If you feel compelled to take data on something, take data on the amount of fun you find. Make fun a goal.

10. Establish a Good Working Relationship with the Person's Primary Health Care Physician

Mark Durand has said, "People tend to get immature when they don't feel well." How often have you experienced a general decline in your mood or your ability to empathize with the needs of others when you don't feel well? When we are sick, we are not ourselves.

Many people who exhibit difficult behaviors do so because they don't feel well. The sudden appearance of behavior problems may be a signal that the person does not feel well. Illnesses as common as a cold or earache can result in behaviors as inconsequential as grumpiness or as serious as head banging.

It is important to establish a working relationship with a good primary health care physician. Although this is easier said than done, the person will—especially if he has difficulty communicating—need a doctor who can help him or her to stay healthy and well.

Remember that physicians, like many other people who grew up in our separate society do not always understand (and may even fear) a person with substantial disabilities.

Don't be afraid of telling the person's doctor that you don't understand a recommendation or finding. It is important to get a clear and straightforward answer to all of your questions.

Remember too that it is important to go beyond a concept of health as the absence of a disease or illness. Feeling well and being healthy involves everything from a balanced diet to a good night's sleep. Help the person to achieve a state of wellness.

For More Information

Imagine
3694 Mt. Tabor Road
Blacksburg, VA 24060
Phone: 540-552-5629
Website: http://www.dimagine.com
E-mail: Dimagine@aol.com.

Dr. Pitonyak's website offers a variety of resources and information dedicated to supporting people who experience disabilities.

Chapter 63

Tips to Help Your Child with Learning Disabilities Transition to School and Work

Chapter Contents

Section 63.1

Planning for Your Child's Transition from Adolescence to Adulthood

Planning for your child's transition from adolescence to adulthood is one of the most important things you can do to pave the way to a successful future. In Minnesota, special education transition planning and services begin when your child with a disability is 14. From then on, you and your child will start learning new skills side-by-side. Your child will begin to take on more responsibility, and you will find new ways to provide support. It can be a challenge. Depending on your child's disability, you may need to consider everything from post-secondary education to employment, from housing to finances. As you and your son or daughter plan for the future, consider these tips to help build a successful transition.

1. Help build your son's or daughter's self-determination and self-advocacy skills.

All young people should have a strong sense of their strengths, abilities, and interests. If students have a disability, they should also be aware of how it might affect them at work, in the community, and in their educational pursuits. Transition is a wonderful time to explore how youth will talk about their disability in different settings and ask for any support or accommodation they will need.

2. Help develop your child's social outlets.

Social relationships and recreation are more than fun; they are important tools that help tie people into the community and provide a wider network of support. Although social isolation can be an issue for many young adults with disabilities, transition planning that addresses opportunities for social relationships and recreation can build a bridge to success.

3. Expand your network and explore community supports.

As children with disabilities become adults with disabilities, they may need support from a variety of sources. Start now to develop helpful networks for your child. Who do you know in your family, social group, professional circle, religious community, or other sphere who could help provide social, recreational, work, or volunteer experiences for your young adult? Look, too, at adults in the community who have the same disability as your child to learn what kinds of supports they use.

4. Make sure your son registers with Selective Service at age 18.

All males—including those with disabilities—must register with Selective Service within 30 days of their 18th birthday. (Exceptions are made for young men in institutional care.) Failure to do so can affect a person's ability to receive federal and state benefits, including student loans, job training, and government jobs. Learn more at http://www.sss.gov.

5. Explore post-secondary accommodations.

Students who receive academic programming and support in high school through individualized education programs (IEP) and 504 plans will not automatically have the same support after they graduate. Although post-secondary institutions are required to provide reasonable accommodations to students with disabilities, they are not required to modify course work, if it would substantially change program requirements. When you and your student visit a prospective school, visit the campus's disability services office to:

* explore how to document your student's disability;

* ask if you can talk with other students and families about their experiences in this particular program;

* inquire about what accommodations are available. In addition to note takers, extended time, and alternative testing environments, are other, less common services offered?

6. Investigate Supplemental Security Income (SSI) programs.

Financial planning is an important part of transition. Many people with disabilities are beneficiaries of SSI, a federal program that provides a monthly benefit check that can help pay for living expenses. A lesser-known program of SSI, called Plan for Achieving Self-Support (PASS), may be helpful to some SSI recipients. It allows a person with disabilities to set aside income and resources in order to reach a work goal. These goals could include such things as enrolling in an educational or training program; obtaining supported employment; starting a business; or purchasing a vehicle to commute to work.

7. Encourage your child to build a résumé by volunteering.

Many young people struggle to find work experiences that help them compete in the job market. Volunteering is a great solution. Young adults can gain skills and build a résumé that shows a prospective employer their abilities, initiative, and dedication to work. Volunteering can also help develop additional social skills, especially if it is done along with a parent, friend, or group of peers.

8. Help your child learn soft employment skills.

In addition to the work skills people need for their jobs, they also need soft skills. These include such things as being able to accept direction, ask for help, deal with conflict, and engage in interpersonal communication. They also include being prompt, having appropriate hygiene, and dressing properly for the workplace. An employer is more likely to be patient with an employee learning the technical aspects of a job if soft skills are in place. You can help your young adult develop these skills by practicing them at home.

9. Plan for health care management.

Like most people, young adults with disabilities need to manage their health care and insurance. You should develop a clear plan on how to address health care needs once your child reaches adulthood.

10. Call PACER Center for information and resources.

The transition staff at PACER Center can help you prepare your son or daughter for the adult world. Trained advocates can help you understand your rights and find resources to help with all aspects of transition. To speak with a transition expert, call PACER at 952-838-9000, or visit http://www.pacer.org online.

Section 63.2

Transitioning from College to Work

Transitioning from college to work, like transitioning through secondary education, is a process. Students must begin this process early and transfer their knowledge of the disability into the world of employment. Students should consider the following:

- What is the impact of the learning disability (LD) on job performance?

- How or when does one disclose a disability?

- What are typical accommodations made in the workforce?

- What kinds of social demands and interactions are needed?

Students must recognize the disability's impact on both educational and career choices. An important variable in relation to job satisfaction is a clear understanding of one's disability. Knowledge of one's disability and how it affects work are critical to satisfying employment. In addition to clearly understanding their disability, students need to identify their goals. They must analyze vocational goals in relation to their disability. What kind of tasks will the job entail? What will be the interaction between the job tasks and the disability? When answering these questions, the individual should evaluate the work environment, the type and amount of colleague interaction, specific tasks one must perform, and how one is evaluated.

At the College Level

Choosing a Major and Career

Choosing a major, and the career that ensues, is a difficult and anxiety provoking task for most students. Students can seek help with this process:

531

- Read the catalog and course descriptions carefully.

- Work with your academic adviser and discuss the requirements for different majors.

- Make an appointment with faculty members in the departments that interest you. Learn what kinds of jobs people who have graduated from these programs have gotten.

- Investigate whether your school has any job shadowing or mentoring programs.

- Consider doing an internship.

- Meet with the disability service provider and discuss how your disability might be an issue in the work setting.

Skill Development

Students strengthen the likelihood for successful, satisfying employment by developing their basic skills and learning strategies. It is important for students to take advantage of reading and writing laboratories, and any other academic resources to enhance skills. One of the most important areas to develop is an understanding of available technologies. Many facets of the employment world rely on technology. The new technologies also offer many advances that can be useful accommodations for some individuals.

The Laws That Govern Employment

It is important for students to learn about the laws that recognize their rights to equal access and non-discrimination. They should clearly understand the aspects of the Americans with Disabilities Act (ADA) and the Rehabilitation Act of 1973, Section 504, which assure equal access and non-discrimination. It is not enough to merely know one's legal rights. Students must recognize how equal access applies to them individually, within that particular setting, and in relation to the disability. They need to ask themselves the following questions:

- Is it necessary for me to disclose my disability in order to perform more efficiently?

- To whom do I disclose?

- How do I disclose?

- When do I disclose?

- How do I negotiate accommodations?

Being able to articulate the effect of the disability in relation to the work environment is central to successful employment.

Steps to Successful Employment

Develop a History of Work Experience

Look for opportunities to gain work experience. Some examples include:

- campus leadership opportunities (for example: student government, mentoring programs, organization involvement);
- work study positions on campus;
- internships;
- off-campus jobs that may be listed in the college career center;
- summer jobs; and,
- networking with family and friends about job opportunities.

Understand the Job Culture

Every company or organization has its own unique culture. The culture consists of company rules, values, and beliefs, which are widely held but often unspoken.

- Observe your co-workers.
- Know what is expected of you.
- Watch how others communicate and interact.

Job Accommodations

Match job tasks with individual strengths and weaknesses to identify specific accommodations that will enhance job performance. Accommodations that may be used in the workplace include the following:

- Tape recorders
- Taped materials
- Dictation
- Written instructions
- Demonstration of tasks and assignments
- Diagrams to explain an assignment

- Extended time on projects
- Separate work space
- Spelling and grammar check software for computers
- A word processor
- Color coding of files
- Talking computers or spell checkers

Identify and Tap into Your Support System

- Family, loved ones, friends, and co-workers can be a critical variable to successful employment.
- Devise an individualized plan for employment (IPE): Clients of the Office of Vocational Rehabilitation (OVR—in some states called Rehabilitative Services Administration, or RSA) can work with counselors to design an individualized plan regarding employment, assessments, and services related to employment.

Ways to Develop Job Skills

- Job shadowing
- Coaching and mentoring
- Seeking assistance from the following:
    - Office of Vocational Rehabilitation
    - Equal Employment Opportunity Commission at 800-669-4000 or online at http://www.eeoc.gov
    - HEATH Resource Center at http://www.heath.gwu.edu
    - Job Accommodation Network (JAN) at http://www.jan.wvu.edu
    - National Rehabilitation Information Center at 800-346-2742 or http://www.naric.com
    - *Peterson's Internships*. Published by Peterson's Guides at http://www.petersons.com

Chapter 64

Finding a Job If You Have a Disability

Chapter Contents

Section 64.1

Elements and Strategies of an Effective Job Search

This section includes text from "Ed Kit 1997: Essential Elements of an Effective Job Search," U.S. Department of Labor, 1997; and "Strategies to Consider in Seeking Employment," Job Accommodation Network (JAN), U.S. Department of Labor, August 4, 2007.

What Job Seekers with Disabilities Need to Know

Whether you are entering the workforce for the first time, returning to the job market, or seeking advancement, the challenges of a job search are similar. Your goal is to find the position that best meets your needs. You must be qualified and able to sell yourself as the best applicant for the job(s) for which you apply. Here are some tips that can help you in meeting your job search goal.

Know Thyself

Have a strong sense of who you are. Know your assets and how to market them to employers.

Be Committed to Lifelong Change

Follow job trends. Take the initiative to maintain cutting edge skills that match changing employer requirements.

Be Computer Literate

Increasing your technical computer skills increases your marketability in the job market. Conduct online job searches. Visit employer web pages and key job sites such as:

- Careerbuilder.com at http://www.careerbuilder.com;
- CareerPath at http://www.careerpath.com;
- Monster Board at http://www.monster.com.

536

Update Your Resume Often

Customize your resume to reflect the assets you bring to each job. Use key words that can be electronically scanned by potential employers to positions you want. Reflect continuous employment in your skill area. Summer employment should support your field of interest. Volunteer or obtain temporary jobs if you are unemployed. Select a resume format that minimizes any gaps in employment.

Be Your Best

Locating a job is a full time endeavor. Give full attention to all that you do. Errors will knock you out of the running.

Be Organized

Have a written personal plan for vertical and lateral growth opportunities. Know what you must do each day to move closer to your goal. Stay focused.

Expand Your Network

Maintain and continuously strive to broaden your network. If you are working, network inside the company. Join professional groups.

Research Job Trends and Companies

Select targets of opportunity that match your skill areas. Request and study annual reports of select companies. Reflect each company's image in all communications with each company's representatives. Make good use of library resources. Read trade journals and business publications.

Have a Positive Attitude

A pleasant personality is a necessary asset. Your eagerness to adapt and to be a team player is essential. Show that you are flexible. A sense of humor and positive attitude are pluses.

Disclose a Disability Only as Needed

The only reason to disclose a disability is if you require an accommodation for an interview or to perform the essential functions of a particular job. Your resume and cover letter should focus on the abilities you bring to the job, not on your disability.

537

Be Prepared to Conduct an Effective Interview

Look your best from head to toe. Dress conservatively. Be brief and to the point when answering interview questions. Maintain a demeanor of success and reflect the company image when you respond. Have full confidence in what you bring to the employer and show how your skills meet the company's specific hiring needs. Ask thoughtful questions about the job and the company. Never say anything negative. Follow up immediately with a thank-you letter or e-mail transmission.

Remember

Push yourself to go the extra mile in your job search and you will find the opportunity you are seeking.

Strategies to Consider in Seeking Employment

- Use personal contacts to find out about possible jobs. Personal contacts could be friends or family; former co-workers or employers; members of your religious organization; local community members such as doctors, physical therapists, counselors; members of professional organizations or social clubs, and so forth.

- Visit or set up informational interviews with as many employers as you can. You may need to visit or telephone many employers in order to know who is hiring and when.

- College, university, or vocational-technical school placement offices offer job placement and career development services.

- The public library may be able to provide employment information.

- Independent living centers may provide employment leads and job club services for individuals with disabilities.

- Classified ads found in the newspaper, local bulletin boards, or professional magazines may be useful.

- Advocacy and support groups may provide employment assistance.

- Public and private employment agencies circulate resumes and match appropriate job candidates.

- Job banks provide computerized listings of jobs that you can be matched up with nationwide openings.

- Use the internet to find employment opportunities. Local libraries usually have computers to access the internet.

- Volunteer activities can sometimes lead to paid employment and can provide good work experience to include on a resume.

- Temporary staffing agencies may work for you. Temporary staffing agencies work with people with disabilities in the same way they work with people without disabilities. Temporary work can help you to build a work history, experience different types of jobs, increase your skills, and the amount of money you can earn.

- These strategies may help to find a job. However, these suggestions are not all inclusive.

Section 64.2

A Practical Approach to Looking for a Job as a Person with Disability

Text is this section is excerpted from "Finding a Job That Is Right for You: A Practical Approach to Looking for a Job as a Person with Disability, Steps 1–4," Job Accommodation Network (JAN), U.S. Department of Labor, August 2006.

What Kind of Job Is Right for You?

Where are the jobs?

The U.S. Department of Labor, Bureau of Labor Statistics *Occupational Outlook Handbook* is a nationally recognized information source describing tasks workers do on the job, working conditions, training and education needed, earnings, and expected job prospects now and in the future.

Additionally, the U.S. Department of Labor, Bureau of Labor Statistics provides up-to-date information on largest employment declines, occupations with the largest job growth, and fastest growing occupations. It is available on the internet at http://www.bls.gov.

- A specific job and general job descriptions can be found in the U.S. Department of Labor's occupational information O*Net website at http://online.onetcenter.org.

- To determine if you have the skills to perform the job, review the Princeton Review Career Quiz—a free online career assessment tool at http://www.princetonreview.com/login3.aspx?RDN=1&uidbadge=%07.

- Other online tools and worksheets to assist you with finding the kind of job you are looking for are available at http://www.jan.wvu.edu/job/Step1.htm.

Does this job meet your financial needs?

One question often asked is "How much does the job pay?" A good online resource to answer this question comes from http://www.salary.com. This site takes the job, location, and cost of living for a region to provide a customized report of salary expectations. Once you know the expected salary, compare this with your budget.

What other options are there to help me enter the workforce?

An employment option many people choose is a temporary agency. The U.S. Department of Labor, Office of Disability Employment Policy has a publication, *People with Disabilities—Temporary Employment Options* designed to explore this option. Temporary agency employment is an excellent way to get back into the workforce, gain skills, and reorient you to the job market.

Two of the largest temporary agencies are:

- Manpower at http://www.manpower.com; and,

- Kelly Services at http://www.kellyservices.us.

Are there any special federal government programs to hire people with disabilities?

Selective placement gives federal agencies incentives for hiring people with disabilities. Qualified applicants can be placed into federal agency jobs without going through the competitive placement process. Additional information about federal employment for people with disabilities can be found through the U.S. Office of Personnel Management online at http://www.opm.gov/disability/PeopleWithDisabilities.asp.

Is self-employment right for you?

The Research and Training Center on Disability in Rural Communities has a self-assessment for individuals considering self-employment available at http://selfemploymenttraining.ruralinstitute.umt.edu/chapter4.htm. If you determine self-employment is for you, the U.S. Department of Labor Office of Disability Employment Policy's Small Business and Self-Employment Service (SBSES) housed at the Job Accommodation Network can help identify resources in your area to assist you.

What about work-from-home?

Work-from-home is an employment option especially for individuals who have difficulty with transportation, fatigue, or specific schedules.

Can you turn a volunteer position into gainful employment?

Volunteering at community service organizations can sometimes lead to employment opportunities. Volunteering allows you the opportunity to showcase your skills and abilities to business and civic leaders in your area. Volunteer Match at http://www.volunteermatch.org is dedicated to matching a volunteer with organizations who need volunteers in a geographical area.

What internships may be available?

Internships can help launch a college student or recent graduate into the job market. Several websites post intern opportunities such as InternJobs.com; StudentJobs.gov, which provides information on federal government job opportunities; InternshipPrograms.com; and Rising Star Internships.

Certain internship programs were specifically developed for students and recent graduates with disabilities.

- The Workforce Recruitment Program from the U.S. Department of Labor, Office of Disability Employment Policy actively recruits students with disabilities on college campuses (http://www.dol.gov/odep/pubs/brochures/wrp1.html).

- Career Opportunities for Students with Disabilities (COSD) is a unique consortium composed of large and small universities, well known national employers, and U.S. Government agencies focused on the career employment of college graduates with disabilities (http://www.cosdonline.org).

- Emerging Leaders helps college students with disabilities find and secure fulfilling internship and leadership opportunities. Emerging Leaders helps corporate and nonprofit employers find outstanding young talent for their business ventures and helps managers understand the benefits of considering diversity and inclusion in their hiring practices (http://www.emerging-leaders.com).

- Entry Point is a program of the American Association for the Advancement of Science (AAAS) offering outstanding internship opportunities for students with disabilities in science, engineering, mathematics, computer science, and some fields of business (http://ehrweb.aaas.org/entrypoint).

- The National Science Foundation's Facilitation Awards for Scientists and Engineers with Disabilities lists opportunities for scientists and engineers with disabilities (http://www.nsf.gov/pubs/2002/nsf02115/nsf02115.htm).

I am a young adult with a disability. Are there any programs to help me get the training I need to enter the workforce?

If you are a young person with a disability, then you may want to check out the Job Corps Program. The Job Corps Program is a no-cost education and vocational training program administered by the U.S. Department of Labor for young U.S. citizens ages 16 through 24 who meet income guidelines. Job Corps helps young people learn a trade, earn a high school diploma or general educational development (GED), and get help finding a good job.

Job Corps
Toll-Free: 800-733-5627
Website: http://jobcorps.doleta.gov

Who Can Help You to Find the Right Job?

As a person with a disability, who can help me find a job?

Your state rehabilitation agency can provide you with a counselor and can help you get a vocational assessment, get training or education, prepare your resume, and assist with your job search.

I am receiving social security benefits. Are there any programs designed to help me find work?

If you receive benefits from the Social Security Administration (SSA), then you may want to ask for help from an Employment Network. These Employment Networks work with the Social Security's Ticket-to-Work Program to find jobs for people who receive social security benefits. These employment networks, like the state vocational rehabilitation agencies, are funded to help you get a job.

If you are receiving Social Security benefits, then you may also want to talk with a Benefits Planning Assistance and Outreach (BPAO) counselor about how working will affect your social security benefits. People often fear losing Medicare/Medicaid coverage and SSI/SSDI benefits before their work income is high enough to cover living expenses.

Are there local resources where I can go to find a job?

If you are looking for local help, you will definitely want to visit your local One-Stop Career Center. One-Stop Centers are local employment or career offices throughout the country. The U.S Department of Labor funds these Centers. To find a One-Stop Center anywhere in the country go online to http://www.servicelocator.org. Many One Stop Centers have Disability Navigators who can help you navigate through the variety of programs and services.

Are there companies that have interest in hiring people with disabilities?

eSight, a global, cross-disability, cross-generational online community addressing disability employment issues, maintains a directory of disability-friendly companies that have indicated interest in recruiting and hiring qualified individuals with disabilities. You can find the list at http://www.esight.org/OverviewByType.cfm?type=profile.

What is a job bank?

A job bank allows you to post your resume on the internet for employers to see. Following are a number of job banks where you may want to post your resume. The first group of job banks is for everyone. The second group is specifically designed for job searchers with disabilities.

Many of these websites also have other information that may be helpful during your search for the right job. For a complete guide to looking for a job online, please go to the Riley Guide Employment Opportunities and Job Resources website at http://www.rileyguide.com.

Job Banks for Everyone

- Monster at http://www.monster.com
- Careerbuilders at http://www.careerbuilder.com
- Yahoo Hotjobs at http://hotjobs.yahoo.com
- U.S. Office of Personnel Management Federal Job website at http://www.usajobs.opm.gov
- Indeed Job Metasearch Engine at http://www.indeed.com
- Career Magazine at http://www.careermag.com
- Net-Temps at http://www.net-temps.com

Disability Related Job Banks

- Career Opportunities for Students with Disabilities (COSD) at http://www.cosdonline.org
- RecruitABILITY at http://www.disabledperson.com/recruitability.asp
- Hireability at http://www.HireAbility.com

Are You Prepared for the Job Interview?

What should be my first step in looking for a job?

It is important to know the job market—what jobs are out there and where—as well as to know yourself, your skills, abilities, knowledge, and experience.

If I know where the jobs are and what jobs are available, now what?

Next, develop a resume presenting your qualifications to an employer. Remember, a resume is usually what the employer sees first.

A resume provides the employer with the skills, abilities, knowledge and experience you have developed to date. So, if you have not already created a list of these, now is the time.

Next, you should define your skills and abilities gathered from life or work experiences. This will help you examine your job experience, paid and unpaid, as well as your academic and personal activities to create a list. The key to this exercise is to not underestimate yourself or your abilities.

Then, document your work history in a resume format. Organize the information you have completed. Once you have built your resume, review it and ask someone else to review it before sending it to employers.

If I want to submit my resume online, is there anything special I need to know?

If submitting your resume directly to a company online or posting it to a job bank, your resume may be computer scanned for key words. U.S. Department of Labor, ODEP's Writing and Formatting a Scannable Resume publication available at http://www.dol.gov/odep/pubs/ek99/resume.htm, will help put your resume in a format readable by a computer.

What else do I need to prepare beside the resume?

A good cover letter is essential to submitting your resume to an employer. Again, the cover letter and resume give the employer a first impression of you so you want both to be perfect.

If I have my cover letter and resume complete, what is next?

You will need to scan the newspaper want ads and job bank websites. Be sure you also let your friends, teachers, community members, church members, and others know that you are looking for a job. Many positions are filled with people the employer knows. Telling everyone you know that you are job hunting may open a job opportunity through this informal network.

What if an employer I am interested in working for is not currently hiring?

If you know an employer that you would like to work for but the employer is not currently hiring, ask for an informational interview so you can be considered for employer's future job openings. This informational interview can be the start of a relationship leading to a future job.

If I found a job opening that I am qualified for, it is in the area I want to live, the pay is enough to support me, I have sent my cover letter and resume, and I have been called for the job, how should I prepare?

Being prepared shows an employer you are motivated. Prepare for your interview by reviewing techniques and things to do and things to avoid in interviews. Next, because some employers require a completed application before hiring, gather all the information typically needed to fill out a job application. Much of the information will be found in your resume, but some may not. For example, you may be asked to provide all of your education, even from elementary school, including addresses.

Finally, research the company offering you an interview. Learn what the company does, who the company's customers are, and who is involved with the company. If you know someone who has worked for or is still working for the company, talk to them in person. Search the internet for the company name to get additional information. By knowing this information, you will be better able to tell the employer what you can do for the company. You will also be able to ask relevant questions about the company and the job during the interview.

Should I have references available at the interview?

Many recruiting professionals suggest having your references ready to provide to the interviewer. Most of the time three references will be sufficient. References should include people who can provide positive feedback about your work history or your character. Remember to ask permission from the people you want to use as references before giving the list to a potential employer. This will prevent your references from being surprised by a call from the employer and give your references time to prepare accordingly.

The day of the interview, what is expected of me and what should I expect?

Generally, the company will explain the procedure before your interview so you will have time to prepare. Remember, preparation is the most important thing. Plan ahead for what you will say and take the time to present your qualifications in a professional manner.

Being on time for an interview is very important. If late, it will reflect poorly on how the interviewer sees you. Few excuses will work if you are late. However, if you plan ahead and scout the interview location before, check traffic reports, check bus or train schedules, and follow weather reports, being late will not be a problem. If you find that you are going to be late, call the employer and explain that you have been delayed. While this is not the best situation, a call may show you are responsible and determined to meet your commitments.

You will face different types of interviews during your job search. At times you will be part of a short interview called a screening interview. During this interview, the employer is checking to see if you have the qualifications the employer needs and what you say in the interview is consistent with your resume. If you meet the employer's requirements, you may be invited to a longer interview. These interviews may be one-on-one or by a group of people. But whether the interview is with one person or a few, be prepared to discuss why you should be hired.

Finally, first impressions are very important. An employer can make a snap judgment about you even before you have a chance to say anything. Therefore, personal grooming is very important on the day of the interview. A shower, a shave (for men), brushed teeth, and brushed or combed hair are all good grooming habits. Applicants are urged not to wear any perfume products including after shave cologne as many individuals have allergies and find scented products offensive. The person interviewing you may be one of these individuals.

Always remember interviewers will see a messy person as someone who may not be able to handle the job. Personal grooming takes little time, but it can make a lasting impression. Also keep good eye contact for the greeting. You want to present yourself as a strong person who can work individually and as a team member. Remember to smile when you first greet anyone. You are happy for this opportunity to show an employer that you are the right person for the job.

If I have an obvious disability, how can I positively address this in the interview?

How you present yourself at an interview helps an interviewer decide whether to hire you. For example, how you sit or how you walk promotes to the interviewer a perception of the kind of person you are. If, because of an obvious disability, you walk with a limp or are unable to sit straight, you may want to develop a positive strategy for addressing your limitations. For example, an individual without arms shared that when he was interviewing he would ask the interviewer if it was appropriate to take notes. He would then pull his notepad and pen out of his pocket with his foot and start writing with his toes.

It was not as important to the applicant to take specific notes as it was to let the interviewer see him taking the notes.

Another suggestion, if you use a piece of assistive technology, would be to bring the equipment into the interview. For example, if you have a vision impairment and use a screen reading software, bring in the software on a laptop to show the interviewer the notes used to prepare for the interview.

Are there questions an interviewer should not ask?

Questions are the main part of the interview and are one of the main ways the interviewer can know if a candidate is right for the job. You can expect lots of different questions from discussion about your education to your last job. However, there are questions that an interviewer cannot legally ask. An employer may not ask or require a job applicant to take a medical examination before making a job offer. An interviewer cannot make any pre-employment inquiry about a disability or the nature or severity of a disability. However, during the post-offer, pre-employment stage of the process, an employer can ask medical questions not related to the job as long as everyone going into the position is asked the questions. An employer may, however, ask questions about the ability to perform specific job functions and may, with certain limitations, ask an individual with an obvious disability to describe or demonstrate how he or she would perform a specific function.

How do I explain recent gaps in my work history because of my disability?

One of the questions often asked of candidates is their work history from most recent to first experience. Individuals can be asked to explain gaps in employment history. While there is not a perfect answer, JAN Consultant Kendra Duckworth suggests: "The best way to handle difficult questions during the interview is to be prepared for them. Make a list of the questions you know you are going to have trouble with and formulate an answer, then practice your delivery of these answers so you will be ready from them." For example, "I see that there is a two year gap in your work history. What have you been doing during this time?" This is an opportunity to talk about what you have been doing, not what you have not been doing. Think about valuable life experiences that you have gained during this time. Have you been taking care of children or a parent, going to school, taking art classes, or volunteering? This question may prompt you to disclose your disability if you have not already done so. Be sure to do it in a way that shows how you have dealt with a difficult situation in a positive manner. Remember to keep the past in the past, stating that you are ready to move forward and are qualified and able to do the job you want." If and when this question arises, it is also wise to have researched the position for which you have applied as well as the organization's focus, mission, and history. Using the information you found during the research, you can transition the conversation back to why an employer should hire you.

Can an employer require medical examinations or ask questions about a disability?

If you are applying for a job, an employer cannot ask you if you are disabled or ask about the nature or severity of your disability. An employer can ask if you can perform the duties of the job with or without reasonable accommodation. An employer can also ask you to describe or to demonstrate how, with or without a reasonable accommodation, you will perform the job duties.

An employer cannot require you to take a medical examination before you are offered a job. Following a job offer, an employer can condition the offer on your passing a required medical examination, but only if all entering employees for the job category have to take the examination. However, an employer cannot reject you because of information about your disability revealed by the medical examination, unless the reasons for rejection are job-related and necessary for the conduct of the employer's business. The employer will also have to consider reasonable accommodation, barring an undue hardship, to allow an applicant the ability to perform the essential functions of the job up to the expectations of anyone entering the position. Finally, the results of all medical examinations must be kept confidential and maintained in separate medical files.

At this point, do I tell the employer I may have a disability?

Disclosing a disability is voluntary during the application and interview stages of the employment process. Some individuals decide to disclose to a potential employer at that time. Disclosure during the application or interview stage may be because the disability is not hidden or the individual decides this is the right time. Many, including the U.S. Department of Labor's Office of Disability Employment

Policy (ODEP), suggest a positive approach to disclosing before a job offer has been made. This approach would anticipate the concerns of the employer, have innovative accommodation suggestions available, practice demonstrating how you would perform difficult functions, and keep the focus on your abilities. This approach should send a message to the interviewer that you are an innovative individual who can anticipate job changes.

Kendra Duckworth, JAN Consultant, suggests in her *Consultants' Corner* article "Disability Disclosure and Interviewing Techniques for Persons with Disabilities," if you need to disclose during an interview "remember to talk about your abilities, not your disabilities. Employers need qualified, capable individuals to fill positions. Find a way to show that you are that person. Sell them on what you can do, not on what you cannot do, and the interview will go better than you expect. Be positive about yourself and be honest."

John Williams, an award-winning columnist, who has been writing about disability issues for 22 years wrote in a 2001 National Organization on Disability article, "It is your choice whether or not to mention your disability; by law, interviewers cannot ask candidates disability-related questions. And it is best not to discuss specific medical problems during your interview. However, if you use assistive technology, describing what you use and how it helps your performance can make a positive impression on the interviewer. This indicates problem-solving ability and self-confidence. Remind the person interviewing you that any purchase of assistive technology products is a capital investment."

Job candidates should be aware that once disclosure of a disability or an accommodation request is made employers may ask the employee about the limitations related to the job and are permitted to make medical inquiries.

Disclosing a disability requires a lot of thought and planning. Candidates with disabilities should plan how they will disclose and assess the consequences of sharing this intimate information with a prospective employer. Ultimately, the job candidate must decide the time, place, and degree of information to share with others.

How do I ask for help when filling out the application and for the interview?

If you think you will need assistance in order to participate in the application and hiring process, you should inform the employer. Assistance needed to reduce the barrier a disability creates is called reasonable accommodation. Employers are required to provide reasonable accommodation only for the known physical or mental limitations of a qualified individual with a disability. Generally, you, as the applicant, have the responsibility to request an accommodation from the employer.

How do I ask for help?

An accommodation may be requested orally or in writing.

I have submitted a request for accommodation and the employer is asking for medical records. What do I do?

In asking for help, you are disclosing to the employer that you have an impairment. When a job applicant requests help, or a reasonable accommodation, an employer may require that the employee provide medical documentation to establish whether the employee has an Americans with Disabilities Act (ADA) disability and needs the requested accommodation.

The employer wants me to have a drug test. Do I have to test?

According to the U.S. Equal Employment Opportunity Commission (EEOC), employers do the have right to request a drug test. The ADA specifically states that tests to determine the current illegal use of controlled substances are not considered medical examinations and can be administered prior to a job offer.

I am applying for a safety sensitive job requiring a polygraph test, and because of my disability I am concerned I will not be able to pass this test. What are my options?

The Employee Polygraph Protection Act allows some employers in safety sensitive industries to administer polygraphs, lie detector tests, to potential employees.

After the interview, are there things that I should do?

After the interview, don't forget to send a thank-you letter to the interviewer. If you have not heard from a company from ten days to two weeks after you sent your thank-you letter, you can follow-up with a phone call. During this call, state your name, the date of the interview, and the position. Let the employer know you are still interested in the position and ask if there is a timetable for making a decision. Generally, an interviewer will tell you when the decision will be made.

Another thing that should be done is your self-evaluation of the interview. How did you do? Do you know? Can you take a step back and evaluate yourself on how you did during the interview? You should take some time and review what happened at the interview. Did you take notes? If you did, they are a good sign you were paying attention. Do you remember if you stumbled over your words? Did you delay answering a question? Did you sit up straight and ask appropriate questions? Did you give the interviewer the extra resume asked for? If you felt you did something wrong, what was it? How would you handle it differently? Think of corrections and if you do not get the job, be better prepared for your next interview. In addition, by reviewing the interview you may discover additional questions for the employer you can ask during your follow-up call or second interview.

Should I wait to hear back after an interview before considering other jobs?

While you are waiting for word from the employer about the job, you can be getting ready for other interviews or continue searching for other positions. You should not wait until you hear back from an employer. If you wait and do not get the position, you will have wasted valuable search and possible interview time.

Effective interviewing is essential to getting the job. Job openings occur every day. Being prepared for these opportunities and being at the right place at the right time, often makes the difference in who is hired.

What should I do if I feel the interviewer has asked an illegal question?

Should you be asked an illegal question, you do not have to answer it. However, you do not want to point out to the interviewer the question is illegal and possibly ruin your chances to be hired. You can change the subject or politely explain that you are not comfortable answering the question. Also, do not dwell on the interviewer's mistake. This may be just a mistake and will have nothing to do with your being hired.

What do I do if I think I was discriminated against during the interview?

If at anytime you feel the employer has discriminated against you based on your disability, then you can file a complaint. Information about filing a claim on the federal level with the EEOC can be found at the website at http://www.eeoc.gov/facts/howtofil.html. Information about filing a claim on the state level can be found at http://www .jan.wvu.edu/cgi-win/TypeQuery.exe?037.

You Got the Job, Now What?

Congratulations. Obviously you have the skills and abilities the employer was seeking. After settling into the new job you may decide you want to advance in the company and need help to do so. This section provides information about what you can do to advance and grow in the new job.

How can I learn the ropes of the company?

A mentor is someone at work who has experience, knowledge, and is willing to share this with you. There is never a time when a mentor cannot help you. Look for and find someone who can give you knowledge, expertise, and access to information at your new job you would not get otherwise.

What can I do to get to know my co-workers?

- Look and see who of your new co-workers helps others. Know that they may be a resource for you.

- Be matter of fact about your disability but do not focus on it.

- Understand that your new co-workers may know little about disability so be understanding about mistakes they may make.

- Make the effort to go around the workplace and introduce yourself.

- Go to work with confidence and a smile.

- Be yourself—some people will be comfortable around you after a while and other may never be no matter what you do.

I am having problems doing my job due to my disability. What do I do?

If, due to a disability, your productivity is below what is expected of your job, you may wish to ask for a reasonable accommodation. Reasonable accommodation is any change in the work environment or in the way things are usually done resulting in an equal employment opportunity for you as an individual with a disability.

Reasonable accommodations can include modifications to the facility, changes in the job process, and assistive technology allowing you to perform at the expected performance standards. Because your employer would not have to excuse poor performance, it is advisable for you to know your limitations and expectations.

Asking for an accommodation before there is a continuing performance problem can help you from being disciplined on the job. An accommodation request is usually initiated by you and may be requested verbally or in writing.

The EEOC, the federal agency charged with enforcing the ADA, discusses requesting reasonable accommodation in its enforcement guidance regarding psychiatric disabilities. This guidance states, "when an individual decides to request accommodation, the individual or his/her representative must let the employer know that s/he needs an adjustment or change at work for a reason related to a medical condition." To request accommodation, an individual may use plain English and need not mention the ADA or use the phrase reasonable accommodation. However, the EEOC suggests individuals with disabilities might find it useful to document accommodation requests in the event there is a dispute about whether or when they requested accommodation. Further, the guidance states requests for accommodation "may be requested on behalf of an individual with a disability . . . by a family member, friend, health professional, or other representative."

If I did not disclose a disability when I was hired, can I still ask for a reasonable accommodation?

You always have the right to request an accommodation. Often people with disabilities do not need an accommodation when first hired for a job. If the job or the employee's condition changes, then there may be a need for an accommodation. An employer could not deny you this request solely because you have not previously disclosed your disability. However, employers could refuse to accommodate if there is an undue hardship or if they feel you are not a person with a disability.

What kind of medical questions can my employer ask after I have requested an accommodation?

When an employee requests an accommodation and the disability or need for accommodation is not obvious, an employer may require that the employee provide medical documentation to establish that the employee has an ADA disability and needs the requested accommodation. According to guidance from the Equal Employment Opportunity Commission, requests for medical information unrelated to the accommodation request are not permitted.

If I am not sure I want to tell my employer about my disability, do I have to?

If you need a reasonable accommodation in order to perform essential job functions, you should inform the employer an accommodation will be needed. Employers are required to provide reasonable accommodation only for the known physical or mental limitations of a qualified individual with a disability. Generally, under the ADA it is an individual's responsibility to inform an employer that an accommodation is needed.

Voluntary disability disclosure is a personal choice and refers to telling your employer and/or fellow co-workers about your physical, sensory, intellectual, or mental health disability. Once employed, many people with disabilities disclose when their disability is affecting work performance. Other people disclose when their disability begins affecting their relationships with co-workers or supervisors, while others make the choice to disclose in order to reduce the stress caused by hiding their disability.

Disclosure can be an opportunity to provide an employer, manager, or co-worker with accurate, first-hand information about the disability as well as strategies successfully used to accommodate a particular disability. This discussion with the employer, supervisor, or other employees may also serve to dispel myths and misconceptions concerning a particular disability.

Many employees choose not to disclose. Some are not yet comfortable talking about their disabilities or have had a bad experience—discrimination, prejudice, or rejection—when disclosing. Others fear future progress in the organization will be limited. Some do not disclose because their disabilities are not affecting either their work performance or their relationships in the workplace.

How do I know what kind of reasonable accommodation I need?

Reasonable accommodation ideas may come from personal, educational, or professional experiences. For example, you may use a reaching device at home better enabling you to reach high and low objects; or possibly you had used a software program in college helping you organize your work; or maybe you had a different mouse at another job increasing the information you were able to enter into the computer. If you have developed strategies or have used equipment to successfully accommodate your disability, then you may want to share this with your employer. However, if you have not needed an accommodation before and do not know where to start, contact the Job Accommodation Network (JAN).

Job Accommodation Network (JAN)
P.O. Box 6080
Morgantown, WV 26506-6080
Toll-Free: 800-526-7234
Toll-Free TTY: 877-781-9403
Phone: 304-293-7186
Fax: 304-293-5407
Website: http://www.jan.wvu.edu

Is there a typical process followed for accommodating employees with disabilities at work?

Every workplace is different. Large corporations have human resource departments and policy and procedures designed to inform employees of how certain things are done. Other businesses are smaller and may not be as detailed in terms of rules and processes to follow. Look through any materials you were given upon hire to see if a reasonable accommodation process is mentioned.

Chapter 65

Personal Coaching for Adults with AD/HD

Coaching is a relatively new field that has become more prominent in recent years. In general, coaches help individuals reach their fullest potential in life. As a specialty within the broader field of coaching, AD/HD coaching has emerged among the many approaches, services, and treatments for AD/HD. This chapter will:

- describe AD/HD coaching and how it may help;
- discuss who may benefit from AD/HD coaching;
- describe the credentialing process available to AD/HD coaches;
- provide practical suggestions for selecting a coach.

Coaching in General

Coaching is an emerging field that seeks to help individuals accomplish their life goals. The coaching relationship is intended to help people achieve better results in their lives: academically, professionally, socially, or in any area of life they want to improve. Through individualized assistance and support, coaches help people concentrate on where they are now, where they want to be, and how they can get there.

Currently, there is no published research evaluating the effectiveness of coaching as an intervention for individuals with AD/HD. There is anecdotal evidence (reports based on individual cases rather than a research study) suggesting that coaching may be a helpful supplement to other interventions for which there is a more established evidence base. This chapter and the suggestions it offers are based upon the emerging standards of coaching practice and the principles of behavior change, not on scientific literature.

What Is AD/HD Coaching?

Although the concepts of professional and personal coaching have been around for several decades, the concept of AD/HD coaching was first addressed in the 1994 book, *Driven to Distraction*,[1] by Edward M. Hallowell, M.D., and John J. Ratey, M.D.

AD/HD coaching seeks to address the daily challenges of living with AD/HD. A coach helps people with AD/HD carry out the practical activities of daily life in an organized, goal-oriented, and timely fashion. Through a close partnership, an AD/HD coach helps the client learn practical skills and initiate change in his or her daily life. A coach may help an adult with AD/HD:

- maintain focus to achieve identified goals;
- translate abstract goals into concrete actions;
- build motivation and learn to use rewards effectively.

Through regular interactions, coaches learn how the symptoms of AD/HD play out in the daily lives of their clients and then provide encouragement, recommendations, feedback, and practical techniques to address specific challenges. They may offer reminders, raise questions, or suggest time management methods. Coaches ask questions to help the client come up with strategies and act on them. Examples of such questions are:

- What can you do about it?
- How can you motivate yourself to take action towards this goal?
- When must this action be completed?
- What steps have you taken already, and when will you take the remaining steps?

Regular meetings and check-ins are an essential part of the coaching process. These sessions can be conducted in person, by phone, or by e-mail, depending on the client's preference. However, before the coaching process begins, the client and the coach should have an initial session that addresses issues such as client needs, expectations of the client and of the coach, and fees and payments (coaching services are often not covered by traditional health insurance). The first coaching session is typically an in-depth, 1–2 hour meeting to develop a step-by-step plan for identifying and achieving the client's goals.

Who Benefits from AD/HD Coaching?

AD/HD coaching may be beneficial particularly for adults with AD/HD. It is important that clients are ready for coaching before they commit to the process. Clients are ready for coaching when they are able to admit that they have a problem, can spend the time necessary to create strategies for improving their behavior, and can adhere to those strategies to the best of their ability.

Obstacles to Effective Coaching

There are several issues that can complicate the coaching process and often require a referral to a medical or mental health professional:

- The client cannot use simple self-management or organizational strategies to achieve goals, despite the coach's resources and reminders.

- The client has a co-existing psychiatric condition such as depression, bipolar disorder, anxiety disorder, substance abuse, or personality disorder.

- The client has stressful life circumstances such as marital problems, divorce, or death of a loved one.

- The client has a serious physical illness or other chronic medical condition.

Under such circumstances, the coach should work collaboratively with the medical or mental health professionals involved in the client's care. In such cases, the client may benefit from the addition of traditional treatments such as medication and psychological therapy.

AD/HD Coaching Credentials

There is currently no specialized schooling or licensing required to become a coach or a coach who specializes in AD/HD. AD/HD coaches often have different educational and professional backgrounds and diverse knowledge about AD/HD. Many coaches, including those who work with individuals with AD/HD, seek credentialing through the International Coach Federation (ICF), an international association of personal and business coaching that is evolving as the principal governing body for this field. General requirements and more information on guidelines and accredited coach training programs can be found on the ICF website (www.coachfederation.org). The ICF recognizes AD/HD coaching as a special area of expertise. Because coaching is a very broad field with many areas of subspecialty, adults with AD/HD should ask potential coaches about their experience with AD/HD and coach-specific training in AD/HD as well as their credential status.

Because the coaching field is still in its infancy, much remains to be done to establish practice standards and ethics. In 2002, a task force of coaches organized by the Attention Deficit Disorder Association (ADDA) wrote "The Guiding Principles for Coaching Individuals with Attention Deficit Disorder." [2] This document proposes the essential elements of AD/HD coaching, establishes standards, and outlines ethical principles to help people better understand AD/HD coaching and field standards.

The Institute for the Advancement of AD/HD Coaching (IAAC) was formed late in 2006 to advance the field of AD/HD coaching through the development and delivery of credentialing and certification for AD/HD coaches worldwide. This adds a new option for those wishing to become AD/HD coaches, and offers people with AD/HD new options when seeking coaches.

Finding and Choosing an AD/HD Coach

Step one: Coaching is a collaborative process so it is important to find the right match in a coach. First, ask yourself the following questions before contacting prospective coaches:

- Is it important that my coaching sessions be face-to-face? (If so, look for a coach who is geographically close and offers this as part of a service package. Many coaches conduct the initial session in person, and then do weekly check-ins by phone and/or e-mail.)

- Do I prefer to be coached by a man or a woman?

- In addition to the coach's knowledge of AD/HD, would I benefit from a coach who has a background in business, academia, or gender issues?

- Am I looking for someone who has expertise in an area such as organization or family issues?

- Do I want someone who has a lot of energy, or someone who takes a more subtle approach?

- Is a sense of humor important? Would a more serious person make a better match?

Step two: Compile a list of potential coaches with training in AD/HD coaching and interview them, using the following types of questions:

- How long have you been a coach?

- What is your approach to coaching adults with AD/HD?

- How many clients with AD/HD have you coached?

- Have you received formal training in coaching? Did this include certification or credentialing of any kind?

- What coach training courses or conferences have you attended? Were they AD/HD-specific?

- Are you involved in any local professional coaching groups? Are they AD/HD-related?

- In what ways are you contributing to the development of the field of AD/HD coaching?

- What is your confidentiality and privacy policy?

Step three: Take notes on each coach's answers to these questions as well as your own overall reaction to the personality and style of each coach.

Step four: Review all of the information and select the coach that best meets your needs.

Coaching Is Not Therapy

Coaches deal with problems in everyday living such as organization, time management, memory, follow-through, and motivation. Coaches focus on what, when, and how—never why. They are not trained to address psychiatric, emotional, and interpersonal problems, which should be addressed by mental health professionals. Through formal educational programs, mental health professionals (psychiatrists, psychologists, clinical social workers, psychiatric nurse practitioners, marriage and family therapists) are trained to diagnose and treat mental health issues such as depression, anxiety, personality disorders, and interpersonal difficulties. They also must have a license to practice. Therapists work primarily through face-to-face contacts while many coaches also work by telephone or e-mail.

Depending on an individual's diagnosis, the mental health professional may employ a number of psychotherapeutic approaches such as cognitive-behavior therapy and behavior modification. The goal of therapy is generally to help clients address the symptoms and problems that brought them to therapy in the first place. Often, mental health professionals take a "problem-centered" approach to therapy rather than a "client-centered" approach; treatment lasts until the specific problem is no longer causing significant impairment and disruption to the client.

If an adult with AD/HD needs assistance primarily in dealing with the practical challenges in daily life, a coach may be a good person to help. If the adult needs assistance with emotional, psychiatric, or interpersonal problems, then a therapist should be consulted. If an adult with AD/HD needs both types of assistance, it may be helpful to select a coach and a therapist, and ask them to work with each other.

Summary

Although the field of coaching is still developing and does not yet have a research base that demonstrates its effectiveness as an intervention for adults with AD/HD, many adults find that having a coach who is familiar with AD/HD can be helpful in facing the challenges of daily life. Because there is a great need for research evaluating the effectiveness of AD/HD coaching, coaches and other professionals are strongly encouraged to pursue research on this emerging form of support for those dealing with AD/HD-related challenges.

References

1. Hallowell, E.M., and Ratey, J.J. (1994). *Driven to distraction*. New York: Pantheon Books.

2. ADDA Subcommittee on ADD Coaching. (2002). *The ADDA Guiding Principles for Coaching Individuals with Attention Deficit Disorder*. Hyde Park, IL.: Nancy Ratey and Peter Jaksa (Eds.).

Part Eight

Additional Help and Information

Chapter 66

Glossary of Terms Related to Learning Disabilities

American Sign Language (ASL): A manual language with its own syntax and grammar, used primarily by people who are deaf.

aphasia: Total or partial loss of the ability to use or understand language; usually caused by stroke, brain disease, or injury.

apraxia: Inability to execute a voluntary movement despite being able to demonstrate normal muscle function.

articulation disorder: Inability to correctly produce speech sounds (phonemes) because of imprecise placement, timing, pressure, speed, or flow of movement of the lips, tongue, or throat.

Asperger disorder: A pervasive developmental disorder characterized by severe and enduring impairment in social skills and restrictive and repetitive behaviors and interests, leading to impaired social and occupational functioning but without significant delays in language development.[1]

assistive devices: Technical tools and devices such as alphabet boards, text telephones, or text-to-speech conversion software used to

Terms in this chapter are excerpted from "Glossary," National Institute on Deafness and Other Communication Disorders (NIDCD), April 2008. Terms marked with a [1] are from *Stedman's Medical Dictionary, 27ᵗʰ Edition*, Copyright © 2000 Lippincott Williams & Wilkins. All rights reserved. Terms marked with a [2] are from "The Condition of Education," National Center for Education Statistics, U.S. Department of Education, 2008.

aid individuals who have communication disorders perform actions, tasks, and activities.

attention deficit/hyperactivity disorder: A disorder manifested at home, in school, and in social situations by developmentally inappropriate degrees of inattention, impulsiveness, and hyperactivity.[1]

audiologist: Health care professional who is trained to evaluate hearing loss and related disorders, including balance (vestibular) disorders and tinnitus, and to rehabilitate individuals with hearing loss and related disorders. An audiologist uses a variety of tests and procedures to assess hearing and balance function and to fit and dispense hearing aids and other assistive devices for hearing.

auditory brainstem response (ABR) test: A test for brain functioning in comatose, unresponsive, etc., patients, and for hearing in infants and young children; involves attaching electrodes to the head to record electrical activity from the hearing nerve and other parts of the brain.

auditory nerve: Eighth cranial nerve that connects the inner ear to the brainstem and is responsible for hearing and balance.

auditory perception: Ability to identify, interpret, and attach meaning to sound.

auditory prosthesis: Device that substitutes or enhances the ability to hear.

augmentative devices: Tools that help individuals with limited or absent speech to communicate, such as communication boards, pictographs (symbols that look like the things they represent), or ideographs (symbols representing ideas).

aural rehabilitation: Techniques used with people who are hearing impaired to improve their ability to speak and communicate.

autism: Brain disorder that begins in early childhood and persists throughout adulthood; affects three crucial areas of development: communication, social interaction, and creative or imaginative play.

bilateral hearing loss: Hearing loss in both ears.

captioning: Text display of spoken words, presented on a television or a movie screen, that allows a deaf or hard-of-hearing viewer to follow the dialogue and the action of a program simultaneously.

carrier: A person who has only one copy of a recessive disorder gene with a change in it. The person "carries" the changed gene but shows no symptoms of the disorder. If both parents are carriers, each child has a one in four chance of inheriting two changed genes and showing the disorder.

central auditory processing disorder: Inability to differentiate, recognize, or understand sounds; hearing and intelligence are normal.

cochlear implant: Medical device that bypasses damaged structures in the inner ear and directly stimulates the auditory nerve, allowing some deaf individuals to learn to hear and interpret sounds and speech.

cognition: Thinking skills that include perception, memory, awareness, reasoning, judgment, intellect, and imagination.

computed tomography (CT or CAT): A procedure for taking x-ray images from many different angles and then assembling them into a cross-section of the body. This technique is generally used to visualize bone.

cued speech: Method of communication that combines speech reading with a system of handshapes placed near the mouth to help deaf or hard-of-hearing individuals differentiate words that look similar on the lips (for example, bunch versus punch) or are hidden (for example, gag).

decibel: Unit that measures the intensity or loudness of sound.

dysarthria: Group of speech disorders caused by disturbances in the strength or coordination of the muscles of the speech mechanism as a result of damage to the brain or nerves.

disfluency: Disruption in the smooth flow or expression of speech.

dyscalculia: Difficulty in performing simple mathematical problems; commonly seen in parietal lobe lesions.[1]

dyslexia: Learning disability characterized by reading difficulties. Some individuals may also have difficulty writing, spelling, or working with numbers.

dysphagia: Difficulty swallowing.

dysphonia: Any impairment of the voice or speaking ability.

dyspraxia of speech: In individuals with normal muscle tone and speech muscle coordination, partial loss of the ability to consistently pronounce words.

dystonia: Abnormal muscle tone of one or more muscles.

genetic counselor: A health professional who provides information and support to individuals and families who have a genetic disease or who are at risk for such a disease.

geneticist: A scientist or physician who specializes in genetics (how children inherit traits from their parents).

hearing: Series of events in which sound waves in the air are converted to electrical signals, which are sent as nerve impulses to the brain, where they are interpreted.

hearing aid: Electronic device that brings amplified sound to the ear. A hearing aid usually consists of a microphone, amplifier, and receiver.

hearing disorder: Disruption in the normal hearing process that may occur in outer, middle, or inner ear, whereby sound waves are not converted to electrical signals and nerve impulses are not transmitted to the brain to be interpreted.

hereditary hearing impairment: Hearing loss passed down through generations of a family.

Landau-Kleffner syndrome: Childhood disorder of unknown origin which often extends into adulthood and can be identified by gradual or sudden loss of the ability to understand and use spoken language.

language: System for communicating ideas and feelings using sounds, gestures, signs, or marks.

language disorders: Any of a number of problems with verbal communication and the ability to use or understand a symbol system for communication.

learning disabilities: Disorders characterized by difficulty with certain skills such as reading or writing in individuals with normal intelligence.

magnetic resonance imaging (MRI): A scanning procedure that uses radio waves and magnets to show images of body parts. This technique is generally used to visualize soft tissues.

misarticulation: Inaccurately produced speech sound (phoneme) or sounds.

motor speech disorders: Group of disorders caused by the inability to accurately produce speech sounds (phonemes) because of muscle weakness or incoordination or difficulty performing voluntary muscle movements.

neural plasticity: Ability of the brain or certain parts of the nervous system to adapt to new conditions, such as an injury.

neural prostheses: Devices that substitute for an injured or diseased part of the nervous system, such as the cochlear implant.

neural stimulation: To activate or energize a nerve through an external source.

neurogenic communication disorder: Inability to exchange information with others because of hearing, speech, or language problems caused by impairment of the nervous system (brain or nerves).

open-set speech recognition: Understanding speech without visual clues (speech reading).

otitis media: Inflammation of the middle ear caused by infection.

otoacoustic emissions: Low-intensity sounds produced by the inner ear that can be quickly measured with a sensitive microphone placed in the ear canal.

pervasive developmental disorders: Disorders characterized by delays in several areas of development that may include socialization and communication.

phonology: Study of speech sounds.

postlingually deafened: Individual who becomes deaf after having acquired language.

presbycusis: Loss of hearing that gradually occurs because of changes in the inner or middle ear in individuals as they grow older.

reading disorders: Any of a group of problems characterized by difficulty using or understanding the symbol system for written language.

sign language: Method of communication for people who are deaf or hard of hearing in which hand movements, gestures, and facial expressions convey grammatical structure and meaning.

sound vocalization: Ability to produce voice.

spasmodic dysphonia: Momentary disruption of voice caused by involuntary movements of one or more muscles of the larynx or voice box.

special education schools: A public elementary or secondary school that (1) focuses primarily on special education, including instruction for any of the following: hard of hearing, deaf, speech impaired, health impaired, orthopedically impaired, mentally retarded, seriously emotionally disturbed, multi-handicapped, visually handicapped, deaf and blind; and the learning disabled; and (2) adapts curriculum, materials, or instruction for students served. About two percent of schools in the Common Core of Data files at the National Center for Education Statistics are special education schools.[2]

specific learning disability: A specific learning disability is a disorder of one or more of the basic psychological processes involved in understanding or in using language, spoken or written, that may manifest itself in an imperfect ability to listen, think, speak, read, write, spell, or to do mathematical calculations. This includes conditions such as perceptual disabilities, brain injury, minimal brain dysfunction, dyslexia, and developmental aphasia.[2]

specific language impairment (SLI): Difficulty with language or the organized-symbol system used for communication in the absence of problems such as mental retardation, hearing loss, or emotional disorders.

speech: Spoken communication.

speech disorder: Any defect or abnormality that prevents an individual from communicating by means of spoken words. Speech disorders may develop from nerve injury to the brain, muscular paralysis, structural defects, hysteria, or mental retardation.

speech processor: Part of a cochlear implant that converts speech sounds into electrical impulses to stimulate the auditory nerve, allowing an individual to understand sound and speech.

speech-language pathologist: Health professional trained to evaluate and treat people who have voice, speech, language, or swallowing disorders (including hearing impairment) that affect their ability to communicate.

speech or language impairments: A communication disorder such as stuttering, impaired articulation, a language impairment, or a voice impairment that adversely affects a child's educational performance.[2]

stroke: Also known as a cerebrovascular accident (CVA); caused by a lack of blood to the brain, resulting in the sudden loss of speech, language, or the ability to move a body part, and, if severe enough, death.

stuttering: Frequent repetition of words or parts of words that disrupts the smooth flow of speech.

tactile: Related to touch or the sense of touch.

tactile devices: Mechanical instruments that make use of touch to help individuals who have certain disabilities, such as deaf-blindness, to communicate.

touch: Tactile sense; the sense by which contact with the skin or mucous membrane is experienced.

Tourette syndrome: Neurological disorder characterized by recurring movements and sounds (called tics).

vibrotactile aids: Mechanical instruments that help individuals who are deaf to detect and interpret sound through the sense of touch.

voice disorders: Group of problems involving abnormal pitch, loudness, or quality of the sound produced by the larynx (voice box).

Chapter 67

Finding Local Resources for a Child with Learning Disabilities or AD/HD

The first steps to take when you notice your child is struggling to learn are pre-referral, assessment, or diagnosis. Once the reason for your child's learning problem has been identified, you'll know more precisely what he needs in order to learn. Where do you look and how do you begin this search? This chapter will help guide you through the four steps to discovering local resources:

1. Summarize your child's needs.
2. Contact national sources for local referrals.
3. Research your local options.
4. Contact local resources.

Summarizing Your Child's Needs

Whatever type of specialist you're seeking for your child, you can turn to a variety of resources (people, organizations, and directories) for contact information. Before you start calling people, make a list summarizing your child's situation. This will help you describe your child's needs in a succinct way. List these facts:

• Child's name

- Gender
- Age
- Grade in school
- Name and type of school (public or private)
- Identification/Diagnosis: For example, "He has an auditory processing problem."
- Observations: For example, "My son can't remember what he has heard after the teacher gives instructions."
- Type of specialist needed (for example, tutor, advocate); be as specific as possible. It may also be helpful to set up a resource notebook to organize all the information you will be gathering.

Contacting National Sources for Local Referrals

Some national organizations have systems in place to help you search for state or local referrals. The referrals are free, but the professionals to whom you are referred usually charge for their services. Check with these national organizations for:

Educational Therapists and Tutors

Association of Educational Therapists (AET)
11300 W. Olympic Blvd., Suite 600
Los Angeles, CA 90064
Toll-Free: 800-286-4267
Phone: 310-909-1490
Fax: 310-437-0585
Website: http://www.aetonline.org

AET provides online referrals to educational therapists who tutor children with learning disabilities.

Scottish Rite Clinics, Centers, and Programs for Childhood Language Disorders
The Supreme Council, 33
1733 16th St. N.W.
Washington, DC 20009-3103
Phone: 202-232-3579
Fax: 202-464-0487
Website: http://www.scottishrite.org/what/phil/ritecare.html

Offers both assessment and tutoring services through 150 locations in the United States.

National Association of Children's Hospitals and Related Institutions (NACHRI or N.A.C.H.)
401 Wythe Street
Alexandria, VA 22314
Phone: 703-684-1355
Fax: 703-684-1589
Website: http://www.childrenshospitals.net

Can refer you to any local teaching hospitals that offer learning clinics.

Other Contacts for Educational Therapists and Tutors

- After-school programs can often refer you to local tutors.

- State Department of Education—Special Education Department Ask for a list of private agencies that offer tutoring services.

- Universities Worldwide can refer you to local educational therapy programs for children. It is available online at http://univ.cc.

Speech, Language, and Hearing Therapists

American Speech-Language-Hearing Association (ASHA)
2200 Research Boulevard
Rockville, MD 20850-3289
Toll-Free: 800-638-8255
Phone: 301-296-5700
Fax: 301-296-8580
Website: http://www.asha.org
E-mail: actioncenter@asha.org

ASHA is a national association that can refer you to therapists in your area.

Medical Professionals

American Medical Association (AMA)
515 N. State Street
Chicago, IL 60610
Toll-Free: 800-621-8335
Phone: 312-464-5000
Fax: 312-464-5600
Website for DoctorFinder: http://webapps.ama-assn.org/doctorfinder/home.html

The AMA is a national association that can help you locate pediatricians, behavioral pediatricians, and other medical professionals in your area.

STOMP Specialized Training of Military Parents
Washington PAVE
6316 S. 12th St.
Tacoma, WA 98465
Toll-Free: 800-5-PARENT (727368)
Phone: 253-565-2266
Fax: 253-566-8052
Website: http://www.stompproject.org
E-mail: stomp@washingtonpave.com

U.S. Army medical command military families can obtain medical assistance for special education students living overseas.

Legal Assistance or Advocate

Legal Services Corporation
Website: http://www.rin.lsc.gov/rinboard/rguide/pdir.htm

LSC funds 179 low-cost legal aid programs in the United States.

Consortium for Appropriate Dispute Resolution (CADRE)
P.O. Box 51360
Eugene, OR 97405-0906
3411-A Willamette Street
Eugene, OR 97405-5122
Phone: 541-686-5060
Fax: 541-686-5063
TTY: 541-284-4740
Website: http://www.directionservice.org/cadre/index.cfm

CADRE provides a national database of Special Education Dispute Resolution Professionals at http://www.directionservice.org/cadre/profs.

Council of Parent Attorneys and Advocates (COPAA)
P.O. Box 6767
Towson, MD 21285
Phone: 410-372-0208
Fax: 410-372-0209
Website: http://www.copaa.net/index.html

COPAA is an independent, nonprofit organization founded to improve the quality and quantity of legal assistance to parents of children with disabilities.

PACER Center, Inc.
8161 Normandale Blvd.
Minneapolis, MN 55437
Toll-Free: 888-248-0822
Phone: 952-838-9000
TTY: 952-838-0190
Fax: 952-838-0199
Website: http://www.fape.org
E-mail: fape@fape.org

The Families and Advocates Partnership for Education (FAPE) is located at the PACER Center, Inc. It provides referrals to national, state, and local disability organizations and advocates and to a nationwide network of parent training and information centers and community parent resource centers.

Parent Training

The following national resources may have information about parent training programs in your area.

National Technical Assistance Center
PACER Center, Inc.
8161 Normandale Blvd.
Minneapolis, MN 55437
Toll-Free: 888-248-0822
Phone: 952-838-9000
TTY: 952-838-0190
Fax: 952-838-0199
Website: http://www.taalliance.org
E-mail: alliance@taalliance.org
PACER Parent Center Directory: http://www.taalliance.org/ptidirectory/index.asp

National Parent Teacher Association (PTA)
PTA National Headquarters
541 N. Fairbanks Court, Suite 1300
Chicago, IL 60611-3396
Toll-Free: 800-307-4782

Phone: 312-670-6782
Fax: 312-670-6783
Website: http://www.pta.org

Additional Resources:

- Schwab Learning's List of National LD Services is a comprehensive list of national organizations for individuals with learning disabilities (LD) and/or Attention-Deficit/Hyperactivity Disorder (AD/HD), such as: National Dissemination Center for Children with Disabilities, formerly NICHCY.

- U.S. Department of Education available online at http://www.ed.gov/about/contacts/state/index.html?src=gu. Select your state and find the contact for "Disability-related issues."

- United Way for referrals to social services. To find a local United Way online, visit: http://uwint.org/devfinal/members/locations.aspx?mid=2&chk=1

- The Military Child Education Coalition (MCEC) provides transitioning information for military families.

The Military Child Education Coalition
108 East FM 2410, Suite D
P. O. Box 2519
Harker Heights, TX 76548-2519
Phone: 254-953-1923
Fax: 254-953-1925
Website: http://www.militarychild.org

Researching Your Local Options

When searching for local resources, consider all possible sources of information, including educators and parents in your community. Contact the special education director of your local school district, your child's teachers, speech therapist, school counselor, after-school program director, parks and recreation department, and sympathetic coaches. Check with other parents who have children with LD or attention-deficit/hyperactivity disorder (AD/HD). Those people may refer you to others in the community, and your network will expand.

Print and Online Directories

Whether you're searching through telephone books or online directories (http://local.google.com, http://local.yahoo.com, and so forth.), the following categories will help you locate the specialists your child needs:

- Educational consulting and services
- Speech and language pathologists
- Tutoring
- Marriage, family, and child counselors, or marriage family therapists (counseling services)
- County mental health services
- Physicians and surgeons—behavioral, developmental, pediatric medicine
- Physicians and surgeons—pediatrics (infants, children, and adolescents)
- Physicians and surgeons—(child) psychiatry
- Psychologists
- Social and human services for individuals and families (county health services)
- Social workers (counseling services)

Online Community as a Source of Information

Online parent bulletin boards often contain valuable ideas on where to find help for your child. Here are two message boards to try:

- AD/HD and medications and education available at: http://millermom.proboards107.com.

- International Dyslexia Association Discussion Forum available at: http://www.interdys.org/DiscussionForum.htm.

- Related article: Online Parent Groups: Support at Your Fingertips available at: http://www.schwablearning.org/articles.aspx?g=3&r=62.

Expanding Your Horizons at Lectures and Workshops

Attending parent lectures, workshops, and conferences can expand your knowledge and introduce you to specialists in your community.

Contacting Local Resources

Before you contact a resource, write their name, address, and phone number at the top of one sheet of paper (and date it). It helps to draw or fold a vertical line down the middle of the paper. Then you can write your questions for the person on the left side of the vertical line and add notes on the right side. When you call an organization, be as concise as possible about what you need. This is where the summary sheet describing your child's needs will help. Many nonprofit groups are under-staffed yet are trying to help as many parents as possible. They cannot spend much time, if any, on the phone. Here's a possible script: "Good morning. My name is Mary Jones. My son is 12 years old and has been assessed with a reading comprehension problem. He needs a tutor. Is this something you can help us with? If not, can you recommend someone else to contact?"

Moving Forward with Confidence

This type of research takes time and effort on your part. Your resources are never set in stone; everything changes. What is helpful one year may not help your child the next. As your child grows and schoolwork becomes more complex, he may face new or different challenges. Navigating the LD journey is not an easy trip for anyone. But developing your research skills and learning to make local connections will allow both you and your child to move forward with confidence.

Chapter 68

Literacy Resources for Parents and Teachers

Literacy is knowing how to make meaning from written language by:

- reading,
- writing,
- thinking, and
- communicating.

This includes everything from knowing how to read and write your name and address to reading or writing scholarly works, and everything in between. With appropriate access, active learning, and balanced instruction, every child can gain their own personal literacy level. This chapter provides a listing of a few of the resources available to help parents and professionals find the tools they need so that all children reach their fullest literacy potential.

What does the research have to say about what works in literacy?

National Institute for Literacy (NIFL)
1775 I Street, N.W., Suite 730
Washington, DC 20006-2401

This chapter includes text from "NICHCY Connections to Literacy," National Dissemination Center for Children with Disabilities (NICHCY), April 2006. The complete document is available at http://www.nichcy.org/resources/literacy2.asp. Contact information was verified in August 2008.

Phone: 202-233-2025
Fax: 202-233-2050
Website: http://www.nifl.gov/nifl/index.html

NIFL offers a national database of literacy programs and many publications, including a 58-page teacher's guide for using the findings of the National Reading Panel in the classroom (called *Put Reading First: The Research Building Blocks for Teaching Children to Read*; a Parent's Guide called *Helping Your Child Learn to Read*; and, a series of adult literacy publications entitled *Bridges to Practice*).

National Reading Panel
c/o NICHD Information Resource Center
P.O. Box 3006
Rockville, MD 20847
Toll-Free: 800-370-2943
Fax: 301-984-1471
Website: http://www.nationalreadingpanel.org/Publications/publications.htm

In April 2000, the National Reading Panel (NRP) released its research-based findings in two reports and a video titled, "Teaching Children to Read." The first report is an excellent resource for anyone interested in learning about reading instruction research. The second report (a more technically-written document) reviews the reports of subgroups that assessed the status of research-based knowledge on the effectiveness of various approaches to teaching children to read.

What has NICHD found out about reading development, reading disorders, and reading instruction?

National Center for Learning Disabilities
381 Park Ave. S., Suite 1401
New York, NY 10016
Toll-Free: 888-575-7373
Phone: 212-545-7510
Fax: 212-545-9665
Website: http://www.ld.org/research/keys99_nichd.cfm

During the past 33 years, scientists at NICHD (the National Institute of Child Health and Human Development) have studied the reading development of 34,501 children and adults. This includes 12,641 individuals with reading difficulties, many of whom have been studied for as long as 12 years. The internet link leads to a synthesis at the National Center for Learning Disabilities (NCLD) and authored by Reid Lyon, which is derived from an analysis of over 2,500 publications generated by NICHD scientists since 1965.

NICHCY Research-to-Practice Database
P.O. Box 1492
Washington, DC 20013
Toll-Free (voice and TTY): 800-695-0285
Fax: 202-884-8441
Website: http://research.nichcy.org/search.asp
E-mail: nichcy@aed.org

NICHCY's database has more than a dozen major reading meta-analyses summarized for you, complete with practical examples and links to research-based materials you can use today to improve children's reading skills.

Reading Rockets
WETA Public Television
2775 S. Quincy St.
Arlington, VA 22206
Phone: 703-998-2001
Fax: 703-998-2060
Website: http://www.readingrockets.org/research/topic/phonics
E-mail: readingrockets@weta.org

Reading Rockets' by-line is "Launching Young Readers" and that's exactly what this content-rich site intends to help you do. At the internet link, you'll find selected research studies that investigate issues important to phonics.

Teaching Reading—Is It Rocket Science? Yes, It Is!

American Federation of Teachers
555 New Jersey Ave. N.W.
Washington, DC 20001
Website: http://www.aft.org/edissues/rocketscience.htm

Teaching Reading Is Rocket Science: What Expert Teachers of Reading Should Know and Be Able To Do reviews the reading research. It also describes the knowledge base essential for teacher candidates and practicing teachers to master if they are to be successful in teaching all children to read well. Finally, the report makes recommendations for improving the system of teacher education and professional development.

Council for Exceptional Children
1110 N. Glebe Rd., Suite 300
Arlington, VA 22201
Toll-Free: 888-232-7733
Toll-Free TTY: 866-915-5000
Fax: 703-264-9494
Website: http://www.cec.sped.org

The Council for Exceptional Children offers professional development online workshops in reading instruction. Educators, teaching assistants, administrators, and teachers-in-training can take these online courses whenever it best fits their schedule. The workshops focus on research-based strategies to strengthen students' reading skills.

Read, Write, Think
International Reading Association
800 Barksdale Road
P.O. Box 8139
Newark, DE 19714-8139
Website: http://www.readwritethink.org

The Read-Write-Think website connects theory to practice and was developed by the International Reading Association in partnership with the National Council of Teachers of English. A wide range of free, standards-based lessons and online resources are available to help teachers work with students to learn language, learn about language, and learn through language.

Literacy and Children with Disabilities

Accessible Books

There are a number of notable sources of materials specially designed for individuals with reading or physical disabilities that impede their use of print text.

National Library Service for the Blind and Physically Handicapped
Library of Congress
Toll-Free: 888-657-7323 (to connect to a local library)

Phone: 202-707-5100
TDD: 202-707-0744
Fax: 202-707-0712
Website: http://www.loc.gov/nls
E-mail: nis@loc.gov

Recording for the Blind and Dyslexic
National Headquarters
20 Roszel Road
Princeton, NJ 08540
Toll-Free: 866-RFBD-585 (732-3585)
Website: http://www.rfbd.org

Bookshare.org
The Benetech Initiative
480 S. California Ave., Suite 201
Palo Alto, CA 94306-1609
Website: http://www.bookshare.org
E-mail: info@bookshare.org

Bookshare.org, is a web-based system supplying accessible books in digital formats designed for people with disabilities.

The Access Center
1000 Thomas Jefferson St., N.W.
Washington, DC 20007
Website: http://www.k8accesscenter.org/training_resources/languagearts.asp
E-mail: accesscenter@air.org

The *Access Center: Improving Outcomes for All Students K–8* develops informational resources and tools to help educators ensure that students with disabilities learn through rigorous curriculum across language arts, including reading. This work is based on research findings developed by some of our nation's most respected researchers and is incorporated into classroom tools that can be applied across settings.

For Children with Learning Disabilities

LD OnLine
WETA Public Television
2775 S. Quincy St.
Arlington, VA 22206

Fax: 703-998-2060
Website: http://www.ldonline.org

Along with other resources, LD Online offers a "Tech Works" brief from the National Center for Technology Innovation (NCTI) available at www.ldonline.org/ld_indepth/technology/readingmatrix.html that connects you with four web-based resources containing detailed information on reading software programs that address specific needs of students with special needs in reading.

National Center for Learning Disabilities (NCLD)
381 Park Ave. S., Suite 1401
New York, NY 10016
Toll-Free: 888-575-7373
Phone: 212-545-7510
Fax: 212-545-9665
Website: http://www.ld.org; or, http://www.getreadytoread.org

Learning Disabilities Association of America (LDA)
4156 Library Road
Pittsburgh, PA 15234-1349
Toll-Free: 888-300-6710
Phone: 412-341-1515
Fax: 412-344-0224
Website: http://www.ldaamerica.org
E-mail: info@ldaamerica.org

Chapter 69

Additional Resources for Information about Learning Disabilities

All Kinds of Minds
2800 Meridian Parkway
Suite 100
Durham, NC 27713
Toll-Free: 888-956-4637
Website: http://
www.allkindsofminds.org

Alliance for Technology Access
1304 Southpoint Blvd.
Suite 240
Petaluma, CA 94954
Phone: 707-778-3011
TTY: 707-778-3015
Fax: 707-765-2080
Website: http://www.ataccess.org

American Speech-Language-Hearing Association
2200 Research Blvd.
Rockville, MD 20850
Toll-Free: 800-638-8255
Toll-Free TTY: 800-498-2071
Fax: 301-296-8580
Website: http://www.asha.org
E-mail: actioncenter@asha.org

Association of Educational Therapists
11300 W. Olympic Blvd.
Suite 600
Los Angeles, CA 90064
Toll-Free: 800-286-4267
Phone: 310-909-1490
Fax: 310-437-0585
Website: http://www.aetonline.org

Information in this chapter was compiled from many sources deemed reliable; inclusion does not constitute endorsement and omission does not imply objection. All contact information was updated and verified in August 2008.

Center for Applied Special Technology (CAST)
40 Harvard Mills Square
Suite 3
Wakefield, MA 01880-3233
Phone: 781-245-2212
Website: http://www.cast.org
E-mail: cast@cast.org

Center for Disability Information and Referral (CeDIR)
Indiana Institute on Disability and Community
Indiana University
2853 East Tenth Street
Bloomington, IN 47408-2696
Toll-Free Voice/TTY:
800-437-7924 (Indiana only)
Phone (Voice/TTY):
812-855-9396
Website: http://
www.iidc.indiana.edu/cedir

Center for Learning Disabilities and the Law
P.O. Box 368
Cabin John, MD 20818

Center on Positive Behavioral Interventions and Supports
1761 Alder Street
1235 College of Education
Eugene, OR 97403
Phone: 541-346-2505
Website: http://www.pbis.org
E-mail: pbis@oregon.uoregon.edu

Children and Adults with Attention-Deficit/ Hyperactivity Disorder (CHADD)
8181 Professional Place
Suite 150
Landover, MD 20785
Toll-Free: 800-233-4050
Phone: 301-306-7070
Fax: 301-306-7090
Website: http://www.chadd.org; or http://help4adhd.org

Closing the Gap: Computer Technology in Special Education Rehabilitation
526 Main Street
P.O. Box 68
Henderson, MN 56044
Phone: 507-248-3294
Fax: 507-248-3810
Website: http://
www.closingthegap.com

Council for Exceptional Children
1110 N. Glebe Road
Suite 300
Arlington, VA 22201-5704
Toll-Free: 888-232-7733
Phone: 703-620-3660
TTY (text only): 703-264-9446
Fax: 703-264-9494
Website: http://www.dldcec.org
E-mail: cec@cec.sped.org

Council for Learning Disabilities
11184 Antioch Road
Box 405
Overland Park, KS 66210
Phone: 913-491-1011
Fax: 913-491-1012
Website: http://www.cldinternational.org
E-mail: CLDinfo@ie-events.com

Frostig Center
971 N. Altadena Dr.
Pasadena, CA 91107
Phone: 626-791-1255
Fax: 626-798-1801
Website: http://www.frostig.org

International Dyslexia Association
40 York Rd., 4th Floor
Baltimore, MD 21204
Phone: 410-296-0232
Fax: 410-321-5069
Website: http://www.interdys.org
E-mail: info@interdys.org

Job Accommodation Network
West Virginia University
P.O. Box 6080
Morgantown, WV 26506-6080
Toll-Free: 800-526-7234
Toll-Free TTY: 877-781-9403
Fax: 304-293-5407
Website: http://www.jan.wvu.edu
E-mail: jan@jan.wvu.edu

LD OnLine
WETA Public Television
2775 S. Quincy St.
Arlington, VA 22206
Fax: 703-998-2060
Website: http://www.ldonline.org

Learning Disabilities Association of America
4156 Library Road
Pittsburgh, PA 15234-1349
Toll-Free: 888-300-6710
Phone: 412-341-1515
Fax: 412-344-0224
Website: http://www.ldaamerica.org
E-mail: info@Idaamerica.org

Learning Disabilities Worldwide, Inc.
P.O. Box 142
Weston, MA 02493
Phone: 781-890-5399
International Phone:
001-781-890-5399
Fax: 781-890-0555
Website: http://www.ldworldwide.org

National Center for Learning Disabilities
381 Park Ave. S.
Suite 1401
New York, NY 10016
Toll-Free: 888-575-7373
Phone: 212-545-7510
Fax: 212-545-9665
Website: http://www.ncld.org

National Dissemination Center for Children with Disabilities (NICHCY)
P.O. Box 1492
Washington, DC 20013
Toll-Free Voice/TTY: 800-695-0285
Fax: 202-884-8441
Website: http://www.nichcy.org
E-mail: nichcy@aed.org

National Eye Institute
31 Center Drive, MSC 2510
Bethesda, MD 20892-2510
Phone: 301-496-5248
Website: http://www.nei.nih.gov
E-mail: 2020@nei.nih.gov

National Institute of Child Health and Human Development (NICHD)
P.O. Box 3006
Rockville, MD 20847
Toll-Free: 800-370-2943
Toll-Free TTY: 888-320-6942
Fax: 301-984-1473
Website: http://
www.nichd.nih.gov
E-mail:
NICHDInformationResourceCenter
@mail.nih.gov

National Institute of Mental Health (NIMH)
6001 Executive Blvd.
Rm. 8184, MSC 9663
Bethesda, MD 20892-9663
Toll-Free: 866-615-6464
Phone: 301-443-4513
TTY: 301-443-8431
Fax: 301-443-4279
Website: http://www.nimh.nih.gov
E-mail: nimhinfo@nih.gov

National Library Service for the Blind and Physically Handicapped
Library of Congress
Toll-Free: 888-657-7323 (to connect to a local library)
Phone: 202-707-5100
TDD: 202-707-0744
Fax: 202-707-0712
Website: http://www.loc.gov/nls
E-mail: nis@loc.gov

National Rehabilitation Information Center (NARIC)
8201 Corporate Drive, Suite 600
Landover, MD 20785
Toll-Free: 800-346-2742
Phone: 301-459-5900
TTY: 301-459-5984
Fax: 301-459-4263
Website: http://www.naric.com
E-mail:
naricinfo@heitechservices.com

National Resource Center for Traumatic Brain Injury
Department of Physical Medicine and Rehabilitation
P.O. Box 980542
Richmond, VA 23298-0542
Phone: 804-828-9055
Fax: 804-828-2378
Website: http://
www.neuro.pmr.vcu.edu
E-mail: mbking@vcu.edu

Office for Civil Rights
U.S. Department of Education
Toll-Free: 800-421-3481
Website: http://www.ed.gov/about/
offices/list/ocr/index.html

Office of Disability Employment Policy
200 Constitution Ave., N.W.
Washington, DC 20210
Toll-Free: 866-633-7365
Toll-Free TTY: 877-889-5627
Fax: 202-693-7888
Website: http://www.dol.gov/odep

Office of Special Education Programs
U.S. Department of Education
Phone: 202-245-7468
Website: http://www.ed.gov/
about/offices/list/osers/osep/
index.html

PACER Center
8161 Normandale Blvd.
Minneapolis, MN 55437-1044
Phone: 952-838-9000
Fax: 952-838-0199
TTY: 952-838-0190
Toll-Free in MN:
800-537-2237
Websites: http://www.pacer.org;
http://www.fape.org;
http://www.taalliance.org
E-mail: pacer@pacer.org

President's Committee on Employment of People with Disabilities
1331 F Street, N.W.
Washington, DC 20004
Phone: 202-376-6200
TTY: 202-376-6205
Website: http://www.pcepd.gov

Recording for the Blind and Dyslexic
20 Roszel Road
Princeton, NJ 08540
Toll-Free: 866-732-3585
Phone: 609-452-0606
Website: http://www.rfbd.org
E-mail: custserv@rfbd.org

U.S. Department of Education
Office for Civil Rights
400 Maryland Ave. S.W.
Washington, DC 20202-1100
Toll-Free: 800-421-3481
Toll-Free TDD: 877-521-2172
Fax: 202-245-6840
Website: http://www.ed.gov/ocr
E-mail: ocr@ed.gov

U.S. Department of Justice
950 Pennsylvania Avenue, N.W.
Civil Rights Division
Disability Rights Section–NYA
Washington, DC 20530
ADA Hotline: 800-466-4232
Fax: 202-307-1198
Website: http://www.usdoj.gov/
crt/drssec.htm;
or, http://www.ada.gov

U.S. Equal Employment Opportunity Commission
1801 L Street, N.W.
Washington, DC 20007
Toll-Free: 800-669-4000
Toll-Free TTY: 800-669-6820
Phone: 202-663-4900
TTY: 202-663-4494
Website: http://www.eeoc.gov

Index

Index

595

601

W

X

Y

Z

Health Reference Series

COMPLETE CATALOG

List price $87 per volume. **School and library price $78 per volume.**

Adolescent Health Sourcebook, 2nd Edition

Basic Consumer Health Information about the Physical, Mental, and Emotional Growth and Development of Adolescents, Including Medical Care, Nutritional and Physical Activity Requirements, Puberty, Sexual Activity, Acne, Tanning, Body Piercing, Common Physical Illnesses and Disorders, Eating Disorders, Attention Deficit Hyperactivity Disorder, Depression, Bullying, Hazing, and Adolescent Injuries Related to Sports, Driving, and Work

Along with Substance Abuse Information about Nicotine, Alcohol, and Drug Use, a Glossary, and Directory of Additional Resources

Edited by Joyce Brennfleck Shannon. 683 pages. 2006. 978-0-7808-0943-7.

"It is written in clear, nontechnical language aimed at general readers. . . . Recommended for public libraries, community colleges, and other agencies serving health care consumers."
— *American Reference Books Annual, 2003*

"Recommended for school and public libraries. Parents and professionals dealing with teens will appreciate the easy-to-follow format and the clearly written text. This could become a 'must have' for every high school teacher." — *E-Streams, Jan '03*

"A good starting point for information related to common medical, mental, and emotional concerns of adolescents." — *School Library Journal, Nov '02*

"This book provides accurate information in an easy to access format. It addresses topics that parents and caregivers might not be aware of and provides practical, useable information."
— *Doody's Health Sciences Book Review Journal, Sep-Oct '02*

"Recommended reference source."
— *Booklist, American Library Association, Sep '02*

■

AIDS Sourcebook, 3rd Edition

Basic Consumer Health Information about Acquired Immune Deficiency Syndrome (AIDS) and Human Immunodeficiency Virus (HIV) Infection, Including Facts about Transmission, Prevention, Diagnosis, Treatment, Opportunistic Infections, and Other Complications, with a Section for Women and Children, Including Details about Associated Gynecological Concerns, Pregnancy, and Pediatric Care

Along with Updated Statistical Information, Reports on Current Research Initiatives, a Glossary, and Directories of Internet, Hotline, and Other Resources

Edited by Dawn D. Matthews. 664 pages. 2003. 978-0-7808-0631-3.

"The 3rd edition of the *AIDS Sourcebook*, part of Omnigraphics' *Health Reference Series*, is a welcome update. . . . This resource is highly recommended for academic and public libraries."
— *American Reference Books Annual, 2004*

"Excellent sourcebook. This continues to be a highly recommended book. There is no other book that provides as much information as this book provides."
— *AIDS Book Review Journal, Dec-Jan '00*

"Recommended reference source."
— *Booklist, American Library Association, Dec '99*

■

Alcoholism Sourcebook, 2nd Edition

Basic Consumer Health Information about Alcohol Use, Abuse, and Dependence, Featuring Facts about the Physical, Mental, and Social Health Effects of Alcohol Addiction, Including Alcoholic Liver Disease, Pancreatic Disease, Cardiovascular Disease, Neurological Disorders, and the Effects of Drinking during Pregnancy

Along with Information about Alcohol Treatment, Medications, and Recovery Programs, in Addition to Tips for Reducing the Prevalence of Underage Drinking, Statistics about Alcohol Use, a Glossary of Related Terms, and Directories of Resources for More Help and Information

Edited by Amy L. Sutton. 653 pages. 2006. 978-0-7808-0942-0.

"This title is one of the few reference works on alcoholism for general readers. For some readers this will be a welcome complement to the many self-help books on the market. Recommended for collections serving general readers and consumer health collections."
— *E-Streams, Mar '01*

"This book is an excellent choice for public and academic libraries."
— *American Reference Books Annual, 2001*

"Recommended reference source."
— *Booklist, American Library Association, Dec '00*

"Presents a wealth of information on alcohol use and abuse and its effects on the body and mind, treatment, and prevention." — *SciTech Book News, Dec '00*

"Important new health guide which packs in the latest consumer information about the problems of alcoholism." — *Reviewer's Bookwatch, Nov '00*

SEE ALSO *Drug Abuse Sourcebook*

Allergies Sourcebook, 3rd Edition

Basic Consumer Health Information about Allergic Disorders, Such as Anaphylaxis, Hives, Eczema, Rhinitis, Sinusitis, and Conjunctivitis, and Their Triggers, Including Pollen, Mold, Dust Mites, Animal Dander, Insects, Chemicals, Food, Food Additives, and Medications;

Along with Advice about the Diagnosis and Treatment of Allergy Symptoms, a Glossary of Related Terms, a Directory of Resources for Help and Information, and Suggestions for Additional Reading

Edited by Amy L. Sutton. 598 pages. 2007. 978-0-7808-0950-5.

"This book brings a great deal of useful material together. . . . This is an excellent addition to public and consumer health library collections."
— *American Reference Books Annual, 2003*

"This second edition would be useful to laypersons with little or advanced knowledge of the subject matter. This book would also serve as a resource for nursing and other health care professions students. It would be useful in public, academic, and hospital libraries with consumer health collections." — *E-Streams, Jul '02*

Alternative Medicine Sourcebook

SEE Complementary & Alternative Medicine Sourcebook

Alzheimer's Disease Sourcebook, 3rd Edition

Basic Consumer Health Information about Alzheimer's Disease, Other Dementias, and Related Disorders, Including Multi-Infarct Dementia, AIDS Dementia Complex, Dementia with Lewy Bodies, Huntington's Disease, Wernicke-Korsakoff Syndrome (Alcohol-Related Dementia), Delirium, and Confusional States

Along with Information for People Newly Diagnosed with Alzheimer's Disease and Caregivers, Reports Detailing Current Research Efforts in Prevention, Diagnosis, and Treatment, Facts about Long-Term Care Issues, and Listings of Sources for Additional Information

Edited by Karen Bellenir. 645 pages. 2003. 978-0-7808-0666-5.

"This very informative and valuable tool will be a great addition to any library serving consumers, students and health care workers."
— *American Reference Books Annual, 2004*

"This is a valuable resource for people affected by dementias such as Alzheimer's. It is easy to navigate and includes important information and resources."
— *Doody's Review Service, Feb '04*

"Recommended reference source."
— *Booklist, American Library Association, Oct '99*

SEE ALSO Brain Disorders Sourcebook

Arthritis Sourcebook, 2nd Edition

Basic Consumer Health Information about Osteoarthritis, Rheumatoid Arthritis, Other Rheumatic Disorders, Infectious Forms of Arthritis, and Diseases with Symptoms Linked to Arthritis, Featuring Facts about Diagnosis, Pain Management, and Surgical Therapies

Along with Coping Strategies, Research Updates, a Glossary, and Resources for Additional Help and Information

Edited by Amy L. Sutton. 593 pages. 2004. 978-0-7808-0667-2.

"This easy-to-read volume is recommended for consumer health collections within public or academic libraries." — *E-Streams, May '05*

"As expected, this updated edition continues the excellent reputation of this series in providing sound, usable health information. . . . Highly recommended."
— *American Reference Books Annual, 2005*

"Excellent reference." — *The Bookwatch, Jan '05*

Asthma Sourcebook, 2nd Edition

Basic Consumer Health Information about the Causes, Symptoms, Diagnosis, and Treatment of Asthma in Infants, Children, Teenagers, and Adults, Including Facts about Different Types of Asthma, Common Co-Occurring Conditions, Asthma Management Plans, Triggers, Medications, and Medication Delivery Devices

Along with Asthma Statistics, Research Updates, a Glossary, a Directory of Asthma-Related Resources, and More

Edited by Karen Bellenir. 609 pages. 2006. 978-0-7808-0866-9.

"A worthwhile reference acquisition for public libraries and academic medical libraries whose readers desire a quick introduction to the wide range of asthma information." — *Choice, Association of College & Research Libraries, Jun '01*

"Recommended reference source."
— *Booklist, American Library Association, Feb '01*

"Highly recommended." — *The Bookwatch, Jan '01*

"There is much good information for patients and their families who deal with asthma daily."
— *American Medical Writers Association Journal, Winter '01*

"This informative text is recommended for consumer health collections in public, secondary school, and community college libraries and the libraries of universities with a large undergraduate population."
— *American Reference Books Annual, 2001*

Attention Deficit Disorder Sourcebook

Basic Consumer Health Information about Attention Deficit/Hyperactivity Disorder in Children and Adults,

Including Facts about Causes, Symptoms, Diagnostic Criteria, and Treatment Options Such as Medications, Behavior Therapy, Coaching, and Homeopathy

Along with Reports on Current Research Initiatives, Legal Issues, and Government Regulations, and Featuring a Glossary of Related Terms, Internet Resources, and a List of Additional Reading Material

Edited by Dawn D. Matthews. 470 pages. 2002. 978-0-7808-0624-5.

"Recommended reference source."
— *Booklist, American Library Association, Jan '03*

"This book is recommended for all school libraries and the reference or consumer health sections of public libraries." — *American Reference Books Annual, 2003*

■

Back & Neck Sourcebook, 2nd Edition

Basic Consumer Health Information about Spinal Pain, Spinal Cord Injuries, and Related Disorders, Such as Degenerative Disk Disease, Osteoarthritis, Scoliosis, Sciatica, Spina Bifida, and Spinal Stenosis, and Featuring Facts about Maintaining Spinal Health, Self-Care, Pain Management, Rehabilitative Care, Chiropractic Care, Spinal Surgeries, and Complementary Therapies

Along with Suggestions for Preventing Back and Neck Pain, a Glossary of Related Terms, and a Directory of Resources

Edited by Amy L. Sutton. 633 pages. 2004. 978-0-7808-0738-9.

"Recommended . . . an easy to use, comprehensive medical reference book." — *E-Streams, Sep '05*

"The strength of this work is its basic, easy-to-read format. Recommended." — *Reference and User Services Quarterly, American Library Association, Winter '97*

■

Blood & Circulatory Disorders Sourcebook, 2nd Edition

Basic Consumer Health Information about the Blood and Circulatory System and Related Disorders, Such as Anemia and Other Hemoglobin Diseases, Cancer of the Blood and Associated Bone Marrow Disorders, Clotting and Bleeding Problems, and Conditions That Affect the Veins, Blood Vessels, and Arteries, Including Facts about the Donation and Transplantation of Bone Marrow, Stem Cells, and Blood and Tips for Keeping the Blood and Circulatory System Healthy

Along with a Glossary of Related Terms and Resources for Additional Help and Information

Edited by Amy L. Sutton. 659 pages. 2005. 978-0-7808-0746-4.

"Highly recommended pick for basic consumer health reference holdings at all levels." — *The Bookwatch, Aug '05*

"Recommended reference source."
— *Booklist, American Library Association, Feb '99*

"An important reference sourcebook written in simple language for everyday, non-technical users. " — *Reviewer's Bookwatch, Jan '99*

■

Brain Disorders Sourcebook, 2nd Edition

Basic Consumer Health Information about Acquired and Traumatic Brain Injuries, Infections of the Brain, Epilepsy and Seizure Disorders, Cerebral Palsy, and Degenerative Neurological Disorders, Including Amyotrophic Lateral Sclerosis (ALS), Dementias, Multiple Sclerosis, and More

Along with Information on the Brain's Structure and Function, Treatment and Rehabilitation Options, Reports on Current Research Initiatives, a Glossary of Terms Related to Brain Disorders and Injuries, and a Directory of Sources for Further Help and Information

Edited by Sandra J. Judd. 625 pages. 2005. 978-0-7808-0744-0.

"Highly recommended pick for basic consumer health reference holdings at all levels."
— *The Bookwatch, Aug '05*

"Belongs on the shelves of any library with a consumer health collection." — *E-Streams, Mar '00*

"Recommended reference source."
— *Booklist, American Library Association, Oct '99*

SEE ALSO Alzheimer's Disease Sourcebook

■

Breast Cancer Sourcebook, 2nd Edition

Basic Consumer Health Information about Breast Cancer, Including Facts about Risk Factors, Prevention, Screening and Diagnostic Methods, Treatment Options, Complementary and Alternative Therapies, Post-Treatment Concerns, Clinical Trials, Special Risk Populations, and New Developments in Breast Cancer Research

Along with Breast Cancer Statistics, a Glossary of Related Terms, and a Directory of Resources for Additional Help and Information

Edited by Sandra J. Judd. 595 pages. 2004. 978-0-7808-0668-9.

"This book will be an excellent addition to public, community college, medical, and academic libraries." — *American Reference Books Annual, 2006*

"It would be a useful reference book in a library or on loan to women in a support group." — *Cancer Forum, Mar '03*

"Recommended reference source."
— *Booklist, American Library Association, Jan '02*

"This reference source is highly recommended. It is quite informative, comprehensive and detailed in nature, and yet it offers practical advice in easy-to-read language. It could be thought of as the 'bible' of breast cancer for the consumer." — *E-Streams, Jan '02*

"From the pros and cons of different screening methods and results to treatment options, *Breast Cancer Sourcebook* provides the latest information on the subject." — *Library Bookwatch, Dec '01*

"This thoroughgoing, very readable reference covers all aspects of breast health and cancer.... Readers will find much to consider here. Recommended for all public and patient health collections." — *Library Journal, Sep '01*

SEE ALSO Cancer Sourcebook for Women, Women's Health Concerns Sourcebook

■

Breastfeeding Sourcebook

Basic Consumer Health Information about the Benefits of Breastmilk, Preparing to Breastfeed, Breastfeeding as a Baby Grows, Nutrition, and More, Including Information on Special Situations and Concerns Such as Mastitis, Illness, Medications, Allergies, Multiple Births, Prematurity, Special Needs, and Adoption

Along with a Glossary and Resources for Additional Help and Information

Edited by Jenni Lynn Colson. 388 pages. 2002. 978-0-7808-0332-9.

"Particularly useful is the information about professional lactation services and chapters on breastfeeding when returning to work.... *Breastfeeding Sourcebook* will be useful for public libraries, consumer health libraries, and technical schools offering nurse assistant training, especially in areas where Internet access is problematic." — *American Reference Books Annual, 2003*

SEE ALSO Pregnancy & Birth Sourcebook

■

Burns Sourcebook

Basic Consumer Health Information about Various Types of Burns and Scalds, Including Flame, Heat, Cold, Electrical, Chemical, and Sun Burns

Along with Information on Short-Term and Long-Term Treatments, Tissue Reconstruction, Plastic Surgery, Prevention Suggestions, and First Aid

Edited by Allan R. Cook. 604 pages. 1999. 978-0-7808-0204-9.

"This is an exceptional addition to the series and is highly recommended for all consumer health collections, hospital libraries, and academic medical centers." — *E-Streams, Mar '00*

"This key reference guide is an invaluable addition to all health care and public libraries in confronting this ongoing health issue." — *American Reference Books Annual, 2000*

"Recommended reference source." — *Booklist, American Library Association, Dec '99*

SEE ALSO Dermatological Disorders Sourcebook

Cancer Sourcebook, 5th Edition

Basic Consumer Health Information about Major Forms and Stages of Cancer, Featuring Facts about Head and Neck Cancers, Lung Cancers, Gastrointestinal Cancers, Genitourinary Cancers, Lymphomas, Blood Cell Cancers, Endocrine Cancers, Skin Cancers, Bone Cancers, Metastatic Cancers, and More

Along with Facts about Cancer Treatments, Cancer Risks and Prevention, a Glossary of Related Terms, Statistical Data, and a Directory of Resources for Additional Information

Edited by Karen Bellenir. 1,133 pages. 2007. 978-0-7808-0947-5.

"With cancer being the second leading cause of death for Americans, a prodigious work such as this one, which locates centrally so much cancer-related information, is clearly an asset to this nation's citizens and others." — *Journal of the National Medical Association, 2004*

"This title is recommended for health sciences and public libraries with consumer health collections." — *E-Streams, Feb '01*

"... can be effectively used by cancer patients and their families who are looking for answers in a language they can understand. Public and hospital libraries should have it on their shelves." — *American Reference Books Annual, 2001*

"Recommended reference source." — *Booklist, American Library Association, Dec '00*

SEE ALSO Breast Cancer Sourcebook, Cancer Sourcebook for Women, Pediatric Cancer Sourcebook, Prostate Cancer Sourcebook

■

Cancer Sourcebook for Women, 3rd Edition

Basic Consumer Health Information about Leading Causes of Cancer in Women, Featuring Facts about Gynecologic Cancers and Related Concerns, Such as Breast Cancer, Cervical Cancer, Endometrial Cancer, Uterine Sarcoma, Vaginal Cancer, Vulvar Cancer, and Common Non-Cancerous Gynecologic Conditions, in Addition to Facts about Lung Cancer, Colorectal Cancer, and Thyroid Cancer in Women

Along with Information about Cancer Risk Factors, Screening and Prevention, Treatment Options, and Tips on Coping with Life after Cancer Treatment, a Glossary of Cancer Terms, and a Directory of Resources for Additional Help and Information

Edited by Amy L. Sutton. 715 pages. 2006. 978-0-7808-0867-6.

"An excellent addition to collections in public, consumer health, and women's health libraries." — *American Reference Books Annual, 2003*

"Overall, the information is excellent, and complex topics are clearly explained. As a reference book for the consumer it is a valuable resource to assist them to make informed decisions about cancer and its treatments." — *Cancer Forum, Nov '02*

"Highly recommended for academic and medical reference collections." — *Library Bookwatch, Sep '02*

"This is a highly recommended book for any public or consumer library, being reader friendly and containing accurate and helpful information."
— *E-Streams, Aug '02*

"Recommended reference source."
—*Booklist, American Library Association, Jul '02*

SEE ALSO *Breast Cancer Sourcebook, Women's Health Concerns Sourcebook*

Cancer Survivorship Sourcebook

Basic Consumer Health Information about the Physical, Educational, Emotional, Social, and Financial Needs of Cancer Patients from Diagnosis, through Cancer Treatment, and Beyond, Including Facts about Researching Specific Types of Cancer and Learning about Clinical Trials and Treatment Options, and Featuring Tips for Coping with the Side Effects of Cancer Treatments and Adjusting to Life after Cancer Treatment Concludes

Along with Suggestions for Caregivers, Friends, and Family Members of Cancer Patients, a Glossary of Cancer Care Terms, and Directories of Related Resources

Edited by Karen Bellenir. 6561 pages. 2007. 978-0-7808-0985-7.

Cardiovascular Diseases & Disorders Sourcebook, 3rd Edition

Basic Consumer Health Information about Heart and Vascular Diseases and Disorders, Such as Angina, Heart Attacks, Arrhythmias, Cardiomyopathy, Valve Disease, Atherosclerosis, and Aneurysms, with Information about Managing Cardiovascular Risk Factors and Maintaining Heart Health, Medications and Procedures Used to Treat Cardiovascular Disorders, and Concerns of Special Significance to Women

Along with Reports on Current Research Initiatives, a Glossary of Related Medical Terms, and a Directory of Sources for Further Help and Information

Edited by Sandra J. Judd. 713 pages. 2005. 978-0-7808-0739-6.

"This updated sourcebook is still the best first stop for comprehensive introductory information on cardiovascular diseases."
— *American Reference Books Annual, 2006*

"Recommended for public libraries and libraries supporting health care professionals."
— *E-Streams, Sep '05*

"This should be a standard health library reference."
—*The Bookwatch, Jun '05*

"Recommended reference source."
—*Booklist, American Library Association, Dec '00*

". . . comprehensive format provides an extensive overview on this subject."
— *Choice, Association of College & Research Libraries*

Caregiving Sourcebook

Basic Consumer Health Information for Caregivers, Including a Profile of Caregivers, Caregiving Responsibilities and Concerns, Tips for Specific Conditions, Care Environments, and the Effects of Caregiving

Along with Facts about Legal Issues, Financial Information, and Future Planning, a Glossary, and a Listing of Additional Resources

Edited by Joyce Brennfleck Shannon. 600 pages. 2001. 978-0-7808-0331-2.

"Essential for most collections."
—*Library Journal, Apr 1, 2002*

"An ideal addition to the reference collection of any public library. Health sciences information professionals may also want to acquire the *Caregiving Sourcebook* for their hospital or academic library for use as a ready reference tool by health care workers interested in aging and caregiving." —*E-Streams, Jan '02*

"Recommended reference source."
—*Booklist, American Library Association, Oct '01*

Child Abuse Sourcebook

Basic Consumer Health Information about the Physical, Sexual, and Emotional Abuse of Children, with Additional Facts about Neglect, Munchausen Syndrome by Proxy (MSBP), Shaken Baby Syndrome, and Controversial Issues Related to Child Abuse, Such as Withholding Medical Care, Corporal Punishment, and Child Maltreatment in Youth Sports, and Featuring Facts about Child Protective Services, Foster Care, Adoption, Parenting Challenges, and Other Abuse Prevention Efforts

Along with a Glossary of Related Terms and Resources for Additional Help and Information

Edited by Dawn D. Matthews. 620 pages. 2004. 978-0-7808-0705-1.

"A valuable and highly recommended resource for school, academic and public libraries whether used on its own or as a starting point for more in-depth research." — *E-Streams, Apr '05*

"Every week the news brings cases of child abuse or neglect, so it is useful to have a source that supplies so much helpful information. . . . Recommended. Public and academic libraries, and child welfare offices."
— *Choice, Association of College & Research Libraries, Mar '05*

"Packed with insights on all kinds of issues, from foster care and adoption to parenting and abuse prevention."
—*The Bookwatch, Nov '04*

SEE ALSO: *Domestic Violence Sourcebook*

Childhood Diseases & Disorders Sourcebook

Basic Consumer Health Information about Medical Problems Often Encountered in Pre-Adolescent Children, Including Respiratory Tract Ailments, Ear Infections, Sore Throats, Disorders of the Skin and Scalp, Digestive and Genitourinary Diseases, Infectious Diseases, Inflammatory Disorders, Chronic Physical and Developmental Disorders, Allergies, and More

Along with Information about Diagnostic Tests, Common Childhood Surgeries, and Frequently Used Medications, with a Glossary of Important Terms and Resource Directory

Edited by Chad T. Kimball. 662 pages. 2003. 978-0-7808-0458-6.

"This is an excellent book for new parents and should be included in all health care and public libraries."
—American Reference Books Annual, 2004

SEE ALSO: Healthy Children Sourcebook

■

Colds, Flu & Other Common Ailments Sourcebook

Basic Consumer Health Information about Common Ailments and Injuries, Including Colds, Coughs, the Flu, Sinus Problems, Headaches, Fever, Nausea and Vomiting, Menstrual Cramps, Diarrhea, Constipation, Hemorrhoids, Back Pain, Dandruff, Dry and Itchy Skin, Cuts, Scrapes, Sprains, Bruises, and More

Along with Information about Prevention, Self-Care, Choosing a Doctor, Over-the-Counter Medications, Folk Remedies, and Alternative Therapies, and Including a Glossary of Important Terms and a Directory of Resources for Further Help and Information

Edited by Chad T. Kimball. 638 pages. 2001. 978-0-7808-0435-7.

"A good starting point for research on common illnesses. It will be a useful addition to public and consumer health library collections."
—American Reference Books Annual, 2002

"Will prove valuable to any library seeking to maintain a current, comprehensive reference collection of health resources. . . . Excellent reference."
— The Bookwatch, Aug '01

"Recommended reference source."
— Booklist, American Library Association, Jul '01

■

Communication Disorders Sourcebook

Basic Information about Deafness and Hearing Loss, Speech and Language Disorders, Voice Disorders, Balance and Vestibular Disorders, and Disorders of Smell, Taste, and Touch

Edited by Linda M. Ross. 533 pages. 1996. 978-0-7808-0077-9.

"This is skillfully edited and is a welcome resource for the layperson. It should be found in every public and medical library." *— Booklist Health Sciences Supplement, American Library Association, Oct '97*

■

Complementary & Alternative Medicine Sourcebook, 3rd Edition

Basic Consumer Health Information about Complementary and Alternative Medical Therapies, Including Acupuncture, Ayurveda, Traditional Chinese Medicine, Herbal Medicine, Homeopathy, Naturopathy, Biofeedback, Hypnotherapy, Yoga, Art Therapy, Aromatherapy, Clinical Nutrition, Vitamin and Mineral Supplements, Chiropractic, Massage, Reflexology, Crystal Therapy, Therapeutic Touch, and More

Along with Facts about Alternative and Complementary Treatments for Specific Conditions Such as Cancer, Diabetes, Osteoarthritis, Chronic Pain, Menopause, Gastrointestinal Disorders, Headaches, and Mental Illness, a Glossary, and a Resource List for Additional Help and Information

Edited by Sandra J. Judd. 657 pages. 2006. 978-0-7808-0864-5.

"Recommended for public, high school, and academic libraries that have consumer health collections. Hospital libraries that also serve the public will find this to be a useful resource." *— E-Streams, Feb '03*

"Recommended reference source."
—Booklist, American Library Association, Jan '03

"An important alternate health reference."
— MBR Bookwatch, Oct '02

"A great addition to the reference collection of every type of library." *— American Reference Books Annual, 2000*

■

Congenital Disorders Sourcebook, 2nd Edition

Basic Consumer Health Information about Non-hereditary Birth Defects and Disorders Related to Prematurity, Gestational Injuries, Congenital Infections, and Birth Complications, Including Heart Defects, Hydrocephalus, Spina Bifida, Cleft Lip and Palate, Cerebral Palsy, and More

Along with Facts about the Prevention of Birth Defects, Fetal Surgery and Other Treatment Options, Research Initiatives, a Glossary of Related Terms, and Resources for Additional Information and Support

Edited by Sandra J. Judd. 647 pages. 2006. 978-0-7808-0945-1.

"Recommended reference source."
—Booklist, American Library Association, Oct '97

SEE ALSO Pregnancy & Birth Sourcebook

■

Contagious Diseases Sourcebook

Basic Consumer Health Information about Infectious Diseases Spread by Person-to-Person Contact through

Direct Touch, Airborne Transmission, Sexual Contact, or Contact with Blood or Other Body Fluids, Including Hepatitis, Herpes, Influenza, Lice, Measles, Mumps, Pinworm, Ringworm, Severe Acute Respiratory Syndrome (SARS), Streptococcal Infections, Tuberculosis, and Others

Along with Facts about Disease Transmission, Antimicrobial Resistance, and Vaccines, with a Glossary and Directories of Resources for More Information

Edited by Karen Bellenir. 643 pages. 2004. 978-0-7808-0736-5.

"This easy-to-read volume is recommended for consumer health collections within public or academic libraries." — E-Streams, May '05

"This informative book is highly recommended for public libraries, consumer health collections, and secondary schools and undergraduate libraries."
— American Reference Books Annual, 2005

"Excellent reference." — The Bookwatch, Jan '05

Death & Dying Sourcebook, 2nd Edition

Basic Consumer Health Information about End-of-Life Care and Related Perspectives and Ethical Issues, Including End-of-Life Symptoms and Treatments, Pain Management, Quality-of-Life Concerns, the Use of Life Support, Patients' Rights and Privacy Issues, Advance Directives, Physician-Assisted Suicide, Caregiving, Organ and Tissue Donation, Autopsies, Funeral Arrangements, and Grief

Along with Statistical Data, Information about the Leading Causes of Death, a Glossary, and Directories of Support Groups and Other Resources

Edited by Joyce Brennfleck Shannon. 653 pages. 2006. 978-0-7808-0871-3.

"Public libraries, medical libraries, and academic libraries will all find this sourcebook a useful addition to their collections."
— American Reference Books Annual, 2001

"An extremely useful resource for those concerned with death and dying in the United States."
— Respiratory Care, Nov '00

"Recommended reference source."
—Booklist, American Library Association, Aug '00

"This book is a definite must for all those involved in end-of-life care." — Doody's Review Service, 2000

Dental Care & Oral Health Sourcebook, 2nd Edition

Basic Consumer Health Information about Dental Care, Including Oral Hygiene, Dental Visits, Pain Management, Cavities, Crowns, Bridges, Dental Implants, and Fillings, and Other Oral Health Concerns, Such as Gum Disease, Bad Breath, Dry Mouth, Genetic and Developmental Abnormalities, Oral Cancers, Orthodontics, and Temporomandibular Disorders

Along with Updates on Current Research in Oral Health, a Glossary, a Directory of Dental and Oral Health Organizations, and Resources for People with Dental and Oral Health Disorders

Edited by Amy L. Sutton. 609 pages. 2003. 978-0-7808-0634-4.

"This book could serve as a turning point in the battle to educate consumers in issues concerning oral health."
— American Reference Books Annual, 2004

"Unique source which will fill a gap in dental sources for patients and the lay public. A valuable reference tool even in a library with thousands of books on dentistry. Comprehensive, clear, inexpensive, and easy to read and use. It fills an enormous gap in the health care literature." — Reference & User Services Quarterly, American Library Association, Summer '98

"Recommended reference source."
— Booklist, American Library Association, Dec '97

Depression Sourcebook

Basic Consumer Health Information about Unipolar Depression, Bipolar Disorder, Postpartum Depression, Seasonal Affective Disorder, and Other Types of Depression in Children, Adolescents, Women, Men, the Elderly, and Other Selected Populations

Along with Facts about Causes, Risk Factors, Diagnostic Criteria, Treatment Options, Coping Strategies, Suicide Prevention, a Glossary, and a Directory of Sources for Additional Help and Information

Edited by Karen Bellenir. 602 pages. 2002. 978-0-7808-0611-5.

"Depression Sourcebook is of a very high standard. Its purpose, which is to serve as a reference source to the lay reader, is very well served."
— Journal of the National Medical Association, 2004

"Invaluable reference for public and school library collections alike." — Library Bookwatch, Apr '03

"Recommended for purchase."
— American Reference Books Annual, 2003

Dermatological Disorders Sourcebook, 2nd Edition

Basic Consumer Health Information about Conditions and Disorders Affecting the Skin, Hair, and Nails, Such as Acne, Rosacea, Rashes, Dermatitis, Pigmentation Disorders, Birthmarks, Skin Cancer, Skin Injuries, Psoriasis, Scleroderma, and Hair Loss, Including Facts about Medications and Treatments for Dermatological Disorders and Tips for Maintaining Healthy Skin, Hair, and Nails

Along with Information about How Aging Affects the Skin, a Glossary of Related Terms, and a Directory of Resources for Additional Help and Information

Edited by Amy L. Sutton. 645 pages. 2005. 978-0-7808-0795-2.

"... comprehensive, easily read reference book."
—*Doody's Health Sciences Book Reviews, Oct '97*

SEE ALSO *Burns Sourcebook*

■

Diabetes Sourcebook, 3rd Edition

Basic Consumer Health Information about Type 1 Diabetes (Insulin-Dependent or Juvenile-Onset Diabetes), Type 2 Diabetes (Noninsulin-Dependent or Adult-Onset Diabetes), Gestational Diabetes, Impaired Glucose Tolerance (IGT), and Related Complications, Such as Amputation, Eye Disease, Gum Disease, Nerve Damage, and End-Stage Renal Disease, Including Facts about Insulin, Oral Diabetes Medications, Blood Sugar Testing, and the Role of Exercise and Nutrition in the Control of Diabetes

Along with a Glossary and Resources for Further Help and Information

Edited by Dawn D. Matthews. 622 pages. 2003. 978-0-7808-0629-0.

"This edition is even more helpful than earlier versions. . . . It is a truly valuable tool for anyone seeking readable and authoritative information on diabetes."
— *American Reference Books Annual, 2004*

"An invaluable reference." — *Library Journal, May '00*

Selected as one of the 250 "Best Health Sciences Books of 1999." — *Doody's Rating Service, Mar-Apr '00*

"Provides useful information for the general public."
— *Healthlines, University of Michigan Health Management Research Center, Sep/Oct '99*

". . . provides reliable mainstream medical information . . . belongs on the shelves of any library with a consumer health collection." — *E-Streams, Sep '99*

"Recommended reference source."
— *Booklist, American Library Association, Feb '99*

■

Diet & Nutrition Sourcebook, 3rd Edition

Basic Consumer Health Information about Dietary Guidelines and the Food Guidance System, Recommended Daily Nutrient Intakes, Serving Proportions, Weight Control, Vitamins and Supplements, Nutrition Issues for Different Life Stages and Lifestyles, and the Needs of People with Specific Medical Concerns, Including Cancer, Celiac Disease, Diabetes, Eating Disorders, Food Allergies, and Cardiovascular Disease

Along with Facts about Federal Nutrition Support Programs, a Glossary of Nutrition and Dietary Terms, and Directories of Additional Resources for More Information about Nutrition

Edited by Joyce Brennfleck Shannon. 633 pages. 2006. 978-0-7808-0800-3.

"This book is an excellent source of basic diet and nutrition information." — *Booklist Health Sciences Supplement, American Library Association, Dec '00*

"This reference document should be in any public library, but it would be a very good guide for beginning students in the health sciences. If the other books in this publisher's series are as good as this, they should all be in the health sciences collections."
— *American Reference Books Annual, 2000*

"This book is an excellent general nutrition reference for consumers who desire to take an active role in their health care for prevention. Consumers of all ages who select this book can feel confident they are receiving current and accurate information." — *Journal of Nutrition for the Elderly, Vol. 19, No. 4, 2000*

SEE ALSO *Digestive Diseases & Disorders Sourcebook, Eating Disorders Sourcebook, Gastrointestinal Diseases & Disorders Sourcebook, Vegetarian Sourcebook*

■

Digestive Diseases & Disorders Sourcebook

Basic Consumer Health Information about Diseases and Disorders that Impact the Upper and Lower Digestive System, Including Celiac Disease, Constipation, Crohn's Disease, Cyclic Vomiting Syndrome, Diarrhea, Diverticulosis and Diverticulitis, Gallstones, Heartburn, Hemorrhoids, Hernias, Indigestion (Dyspepsia), Irritable Bowel Syndrome, Lactose Intolerance, Ulcers, and More

Along with Information about Medications and Other Treatments, Tips for Maintaining a Healthy Digestive Tract, a Glossary, and Directory of Digestive Diseases Organizations

Edited by Karen Bellenir. 335 pages. 2000. 978-0-7808-0327-5.

"This title would be an excellent addition to all public or patient-research libraries."
— *American Reference Books Annual, 2001*

"This title is recommended for public, hospital, and health sciences libraries with consumer health collections." — *E-Streams, Jul-Aug '00*

"Recommended reference source."
— *Booklist, American Library Association, May '00*

SEE ALSO *Eating Disorders Sourcebook, Gastrointestinal Diseases & Disorders Sourcebook*

■

Disabilities Sourcebook

Basic Consumer Health Information about Physical and Psychiatric Disabilities, Including Descriptions of Major Causes of Disability, Assistive and Adaptive Aids, Workplace Issues, and Accessibility Concerns

Along with Information about the Americans with Disabilities Act, a Glossary, and Resources for Additional Help and Information

Edited by Dawn D. Matthews. 616 pages. 2000. 978-0-7808-0389-3.

"It is a must for libraries with a consumer health section." — *American Reference Books Annual, 2002*

"A much needed addition to the Omnigraphics *Health Reference Series*. A current reference work to provide people with disabilities, their families, caregivers or those who work with them, a broad range of information in one volume, has not been available until now. . . . It is recommended for all public and academic library reference collections."　　—*E-Streams, May '01*

"An excellent source book in easy-to-read format covering many current topics; highly recommended for all libraries."　　—*Choice, Association of College & Research Libraries, Jan '01*

"Recommended reference source."
　　—*Booklist, American Library Association, Jul '00*

Domestic Violence Sourcebook, 2nd Edition

Basic Consumer Health Information about the Causes and Consequences of Abusive Relationships, Including Physical Violence, Sexual Assault, Battery, Stalking, and Emotional Abuse, and Facts about the Effects of Violence on Women, Men, Young Adults, and the Elderly, with Reports about Domestic Violence in Selected Populations, and Featuring Facts about Medical Care, Victim Assistance and Protection, Prevention Strategies, Mental Health Services, and Legal Issues

Along with a Glossary of Related Terms and Resources for Additional Help and Information

Edited by Dawn D. Matthews. 628 pages. 2004. 978-0-7808-0669-6.

"Educators, clergy, medical professionals, police, and victims and their families will benefit from this realistic and easy-to-understand resource."
　　—*American Reference Books Annual, 2005*

"Recommended for all collections supporting consumer health information. It should also be considered for any collection needing general, readable information on domestic violence."　　—*E-Streams, Jan '05*

"This sourcebook complements other books in its field, providing a one-stop resource . . . Recommended."
　　—*Choice, Association of College & Research Libraries, Jan '05*

"Interested lay persons should find the book extremely beneficial. . . . A copy of *Domestic Violence and Child Abuse Sourcebook* should be in every public library in the United States."
　　—*Social Science & Medicine, No. 56, 2003*

"This is important information. The Web has many resources but this sourcebook fills an important societal need. I am not aware of any other resources of this type."　　—*Doody's Review Service, Sep '01*

"Recommended reference source."
　　—*Booklist, American Library Association, Apr '01*

"Important pick for college-level health reference libraries."　　—*The Bookwatch, Mar '01*

"Because this problem is so widespread and because this book includes a lot of issues within one volume, this work is recommended for all public libraries."
　　—*American Reference Books Annual, 2001*

SEE ALSO Child Abuse Sourcebook

Drug Abuse Sourcebook, 2nd Edition

Basic Consumer Health Information about Illicit Substances of Abuse and the Misuse of Prescription and Over-the-Counter Medications, Including Depressants, Hallucinogens, Inhalants, Marijuana, Stimulants, and Anabolic Steroids

Along with Facts about Related Health Risks, Treatment Programs, Prevention Programs, a Glossary of Abuse and Addiction Terms, a Glossary of Drug-Related Street Terms, and a Directory of Resources for More Information

Edited by Catherine Ginther. 607 pages. 2004. 978-0-7808-0740-2.

"Commendable for organizing useful, normally scattered government and association-produced data into a logical sequence."
　　—*American Reference Books Annual, 2006*

"This easy-to-read volume is recommended for consumer health collections within public or academic libraries."　　—*E-Streams, Sep '05*

"An excellent library reference."
　　—*The Bookwatch, May '05*

"Containing a wealth of information, this book will be useful to the college student just beginning to explore the topic of substance abuse. This resource belongs in libraries that serve a lower-division undergraduate or community college clientele as well as the general public."　　—*Choice, Association of College & Research Libraries, Jun '01*

"Recommended reference source."
　　—*Booklist, American Library Association, Feb '01*

SEE ALSO Alcoholism Sourcebook

Ear, Nose & Throat Disorders Sourcebook, 2nd Edition

Basic Consumer Health Information about Disorders of the Ears, Hearing Loss, Vestibular Disorders, Nasal and Sinus Problems, Throat and Vocal Cord Disorders, and Otolaryngologic Cancers, Including Facts about Ear Infections and Injuries, Genetic and Congenital Deafness, Sensorineural Hearing Disorders, Tinnitus, Vertigo, Ménière Disease, Rhinitis, Sinusitis, Snoring, Sore Throats, Hoarseness, and More

Along with Reports on Current Research Initiatives, a Glossary of Related Medical Terms, and a Directory of Sources for Further Help and Information

Edited by Sandra J. Judd. 659 pages. 2006. 978-0-7808-0872-0.

Eating Disorders Sourcebook, 2nd Edition

Basic Consumer Health Information about Anorexia Nervosa, Bulimia Nervosa, Binge Eating, Compulsive Exercise, Female Athlete Triad, and Other Eating Disorders, Including Facts about Body Image and Other Cultural and Age-Related Risk Factors, Prevention Efforts, Adverse Health Effects, Treatment Options, and the Recovery Process

Along with Guidelines for Healthy Weight Control, a Glossary, and Directories of Additional Resources

Edited by Joyce Brennfleck Shannon. 585 pages. 2007. 978-0-7808-0948-2.

SEE ALSO *Diet & Nutrition Sourcebook, Digestive Diseases & Disorders Sourcebook, Gastrointestinal Diseases & Disorders Sourcebook*

Emergency Medical Services Sourcebook

Basic Consumer Health Information about Preventing, Preparing for, and Managing Emergency Situations, When and Who to Call for Help, What to Expect in the Emergency Room, the Emergency Medical Team, Patient Issues, and Current Topics in Emergency Medicine

Along with Statistical Data, a Glossary, and Sources of Additional Help and Information

Edited by Jenni Lynn Colson. 494 pages. 2002. 978-0-7808-0420-3.

Endocrine & Metabolic Disorders Sourcebook

Basic Information for the Layperson about Pancreatic and Insulin-Related Disorders Such as Pancreatitis, Diabetes, and Hypoglycemia; Adrenal Gland Disorders Such as Cushing's Syndrome, Addison's Disease, and Congenital Adrenal Hyperplasia; Pituitary Gland Disorders Such as Growth Hormone Deficiency, Acromegaly, and Pituitary Tumors; Thyroid Disorders Such as Hypothyroidism, Graves' Disease, Hashimoto's Disease, and Goiter; Hyperparathyroidism; and Other Diseases and Syndromes of Hormone Imbalance or Metabolic Dysfunction

Along with Reports on Current Research Initiatives

Edited by Linda M. Shin. 574 pages. 1998. 978-0-7808-0207-0.

Environmental Health Sourcebook, 2nd Edition

Basic Consumer Health Information about the Environment and Its Effect on Human Health, Including the Effects of Air Pollution, Water Pollution, Hazardous Chemicals, Food Hazards, Radiation Hazards, Biological Agents, Household Hazards, Such as Radon, Asbestos, Carbon Monoxide, and Mold, and Information about Associated Diseases and Disorders, Including Cancer, Allergies, Respiratory Problems, and Skin Disorders

Along with Information about Environmental Concerns for Specific Populations, a Glossary of Related Terms, and Resources for Further Help and Information

Edited by Dawn D. Matthews. 673 pages. 2003. 978-0-7808-0632-0.

Ethnic Diseases Sourcebook

Basic Consumer Health Information for Ethnic and Racial Minority Groups in the United States, Including General Health Indicators and Behaviors, Ethnic Diseases, Genetic Testing, the Impact of Chronic Diseases, Women's Health, Mental Health Issues, and Preventive Health Care Services

Along with a Glossary and a Listing of Additional Resources

Edited by Joyce Brennfleck Shannon. 664 pages. 2001. 978-0-7808-0336-7.

"Recommended for health sciences libraries where public health programs are a priority."
— E-Streams, Jan '02

"Not many books have been written on this topic to date, and the *Ethnic Diseases Sourcebook* is a strong addition to the list. It will be an important introductory resource for health consumers, students, health care personnel, and social scientists. It is recommended for public, academic, and large hospital libraries."
— American Reference Books Annual, 2002

"Recommended reference source."
— Booklist, American Library Association, Oct '01

"Will prove valuable to any library seeking to maintain a current, comprehensive reference collection of health resources.... An excellent source of health information about genetic disorders which affect particular ethnic and racial minorities in the U.S."
— The Bookwatch, Aug '01

Eye Care Sourcebook, 2nd Edition

Basic Consumer Health Information about Eye Care and Eye Disorders, Including Facts about the Diagnosis, Prevention, and Treatment of Common Refractive Problems Such as Myopia, Hyperopia, Astigmatism, and Presbyopia, and Eye Diseases, Including Glaucoma, Cataract, Age-Related Macular Degeneration, and Diabetic Retinopathy

Along with a Section on Vision Correction and Refractive Surgeries, Including LASIK and LASEK, a Glossary, and Directories of Resources for Additional Help and Information

Edited by Amy L. Sutton. 543 pages. 2003. 978-0-7808-0635-1.

". . . a solid reference tool for eye care and a valuable addition to a collection."
— American Reference Books Annual, 2004

Family Planning Sourcebook

Basic Consumer Health Information about Planning for Pregnancy and Contraception, Including Traditional Methods, Barrier Methods, Hormonal Methods, Permanent Methods, Future Methods, Emergency Contraception, and Birth Control Choices for Women at Each Stage of Life

Along with Statistics, a Glossary, and Sources of Additional Information

Edited by Amy Marcaccio Keyzer. 520 pages. 2001. 978-0-7808-0379-4.

"Recommended for public, health, and undergraduate libraries as part of the circulating collection."
— E-Streams, Mar '02

"Information is presented in an unbiased, readable manner, and the sourcebook will certainly be a necessary addition to those public and high school libraries where Internet access is restricted or otherwise problematic." *— American Reference Books Annual, 2002*

"Recommended reference source."
— Booklist, American Library Association, Oct '01

"Will prove valuable to any library seeking to maintain a current, comprehensive reference collection of health resources. . . . Excellent reference."
— The Bookwatch, Aug '01

SEE ALSO Pregnancy & Birth Sourcebook

Fitness & Exercise Sourcebook, 3rd Edition

Basic Consumer Health Information about the Physical and Mental Benefits of Fitness, Including Cardiorespiratory Endurance, Muscular Strength, Muscular Endurance, and Flexibility, with Facts about Sports Nutrition and Exercise-Related Injuries and Tips about Physical Activity and Exercises for People of All Ages and for People with Health Concerns

Along with Advice on Selecting and Using Exercise Equipment, Maintaining Exercise Motivation, a Glossary of Related Terms, and a Directory of Resources for More Help and Information

Edited by Amy L. Sutton. 663 pages. 2007. 978-0-7808-0946-8.

"This work is recommended for all general reference collections."
— American Reference Books Annual, 2002

"Highly recommended for public, consumer, and school grades fourth through college." *— E-Streams, Nov '01*

"Recommended reference source."
— Booklist, American Library Association, Oct '01

"The information appears quite comprehensive and is considered reliable. . . . This second edition is a welcomed addition to the series."
— Doody's Review Service, Sep '01

Food Safety Sourcebook

Basic Consumer Health Information about the Safe Handling of Meat, Poultry, Seafood, Eggs, Fruit Juices, and Other Food Items, and Facts about Pesticides, Drinking Water, Food Safety Overseas, and the Onset, Duration, and Symptoms of Foodborne Illnesses, Including Types of Pathogenic Bacteria, Parasitic Protozoa, Worms, Viruses, and Natural Toxins

Along with the Role of the Consumer, the Food Handler, and the Government in Food Safety; a Glossary, and Resources for Additional Help and Information

Edited by Dawn D. Matthews. 339 pages. 1999. 978-0-7808-0326-8.

"This book is recommended for public libraries and universities with home economic and food science programs." —*E-Streams, Nov '00*

"Recommended reference source."
—*Booklist, American Library Association, May '00*

"This book takes the complex issues of food safety and foodborne pathogens and presents them in an easily understood manner. [It does] an excellent job of covering a large and often confusing topic."
—*American Reference Books Annual, 2000*

■

Forensic Medicine Sourcebook

Basic Consumer Information for the Layperson about Forensic Medicine, Including Crime Scene Investigation, Evidence Collection and Analysis, Expert Testimony, Computer-Aided Criminal Identification, Digital Imaging in the Courtroom, DNA Profiling, Accident Reconstruction, Autopsies, Ballistics, Drugs and Explosives Detection, Latent Fingerprints, Product Tampering, and Questioned Document Examination

Along with Statistical Data, a Glossary of Forensics Terminology, and Listings of Sources for Further Help and Information

Edited by Annemarie S. Muth. 574 pages. 1999. 978-0-7808-0232-2.

"Given the expected widespread interest in its content and its easy to read style, this book is recommended for most public and all college and university libraries."
—*E-Streams, Feb '01*

"Recommended for public libraries."
—*Reference & User Services Quarterly, American Library Association, Spring 2000*

"Recommended reference source."
—*Booklist, American Library Association, Feb '00*

"A wealth of information, useful statistics, references are up-to-date and extremely complete. This wonderful collection of data will help students who are interested in a career in any type of forensic field. It is a great resource for attorneys who need information about types of expert witnesses needed in a particular case. It also offers useful information for fiction and nonfiction writers whose work involves a crime. A fascinating compilation. All levels."
—*Choice, Association of College & Research Libraries, Jan '00*

"There are several items that make this book attractive to consumers who are seeking certain forensic data. . . . This is a useful current source for those seeking general forensic medical answers."
—*American Reference Books Annual, 2000*

Gastrointestinal Diseases & Disorders Sourcebook, 2nd Edition

Basic Consumer Health Information about the Upper and Lower Gastrointestinal (GI) Tract, Including the Esophagus, Stomach, Intestines, Rectum, Liver, and Pancreas, with Facts about Gastroesophageal Reflux Disease, Gastritis, Hernias, Ulcers, Celiac Disease, Diverticulitis, Irritable Bowel Syndrome, Hemorrhoids, Gastrointestinal Cancers, and Other Diseases and Disorders Related to the Digestive Process

Along with Information about Commonly Used Diagnostic and Surgical Procedures, Statistics, Reports on Current Research Initiatives and Clinical Trials, a Glossary, and Resources for Additional Help and Information

Edited by Sandra J. Judd. 681 pages. 2006. 978-0-7808-0798-3.

". . . very readable form. The successful editorial work that brought this material together into a useful and understandable reference makes accessible to all readers information that can help them more effectively understand and obtain help for digestive tract problems."
—*Choice, Association of College & Research Libraries, Feb '97*

SEE ALSO *Diet & Nutrition Sourcebook, Digestive Diseases & Disorders Sourcebook, Eating Disorders Sourcebook*

■

Genetic Disorders Sourcebook, 3rd Edition

Basic Consumer Health Information about Hereditary Diseases and Disorders, Including Facts about the Human Genome, Genetic Inheritance Patterns, Disorders Associated with Specific Genes, Such as Sickle Cell Disease, Hemophilia, and Cystic Fibrosis, Chromosome Disorders, Such as Down Syndrome, Fragile X Syndrome, and Turner Syndrome, and Complex Diseases and Disorders Resulting from the Interaction of Environmental and Genetic Factors, Such as Allergies, Cancer, and Obesity

Along with Facts about Genetic Testing, Suggestions for Parents of Children with Special Needs, Reports on Current Research Initiatives, a Glossary of Genetic Terminology, and Resources for Additional Help and Information

Edited by Karen Bellenir. 777 pages. 2004. 978-0-7808-0742-6.

"This text is recommended for any library with an interest in providing consumer health resources."
—*E-Streams, Aug '05*

"This is a valuable resource for anyone wishing to have an understandable description of any of the topics or disorders included. The editor succeeds in making complex genetic issues understandable."
—*Doody's Book Review Service, May '05*

"A good acquisition for public libraries."
—*American Reference Books Annual, 2005*

Head Trauma Sourcebook

Basic Information for the Layperson about Open-Head and Closed-Head Injuries, Treatment Advances, Recovery, and Rehabilitation

Along with Reports on Current Research Initiatives

Edited by Karen Bellenir. 414 pages. 1997. 978-0-7808-0208-7.

Headache Sourcebook

Basic Consumer Health Information about Migraine, Tension, Cluster, Rebound and Other Types of Headaches, with Facts about the Cause and Prevention of Headaches, the Effects of Stress and the Environment, Headaches during Pregnancy and Menopause, and Childhood Headaches

Along with a Glossary and Other Resources for Additional Help and Information

Edited by Dawn D. Matthews. 362 pages. 2002. 978-0-7808-0337-4.

Healthy Aging Sourcebook

Basic Consumer Health Information about Maintaining Health through the Aging Process, Including Advice on Nutrition, Exercise, and Sleep, Help in Making Decisions about Midlife Issues and Retirement, and Guidance Concerning Practical and Informed Choices in Health Consumerism

Along with Data Concerning the Theories of Aging, Different Experiences in Aging by Minority Groups, and Facts about Aging Now and Aging in the Future; and Featuring a Glossary, a Guide to Consumer Help, Additional Suggested Reading, and Practical Resource Directory

Edited by Jenifer Swanson. 536 pages. 1999. 978-0-7808-0390-9.

SEE ALSO *Physical & Mental Issues in Aging Sourcebook*

Healthy Children Sourcebook

Basic Consumer Health Information about the Physical and Mental Development of Children between the Ages of 3 and 12, Including Routine Health Care, Preventative Health Services, Safety and First Aid,

Healthy Sleep, Dental Care, Nutrition, and Fitness, and Featuring Parenting Tips on Such Topics as Bedwetting, Choosing Day Care, Monitoring TV and Other Media, and Establishing a Foundation for Substance Abuse Prevention

Along with a Glossary of Commonly Used Pediatric Terms and Resources for Additional Help and Information.

Edited by Chad T. Kimball. 647 pages. 2003. 978-0-7808-0247-6.

SEE ALSO *Childhood Diseases & Disorders Sourcebook*

Healthy Heart Sourcebook for Women

Basic Consumer Health Information about Cardiac Issues Specific to Women, Including Facts about Major Risk Factors and Prevention, Treatment and Control Strategies, and Important Dietary Issues

Along with a Special Section Regarding the Pros and Cons of Hormone Replacement Therapy and Its Impact on Heart Health, and Additional Help, Including Recipes, a Glossary, and a Directory of Resources

Edited by Dawn D. Matthews. 336 pages. 2000. 978-0-7808-0329-9.

SEE ALSO *Cardiovascular Diseases & Disorders Sourcebook, Women's Health Concerns Sourcebook*

Hepatitis Sourcebook

Basic Consumer Health Information about Hepatitis A, Hepatitis B, Hepatitis C, and Other Forms of Hepatitis, Including Autoimmune Hepatitis, Alcoholic Hepatitis, Nonalcoholic Steatohepatitis, and Toxic Hepatitis, with

Facts about Risk Factors, Screening Methods, Diagnostic Tests, and Treatment Options

Along with Information on Liver Health, Tips for People Living with Chronic Hepatitis, Reports on Current Research Initiatives, a Glossary of Terms Related to Hepatitis, and a Directory of Sources for Further Help and Information

Edited by Sandra J. Judd. 597 pages. 2005. 978-0-7808-0749-5.

"Highly recommended."
— American Reference Books Annual, 2006

■

Household Safety Sourcebook

Basic Consumer Health Information about Household Safety, Including Information about Poisons, Chemicals, Fire, and Water Hazards in the Home

Along with Advice about the Safe Use of Home Maintenance Equipment, Choosing Toys and Nursery Furniture, Holiday and Recreation Safety, a Glossary, and Resources for Further Help and Information

Edited by Dawn D. Matthews. 606 pages. 2002. 978-0-7808-0338-1.

"This work will be useful in public libraries with large consumer health and wellness departments."
— American Reference Books Annual, 2003

"As a sourcebook on household safety this book meets its mark. It is encyclopedic in scope and covers a wide range of safety issues that are commonly seen in the home." — E-Streams, Jul '02

■

Hypertension Sourcebook

Basic Consumer Health Information about the Causes, Diagnosis, and Treatment of High Blood Pressure, with Facts about Consequences, Complications, and Co-Occurring Disorders, Such as Coronary Heart Disease, Diabetes, Stroke, Kidney Disease, and Hypertensive Retinopathy, and Issues in Blood Pressure Control, Including Dietary Choices, Stress Management, and Medications

Along with Reports on Current Research Initiatives and Clinical Trials, a Glossary, and Resources for Additional Help and Information

Edited by Dawn D. Matthews and Karen Bellenir. 613 pages. 2004. 978-0-7808-0674-0.

"Academic, public, and medical libraries will want to add the *Hypertension Sourcebook* to their collections."
— E-Streams, Aug '05

"The strength of this source is the wide range of information given about hypertension."
— American Reference Books Annual, 2005

■

Immune System Disorders Sourcebook, 2nd Edition

Basic Consumer Health Information about Disorders of the Immune System, Including Immune System Function and Response, Diagnosis of Immune Disorders, Information about Inherited Immune Disease, Acquired Immune Disease, and Autoimmune Diseases, Including Primary Immune Deficiency, Acquired Immunodeficiency Syndrome (AIDS), Lupus, Multiple Sclerosis, Type 1 Diabetes, Rheumatoid Arthritis, and Graves' Disease

Along with Treatments, Tips for Coping with Immune Disorders, a Glossary, and a Directory of Additional Resources.

Edited by Joyce Brennfleck Shannon. 671 pages. 2005. 978-0-7808-0748-8.

"Highly recommended for academic and public libraries." — American Reference Books Annual, 2006

"The updated second edition is a 'must' for any consumer health library seeking a solid resource covering the treatments, symptoms, and options for immune disorder sufferers. . . . An excellent guide."
— MBR Bookwatch, Jan '06

■

Infant & Toddler Health Sourcebook

Basic Consumer Health Information about the Physical and Mental Development of Newborns, Infants, and Toddlers, Including Neonatal Concerns, Nutrition Recommendations, Immunization Schedules, Common Pediatric Disorders, Assessments and Milestones, Safety Tips, and Advice for Parents and Other Caregivers

Along with a Glossary of Terms and Resource Listings for Additional Help

Edited by Jenifer Swanson. 585 pages. 2000. 978-0-7808-0246-9.

"As a reference for the general public, this would be useful in any library." — E-Streams, May '01

"Recommended reference source."
— Booklist, American Library Association, Feb '01

"This is a good source for general use."
— American Reference Books Annual, 2001

■

Infectious Diseases Sourcebook

Basic Consumer Health Information about Non-Contagious Bacterial, Viral, Prion, Fungal, and Parasitic Diseases Spread by Food and Water, Insects and Animals, or Environmental Contact, Including Botulism, E. Coli, Encephalitis, Legionnaires' Disease, Lyme Disease, Malaria, Plague, Rabies, Salmonella, Tetanus, and Others, and Facts about Newly Emerging Diseases, Such as Hantavirus, Mad Cow Disease, Monkeypox, and West Nile Virus

Along with Information about Preventing Disease Transmission, the Threat of Bioterrorism, and Current Research Initiatives, with a Glossary and Directory of Resources for More Information

Edited by Karen Bellenir. 634 pages. 2004. 978-0-7808-0675-7.

"This reference continues the excellent tradition of the *Health Reference Series* in consolidating a wealth of information on a selected topic into a format that is easy to use and accessible to the general public."
— *American Reference Books Annual, 2005*

"Recommended for public and academic libraries."
— *E-Streams, Jan '05*

Injury & Trauma Sourcebook

Basic Consumer Health Information about the Impact of Injury, the Diagnosis and Treatment of Common and Traumatic Injuries, Emergency Care, and Specific Injuries Related to Home, Community, Workplace, Transportation, and Recreation

Along with Guidelines for Injury Prevention, a Glossary, and a Directory of Additional Resources

Edited by Joyce Brennfleck Shannon. 696 pages. 2002. 978-0-7808-0421-0.

"This publication is the most comprehensive work of its kind about injury and trauma."
— *American Reference Books Annual, 2003*

"This sourcebook provides concise, easily readable, basic health information about injuries. . . . This book is well organized and an easy to use reference resource suitable for hospital, health sciences and public libraries with consumer health collections."
— *E-Streams, Nov '02*

"Practitioners should be aware of guides such as this in order to facilitate their use by patients and their families."
— *Doody's Health Sciences Book Review Journal, Sep-Oct '02*

"Recommended reference source."
— *Booklist, American Library Association, Sep '02*

"Highly recommended for academic and medical reference collections."
— *Library Bookwatch, Sep '02*

Kidney & Urinary Tract Diseases & Disorders Sourcebook

SEE Urinary Tract & Kidney Diseases & Disorders Sourcebook

Learning Disabilities Sourcebook, 2nd Edition

Basic Consumer Health Information about Learning Disabilities, Including Dyslexia, Developmental Speech and Language Disabilities, Non-Verbal Learning Disorders, Developmental Arithmetic Disorder, Developmental Writing Disorder, and Other Conditions That Impede Learning Such as Attention Deficit/Hyperactivity Disorder, Brain Injury, Hearing Impairment, Klinefelter Syndrome, Dyspraxia, and Tourette's Syndrome

Along with Facts about Educational Issues and Assistive Technology, Coping Strategies, a Glossary of Related Terms, and Resources for Further Help and Information

Edited by Dawn D. Matthews. 621 pages. 2003. 978-0-7808-0626-9.

"The second edition of Learning Disabilities Sourcebook far surpasses the earlier edition in that it is more focused on information that will be useful as a consumer health resource."
— *American Reference Books Annual, 2004*

"Teachers as well as consumers will find this an essential guide to understanding various syndromes and their latest treatments. [An] invaluable reference for public and school library collections alike."
— *Library Bookwatch, Apr '03*

Named "Outstanding Reference Book of 1999."
— *New York Public Library, Feb '00*

"An excellent candidate for inclusion in a public library reference section. It's a great source of information. Teachers will also find the book useful. Definitely worth reading."
— *Journal of Adolescent & Adult Literacy, Feb 2000*

"Readable . . . provides a solid base of information regarding successful techniques used with individuals who have learning disabilities, as well as practical suggestions for educators and family members. Clear language, concise descriptions, and pertinent information for contacting multiple resources add to the strength of this book as a useful tool."
— *Choice, Association of College & Research Libraries, Feb '99*

"Recommended reference source."
— *Booklist, American Library Association, Sep '98*

"A useful resource for libraries and for those who don't have the time to identify and locate the individual publications."
— *Disability Resources Monthly, Sep '98*

Leukemia Sourcebook

Basic Consumer Health Information about Adult and Childhood Leukemias, Including Acute Lymphocytic Leukemia (ALL), Chronic Lymphocytic Leukemia (CLL), Acute Myelogenous Leukemia (AML), Chronic Myelogenous Leukemia (CML), and Hairy Cell Leukemia, and Treatments Such as Chemotherapy, Radiation Therapy, Peripheral Blood Stem Cell and Marrow Transplantation, and Immunotherapy

Along with Tips for Life During and After Treatment, a Glossary, and Directories of Additional Resources

Edited by Joyce Brennfleck Shannon. 587 pages. 2003. 978-0-7808-0627-6.

"Unlike other medical books for the layperson, . . . the language does not talk down to the reader. . . . This volume is highly recommended for all libraries."
— *American Reference Books Annual, 2004*

". . . a fine title which ranges from diagnosis to alternative treatments, staging, and tips for life during and after diagnosis."
— *The Bookwatch, Dec '03*

Liver Disorders Sourcebook

Basic Consumer Health Information about the Liver and How It Works; Liver Diseases, Including Cancer, Cirrhosis, Hepatitis, and Toxic and Drug Related Diseases; Tips for Maintaining a Healthy Liver; Laboratory Tests, Radiology Tests, and Facts about Liver Transplantation

Along with a Section on Support Groups, a Glossary, and Resource Listings

Edited by Joyce Brennfleck Shannon. 591 pages. 2000. 978-0-7808-0383-1.

"A valuable resource."
—*American Reference Books Annual, 2001*

"This title is recommended for health sciences and public libraries with consumer health collections."
—*E-Streams, Oct '00*

"Recommended reference source."
—*Booklist, American Library Association, Jun '00*

■

Lung Disorders Sourcebook

Basic Consumer Health Information about Emphysema, Pneumonia, Tuberculosis, Asthma, Cystic Fibrosis, and Other Lung Disorders, Including Facts about Diagnostic Procedures, Treatment Strategies, Disease Prevention Efforts, and Such Risk Factors as Smoking, Air Pollution, and Exposure to Asbestos, Radon, and Other Agents

Along with a Glossary and Resources for Additional Help and Information

Edited by Dawn D. Matthews. 678 pages. 2002. 978-0-7808-0339-8.

"This title is a great addition for public and school libraries because it provides concise health information on the lungs."
—*American Reference Books Annual, 2003*

"Highly recommended for academic and medical reference collections." —*Library Bookwatch, Sep '02*

SEE ALSO Respiratory Diseases & Disorders Sourcebook

■

Medical Tests Sourcebook, 2nd Edition

Basic Consumer Health Information about Medical Tests, Including Age-Specific Health Tests, Important Health Screenings and Exams, Home-Use Tests, Blood and Specimen Tests, Electrical Tests, Scope Tests, Genetic Testing, and Imaging Tests, Such as X-Rays, Ultrasound, Computed Tomography, Magnetic Resonance Imaging, Angiography, and Nuclear Medicine

Along with a Glossary and Directory of Additional Resources

Edited by Joyce Brennfleck Shannon. 654 pages. 2004. 978-0-7808-0670-2.

"Recommended for hospital and health sciences

libraries with consumer health collections."
—*E-Streams, Mar '00*

"This is an overall excellent reference with a wealth of general knowledge that may aid those who are reluctant to get vital tests performed."
—*Today's Librarian, Jan '00*

"A valuable reference guide."
—*American Reference Books Annual, 2000*

■

Men's Health Concerns Sourcebook, 2nd Edition

Basic Consumer Health Information about the Medical and Mental Concerns of Men, Including Theories about the Shorter Male Lifespan, the Leading Causes of Death and Disability, Physical Concerns of Special Significance to Men, Reproductive and Sexual Concerns, Sexually Transmitted Diseases, Men's Mental and Emotional Health, and Lifestyle Choices That Affect Wellness, Such as Nutrition, Fitness, and Substance Use

Along with a Glossary of Related Terms and a Directory of Organizational Resources in Men's Health

Edited by Robert Aquinas McNally. 644 pages. 2004. 978-0-7808-0671-9.

"A very accessible reference for non-specialist general readers and consumers." —*The Bookwatch, Jun '04*

"This comprehensive reference and the series are highly recommended."
—*American Reference Books Annual, 2000*

"Recommended reference source."
—*Booklist, American Library Association, Dec '98*

■

Mental Health Disorders Sourcebook, 3rd Edition

Basic Consumer Health Information about Mental and Emotional Health and Mental Illness, Including Facts about Depression, Bipolar Disorder, and Other Mood Disorders, Phobias, Post-Traumatic Stress Disorder (PTSD), Obsessive-Compulsive Disorder, and Other Anxiety Disorders, Impulse Control Disorders, Eating Disorders, Personality Disorders, and Psychotic Disorders, Including Schizophrenia and Dissociative Disorders

Along with Statistical Information, a Special Section Concerning Mental Health Issues in Children and Adolescents, a Glossary, and Directories of Resources for Additional Help and Information

Edited by Karen Bellenir. 661 pages. 2005. 978-0-7808-0747-1.

"Recommended for public libraries and academic libraries with an undergraduate program in psychology."
—*American Reference Books Annual, 2006*

"Recommended reference source."
—*Booklist, American Library Association, Jun '00*

630

Mental Retardation Sourcebook

Basic Consumer Health Information about Mental Retardation and Its Causes, Including Down Syndrome, Fetal Alcohol Syndrome, Fragile X Syndrome, Genetic Conditions, Injury, and Environmental Sources

Along with Preventive Strategies, Parenting Issues, Educational Implications, Health Care Needs, Employment and Economic Matters, Legal Issues, a Glossary, and a Resource Listing for Additional Help and Information

Edited by Joyce Brennfleck Shannon. 642 pages. 2000. 978-0-7808-0377-0.

"Public libraries will find the book useful for reference and as a beginning research point for students, parents, and caregivers."
— American Reference Books Annual, 2001

"The strength of this work is that it compiles many basic fact sheets and addresses for further information in one volume. It is intended and suitable for the general public. This sourcebook is relevant to any collection providing health information to the general public."
— E-Streams, Nov '00

"From preventing retardation to parenting and family challenges, this covers health, social and legal issues and will prove an invaluable overview."
— Reviewer's Bookwatch, Jul '00

Movement Disorders Sourcebook

Basic Consumer Health Information about Neurological Movement Disorders, Including Essential Tremor, Parkinson's Disease, Dystonia, Cerebral Palsy, Huntington's Disease, Myasthenia Gravis, Multiple Sclerosis, and Other Early-Onset and Adult-Onset Movement Disorders, Their Symptoms and Causes, Diagnostic Tests, and Treatments

Along with Mobility and Assistive Technology Information, a Glossary, and a Directory of Additional Resources

Edited by Joyce Brennfleck Shannon. 655 pages. 2003. 978-0-7808-0628-3.

". . . a good resource for consumers and recommended for public, community college and undergraduate libraries." *— American Reference Books Annual, 2004*

Muscular Dystrophy Sourcebook

Basic Consumer Health Information about Congenital, Childhood-Onset, and Adult-Onset Forms of Muscular Dystrophy, Such as Duchenne, Becker, Emery-Dreifuss, Distal, Limb-Girdle, Facioscapulohumeral (FSHD), Myotonic, and Ophthalmoplegic Muscular Dystrophies, Including Facts about Diagnostic Tests, Medical and Physical Therapies, Management of Co-Occurring Conditions, and Parenting Guidelines

Along with Practical Tips for Home Care, a Glossary, and Directories of Additional Resources

Edited by Joyce Brennfleck Shannon. 577 pages. 2004. 978-0-7808-0676-4.

"This book is highly recommended for public and academic libraries as well as health care offices that support the information needs of patients and their families."
— E-Streams, Apr '05

"Excellent reference." *— The Bookwatch, Jan '05*

Obesity Sourcebook

Basic Consumer Health Information about Diseases and Other Problems Associated with Obesity, and Including Facts about Risk Factors, Prevention Issues, and Management Approaches

Along with Statistical and Demographic Data, Information about Special Populations, Research Updates, a Glossary, and Source Listings for Further Help and Information

Edited by Wilma Caldwell and Chad T. Kimball. 376 pages. 2001. 978-0-7808-0333-6.

"The book synthesizes the reliable medical literature on obesity into one easy-to-read and useful resource for the general public."
— American Reference Books Annual, 2002

"This is a very useful resource book for the lay public."
— Doody's Review Service, Nov '01

"Well suited for the health reference collection of a public library or an academic health science library that serves the general population." *— E-Streams, Sep '01*

"Recommended reference source."
— Booklist, American Library Association, Apr '01

"Recommended pick both for specialty health library collections and any general consumer health reference collection." *— The Bookwatch, Apr '01*

Oral Health Sourcebook

SEE Dental Care & Oral Health Sourcebook

Osteoporosis Sourcebook

Basic Consumer Health Information about Primary and Secondary Osteoporosis and Juvenile Osteoporosis and Related Conditions, Including Fibrous Dysplasia, Gaucher Disease, Hyperthyroidism, Hypophosphatasia, Myeloma, Osteopetrosis, Osteogenesis Imperfecta, and Paget's Disease

Along with Information about Risk Factors, Treatments, Traditional and Non-Traditional Pain Management, a Glossary of Related Terms, and a Directory of Resources

Edited by Allan R. Cook. 584 pages. 2001. 978-0-7808-0239-1.

"This would be a book to be kept in a staff or patient library. The targeted audience is the layperson, but the therapist who needs a quick bit of information on a particular topic will also find the book useful."
— Physical Therapy, Jan '02

SEE ALSO *Healthy Aging Sourcebook, Physical & Mental Issues in Aging Sourcebook, Women's Health Concerns Sourcebook*

Pain Sourcebook, 2nd Edition

Basic Consumer Health Information about Specific Forms of Acute and Chronic Pain, Including Muscle and Skeletal Pain, Nerve Pain, Cancer Pain, and Disorders Characterized by Pain, Such as Fibromyalgia, Shingles, Angina, Arthritis, and Headaches

Along with Information about Pain Medications and Management Techniques, Complementary and Alternative Pain Relief Options, Tips for People Living with Chronic Pain, a Glossary, and a Directory of Sources for Further Information

Edited by Karen Bellenir. 670 pages. 2002. 978-0-7808-0612-2.

Pediatric Cancer Sourcebook

Basic Consumer Health Information about Leukemias, Brain Tumors, Sarcomas, Lymphomas, and Other Cancers in Infants, Children, and Adolescents, Including Descriptions of Cancers, Treatments, and Coping Strategies

Along with Suggestions for Parents, Caregivers, and Concerned Relatives, a Glossary of Cancer Terms, and Resource Listings

Edited by Edward J. Prucha. 587 pages. 1999. 978-0-7808-0245-2.

SEE ALSO *Childhood Diseases & Disorders Sourcebook, Healthy Children Sourcebook*

Physical & Mental Issues in Aging Sourcebook

Basic Consumer Health Information on Physical and Mental Disorders Associated with the Aging Process, Including Concerns about Cardiovascular Disease, Pulmonary Disease, Oral Health, Digestive Disorders, Musculoskeletal and Skin Disorders, Metabolic Changes, Sexual and Reproductive Issues, and Changes in Vision, Hearing, and Other Senses

Along with Data about Longevity and Causes of Death, Information on Acute and Chronic Pain, Descriptions of Mental Concerns, a Glossary of Terms, and Resource Listings for Additional Help

Edited by Jenifer Swanson. 660 pages. 1999. 978-0-7808-0233-9.

SEE ALSO *Healthy Aging Sourcebook*

Podiatry Sourcebook, 2nd Edition

Basic Consumer Health Information about Disorders, Diseases, Deformities, and Injuries that Affect the Foot and Ankle, Including Sprains, Corns, Calluses, Bunions, Plantar Warts, Plantar Fasciitis, Neuromas, Clubfoot, Flat Feet, Achilles Tendonitis, and Much More

Along with Information about Selecting a Foot Care Specialist, Foot Fitness, Shoes and Socks, Diagnostic Tests and Corrective Procedures, Financial Assistance for Corrective Devices, a Glossary of Related Terms, and a Directory of Resources for Additional Help and Information

Edited by Ivy L. Alexander. 543 pages. 2007. 978-0-7808-0944-4.

"Recommended reference source."
— Booklist, American Library Association, Feb '02

"There is a lot of information presented here on a topic that is usually only covered sparingly in most larger comprehensive medical encyclopedias."
— American Reference Books Annual, 2002

■

Pregnancy & Birth Sourcebook, 2nd Edition

Basic Consumer Health Information about Conception and Pregnancy, Including Facts about Fertility, Infertility, Pregnancy Symptoms and Complications, Fetal Growth and Development, Labor, Delivery, and the Postpartum Period, as Well as Information about Maintaining Health and Wellness during Pregnancy and Caring for a Newborn

Along with Information about Public Health Assistance for Low-Income Pregnant Women, a Glossary, and Directories of Agencies and Organizations Providing Help and Support

Edited by Amy L. Sutton. 626 pages. 2004. 978-0-7808-0672-6.

"Will appeal to public and school reference collections strong in medicine and women's health. . . . Deserves a spot on any medical reference shelf."
— The Bookwatch, Jul '04

"A well-organized handbook. Recommended."
— Choice, Association of College & Research Libraries, Apr '98

"Recommended reference source."
— Booklist, American Library Association, Mar '98

"Recommended for public libraries."
— American Reference Books Annual, 1998

SEE ALSO Breastfeeding Sourcebook, Congenital Disorders Sourcebook, Family Planning Sourcebook

■

Prostate & Urological Disorders Sourcebook

Basic Consumer Health Information about Urogenital and Sexual Disorders in Men, Including Prostate and Other Andrological Cancers, Prostatitis, Benign Prostatic Hyperplasia, Testicular and Penile Trauma, Cryptorchidism, Peyronie Disease, Erectile Dysfunction, and Male Factor Infertility, and Facts about Commonly Used Tests and Procedures, Such as Prostatectomy, Vasectomy, Vasectomy Reversal, Penile Implants, and Semen Analysis

Along with a Glossary of Andrological Terms and a Directory of Resources for Additional Information

Edited by Karen Bellenir. 631 pages. 2005. 978-0-7808-0797-6.

Prostate Cancer Sourcebook

Basic Consumer Health Information about Prostate Cancer, Including Information about the Associated Risk Factors, Detection, Diagnosis, and Treatment of Prostate Cancer

Along with Information on Non-Malignant Prostate Conditions, and Featuring a Section Listing Support and Treatment Centers and a Glossary of Related Terms

Edited by Dawn D. Matthews. 358 pages. 2001. 978-0-7808-0324-4.

"Recommended reference source."
— Booklist, American Library Association, Jan '02

"A valuable resource for health care consumers seeking information on the subject. . . . All text is written in a clear, easy-to-understand language that avoids technical jargon. Any library that collects consumer health resources would strengthen their collection with the addition of the Prostate Cancer Sourcebook."
— American Reference Books Annual, 2002

SEE ALSO Men's Health Concerns Sourcebook

■

Reconstructive & Cosmetic Surgery Sourcebook

Basic Consumer Health Information on Cosmetic and Reconstructive Plastic Surgery, Including Statistical Information about Different Surgical Procedures, Things to Consider Prior to Surgery, Plastic Surgery Techniques and Tools, Emotional and Psychological Considerations, and Procedure-Specific Information

Along with a Glossary of Terms and a Listing of Resources for Additional Help and Information

Edited by M. Lisa Weatherford. 374 pages. 2001. 978-0-7808-0214-8.

"An excellent reference that addresses cosmetic and medically necessary reconstructive surgeries. . . . The style of the prose is calm and reassuring, discussing the many positive outcomes now available due to advances in surgical techniques."
— American Reference Books Annual, 2002

"Recommended for health science libraries that are open to the public, as well as hospital libraries that are open to the patients. This book is a good resource for the consumer interested in plastic surgery."
— E-Streams, Dec '01

"Recommended reference source."
— Booklist, American Library Association, Jul '01

■

Rehabilitation Sourcebook

Basic Consumer Health Information about Rehabilitation for People Recovering from Heart Surgery, Spinal Cord Injury, Stroke, Orthopedic Impairments, Amputation, Pulmonary Impairments, Traumatic Injury, and More, Including Physical Therapy, Occupational Therapy, Speech/Language Therapy, Massage Therapy, Dance Therapy, Art Therapy, and Recreational Therapy

Along with Information on Assistive and Adaptive Devices, a Glossary, and Resources for Additional Help and Information

Edited by Dawn D. Matthews. 531 pages. 1999. 978-0-7808-0236-0.

"This is an excellent resource for public library reference and health collections."
— American Reference Books Annual, 2001

"Recommended reference source."
— Booklist, American Library Association, May '00

Respiratory Diseases & Disorders Sourcebook

Basic Information about Respiratory Diseases and Disorders, Including Asthma, Cystic Fibrosis, Pneumonia, the Common Cold, Influenza, and Others, Featuring Facts about the Respiratory System, Statistical and Demographic Data, Treatments, Self-Help Management Suggestions, and Current Research Initiatives

Edited by Allan R. Cook and Peter D. Dresser. 771 pages. 1995. 978-0-7808-0037-3.

"Designed for the layperson and for patients and their families coping with respiratory illness. . . . an extensive array of information on diagnosis, treatment, management, and prevention of respiratory illnesses for the general reader."   — Choice, Association of College & Research Libraries, Jun '96

"A highly recommended text for all collections. It is a comforting reminder of the power of knowledge that good books carry between their covers."
— Academic Library Book Review, Spring '96

"A comprehensive collection of authoritative information presented in a nontechnical, humanitarian style for patients, families, and caregivers."
— Association of Operating Room Nurses, Sep/Oct '95

SEE ALSO Lung Disorders Sourcebook

Sexually Transmitted Diseases Sourcebook, 3rd Edition

Basic Consumer Health Information about Chlamydial Infections, Gonorrhea, Hepatitis, Herpes, HIV/AIDS, Human Papillomavirus, Pubic Lice, Scabies, Syphilis, Trichomoniasis, Vaginal Infections, and Other Sexually Transmitted Diseases, Including Facts about Risk Factors, Symptoms, Diagnosis, Treatment, and the Prevention of Sexually Transmitted Infections

Along with Updates on Current Research Initiatives, a Glossary of Related Terms, and Resources for Additional Help and Information

Edited by Amy L. Sutton. 629 pages. 2006. 978-0-7808-0824-9.

"Recommended for consumer health collections in public libraries, and secondary school and community college libraries."
— American Reference Books Annual, 2002

"Every school and public library should have a copy of this comprehensive and user-friendly reference book."
— Choice, Association of College & Research Libraries, Sep '01

"This is a highly recommended book. This is an especially important book for all school and public libraries."
— AIDS Book Review Journal, Jul-Aug '01

"Recommended reference source."
— Booklist, American Library Association, Apr '01

Sleep Disorders Sourcebook, 2nd Edition

Basic Consumer Health Information about Sleep and Sleep Disorders, Including Insomnia, Sleep Apnea, Restless Legs Syndrome, Narcolepsy, Parasomnias, and Other Health Problems That Affect Sleep, Plus Facts about Diagnostic Procedures, Treatment Strategies, Sleep Medications, and Tips for Improving Sleep Quality

Along with a Glossary of Related Terms and Resources for Additional Help and Information

Edited by Amy L. Sutton. 567 pages. 2005. 978-0-7808-0743-3.

"This book will be useful for just about everybody, especially the 40 million Americans with sleep disorders."
— American Reference Books Annual, 2006

"Recommended for public libraries and libraries supporting health care professionals." — E-Streams, Sep '05

". . . key medical library acquisition."
— The Bookwatch, Jun '05

Smoking Concerns Sourcebook

Basic Consumer Health Information about Nicotine Addiction and Smoking Cessation, Featuring Facts about the Health Effects of Tobacco Use, Including Lung and Other Cancers, Heart Disease, Stroke, and Respiratory Disorders, Such as Emphysema and Chronic Bronchitis

Along with Information about Smoking Prevention Programs, Suggestions for Achieving and Maintaining a Smoke-Free Lifestyle, Statistics about Tobacco Use, Reports on Current Research Initiatives, a Glossary of Related Terms, and Directories of Resources for Additional Help and Information

Edited by Karen Bellenir. 621 pages. 2004. 978-0-7808-0323-7.

"Provides everything needed for the student or general reader seeking practical details on the effects of tobacco use."   — The Bookwatch, Mar '05

"Public libraries and consumer health care libraries will find this work useful."
— American Reference Books Annual, 2005

Sports Injuries Sourcebook, 3rd Edition

Basic Consumer Health Information about Sprains and Strains, Fractures, Growth Plate Injuries, Overtraining Injuries, and Injuries to the Head, Face, Shoulders, Elbows, Hands, Spinal Column, Knees, Ankles, and Feet, and with Facts about Heat-Related Illness, Steroids and Sport Supplements, Protective Equipment, Diagnostic Procedures, Treatment Options, and Rehabilitation

Along with a Glossary of Related Terms and a Directory of Resources for Additional Help and Information

Edited by Sandra J. Judd. 651 pages. 2007. 978-0-7808-0949-9.

"This is an excellent reference for consumers and it is recommended for public, community college, and undergraduate libraries."
— *American Reference Books Annual, 2003*

"Recommended reference source."
— *Booklist, American Library Association, Feb '03*

Stress-Related Disorders Sourcebook

Basic Consumer Health Information about Stress and Stress-Related Disorders, Including Stress Origins and Signals, Environmental Stress at Work and Home, Mental and Emotional Stress Associated with Depression, Post-Traumatic Stress Disorder, Panic Disorder, Suicide, and the Physical Effects of Stress on the Cardiovascular, Immune, and Nervous Systems

Along with Stress Management Techniques, a Glossary, and a Listing of Additional Resources

Edited by Joyce Brennfleck Shannon. 610 pages. 2002. 978-0-7808-0560-6.

"Well written for a general readership, the *Stress-Related Disorders Sourcebook* is a useful addition to the health reference literature."
— *American Reference Books Annual, 2003*

"I am impressed by the amount of information. It offers a thorough overview of the causes and consequences of stress for the layperson. . . . A well-done and thorough reference guide for professionals and nonprofessionals alike."
— *Doody's Review Service, Dec '02*

Stroke Sourcebook

Basic Consumer Health Information about Stroke, Including Ischemic, Hemorrhagic, Transient Ischemic Attack (TIA), and Pediatric Stroke, Stroke Triggers and Risks, Diagnostic Tests, Treatments, and Rehabilitation Information

Along with Stroke Prevention Guidelines, Legal and Financial Information, a Glossary, and a Directory of Additional Resources

Edited by Joyce Brennfleck Shannon. 606 pages. 2003. 978-0-7808-0630-6.

"This volume is highly recommended and should be in every medical, hospital, and public library."
— *American Reference Books Annual, 2004*

"Highly recommended for the amount and variety of topics and information covered." — *Choice, Nov '03*

Surgery Sourcebook

Basic Consumer Health Information about Inpatient and Outpatient Surgeries, Including Cardiac, Vascular, Orthopedic, Ocular, Reconstructive, Cosmetic, Gynecologic, and Ear, Nose, and Throat Procedures and More

Along with Information about Operating Room Policies and Instruments, Laser Surgery Techniques, Hospital Errors, Statistical Data, a Glossary, and Listings of Sources for Further Help and Information

Edited by Annemarie S. Muth and Karen Bellenir. 596 pages. 2002. 978-0-7808-0380-0.

"Large public libraries and medical libraries would benefit from this material in their reference collections."
— *American Reference Books Annual, 2004*

"Invaluable reference for public and school library collections alike." — *Library Bookwatch, Apr '03*

Thyroid Disorders Sourcebook

Basic Consumer Health Information about Disorders of the Thyroid and Parathyroid Glands, Including Hypothyroidism, Hyperthyroidism, Graves Disease, Hashimoto Thyroiditis, Thyroid Cancer, and Parathyroid Disorders, Featuring Facts about Symptoms, Risk Factors, Tests, and Treatments

Along with Information about the Effects of Thyroid Imbalance on Other Body Systems, Environmental Factors That Affect the Thyroid Gland, a Glossary, and a Directory of Additional Resources

Edited by Joyce Brennfleck Shannon. 599 pages. 2005. 978-0-7808-0745-7.

"Recommended for consumer health collections."
— *American Reference Books Annual, 2006*

"Highly recommended pick for basic consumer health reference holdings at all levels."
— *The Bookwatch, Aug '05*

Transplantation Sourcebook

Basic Consumer Health Information about Organ and Tissue Transplantation, Including Physical and Financial Preparations, Procedures and Issues Relating to Specific Solid Organ and Tissue Transplants, Rehabilitation, Pediatric Transplant Information, the Future of Transplantation, and Organ and Tissue Donation

Along with a Glossary and Listings of Additional Resources

Edited by Joyce Brennfleck Shannon. 628 pages. 2002. 978-0-7808-0322-0.

"Along with these advances [in transplantation technology] have come a number of daunting questions for potential transplant patients, their families, and their health care providers. This reference text is the best single tool to address many of these questions. . . . It will be a much-needed addition to the reference collections in health care, academic, and large public libraries."
— *American Reference Books Annual, 2003*

"Recommended for libraries with an interest in offering consumer health information." — *E-Streams, Jul '02*

"This is a unique and valuable resource for patients facing transplantation and their families."
— *Doody's Review Service, Jun '02*

Traveler's Health Sourcebook

Basic Consumer Health Information for Travelers, Including Physical and Medical Preparations, Transportation Health and Safety, Essential Information about Food and Water, Sun Exposure, Insect and Snake Bites, Camping and Wilderness Medicine, and Travel with Physical or Medical Disabilities

Along with International Travel Tips, Vaccination Recommendations, Geographical Health Issues, Disease Risks, a Glossary, and a Listing of Additional Resources

Edited by Joyce Brennfleck Shannon. 613 pages. 2000. 978-0-7808-0384-8.

"Recommended reference source."
— *Booklist, American Library Association, Feb '01*

"This book is recommended for any public library, any travel collection, and especially any collection for the physically disabled."
— *American Reference Books Annual, 2001*

SEE ALSO Worldwide Health Sourcebook

Urinary Tract & Kidney Diseases & Disorders Sourcebook, 2nd Edition

Basic Consumer Health Information about the Urinary System, Including the Bladder, Urethra, Ureters, and Kidneys, with Facts about Urinary Tract Infections, Incontinence, Congenital Disorders, Kidney Stones, Cancers of the Urinary Tract and Kidneys, Kidney Failure, Dialysis, and Kidney Transplantation

Along with Statistical and Demographic Information, Reports on Current Research in Kidney and Urologic Health, a Summary of Commonly Used Diagnostic Tests, a Glossary of Related Terms, and a Directory of Resources for Additional Help and Information

Edited by Ivy L. Alexander. 649 pages. 2005. 978-0-7808-0750-1.

"A good choice for a consumer health information library or for a medical library needing information to refer to their patients."
— *American Reference Books Annual, 2006*

Vegetarian Sourcebook

Basic Consumer Health Information about Vegetarian Diets, Lifestyle, and Philosophy, Including Definitions of Vegetarianism and Veganism, Tips about Adopting Vegetarianism, Creating a Vegetarian Pantry, and Meeting Nutritional Needs of Vegetarians, with Facts Regarding Vegetarianism's Effect on Pregnant and Lactating Women, Children, Athletes, and Senior Citizens

Along with a Glossary of Commonly Used Vegetarian Terms and Resources for Additional Help and Information

Edited by Chad T. Kimball. 360 pages. 2002. 978-0-7808-0439-5.

"Organizes into one concise volume the answers to the most common questions concerning vegetarian diets and lifestyles. This title is recommended for public and secondary school libraries." — *E-Streams, Apr '03*

"Invaluable reference for public and school library collections alike." — *Library Bookwatch, Apr '03*

"The articles in this volume are easy to read and come from authoritative sources. The book does not necessarily support the vegetarian diet but instead provides the pros and cons of this important decision. The Vegetarian Sourcebook is recommended for public libraries and consumer health libraries."
— *American Reference Books Annual, 2003*

SEE ALSO Diet & Nutrition Sourcebook

Women's Health Concerns Sourcebook, 2nd Edition

Basic Consumer Health Information about the Medical and Mental Concerns of Women, Including Maintaining Health and Wellness, Gynecological Concerns, Breast Health, Sexuality and Reproductive Issues, Menopause, Cancer in Women, Leading Causes of Death and Disability among Women, Physical Concerns of Special Significance to Women, and Women's Mental and Emotional Health

Along with a Glossary of Related Terms and Directories of Resources for Additional Help and Information

Edited by Amy L. Sutton. 746 pages. 2004. 978-0-7808-0673-3.

"This is a useful reference book, which makes the reader knowledgeable about several issues that concern women's health. It is recommended for public libraries and home library collections." — *E-Streams, May '05*

"A useful addition to public and consumer health library collections."
— *American Reference Books Annual, 2005*

"A highly recommended title."
— *The Bookwatch, May '04*

"Handy compilation. There is an impressive range of diseases, devices, disorders, procedures, and other physical and emotional issues covered . . . well organized, illustrated, and indexed." — *Choice, Association of College & Research Libraries, Jan '98*

SEE ALSO *Breast Cancer Sourcebook, Cancer Sourcebook for Women, Healthy Heart Sourcebook for Women, Osteoporosis Sourcebook*

■

Workplace Health & Safety Sourcebook

Basic Consumer Health Information about Workplace Health and Safety, Including the Effect of Workplace Hazards on the Lungs, Skin, Heart, Ears, Eyes, Brain, Reproductive Organs, Musculoskeletal System, and Other Organs and Body Parts

Along with Information about Occupational Cancer, Personal Protective Equipment, Toxic and Hazardous Chemicals, Child Labor, Stress, and Workplace Violence

Edited by Chad T. Kimball. 626 pages. 2000. 978-0-7808-0231-5.

"As a reference for the general public, this would be useful in any library." — *E-Streams, Jun '01*

"Provides helpful information for primary care physicians and other caregivers interested in occupational medicine. . . . General readers; professionals."
Choice, Association of College & Research Libraries, May '01

"Recommended reference source."
— *Booklist, American Library Association, Feb '01*

"Highly recommended." — *The Bookwatch, Jan '01*

■

Worldwide Health Sourcebook

Basic Information about Global Health Issues, Including Malnutrition, Reproductive Health, Disease Dispersion and Prevention, Emerging Diseases, Risky Health Behaviors, and the Leading Causes of Death

Along with Global Health Concerns for Children, Women, and the Elderly, Mental Health Issues, Research and Technology Advancements, and Economic, Environmental, and Political Health Implications, a Glossary, and a Resource Listing for Additional Help and Information

Edited by Joyce Brennfleck Shannon. 614 pages. 2001. 978-0-7808-0330-5.

"Named an Outstanding Academic Title."
— *Choice, Association of College & Research Libraries, Jan '02*

"Yet another handy but also unique compilation in the extensive *Health Reference Series*, this is a useful work because many of the international publications reprinted or excerpted are not readily available. Highly recommended." — *Choice, Association of College & Research Libraries, Nov '01*

"Recommended reference source."
— *Booklist, American Library Association, Oct '01*

SEE ALSO *Traveler's Health Sourcebook*

Teen Health Series

Helping Young Adults Understand, Manage, and Avoid Serious Illness

List price $65 per volume. **School and library price $58 per volume.**

Alcohol Information for Teens

Health Tips about Alcohol and Alcoholism

Including Facts about Underage Drinking, Preventing Teen Alcohol Use, Alcohol's Effects on the Brain and the Body, Alcohol Abuse Treatment, Help for Children of Alcoholics, and More

Edited by Joyce Brennfleck Shannon. 370 pages. 2005. 978-0-7808-0741-9.

"Boxed facts and tips add visual interest to the well-researched and clearly written text."
— *Curriculum Connection, Apr '06*

Allergy Information for Teens

Health Tips about Allergic Reactions Such as Anaphylaxis, Respiratory Problems, and Rashes

Including Facts about Identifying and Managing Allergies to Food, Pollen, Mold, Animals, Chemicals, Drugs, and Other Substances

Edited by Karen Bellenir. 410 pages. 2006. 978-0-7808-0799-0.

Asthma Information for Teens

Health Tips about Managing Asthma and Related Concerns

Including Facts about Asthma Causes, Triggers, Symptoms, Diagnosis, and Treatment

Edited by Karen Bellenir. 386 pages. 2005. 978-0-7808-0770-9.

"Highly recommended for medical libraries, public school libraries, and public libraries."
— *American Reference Books Annual, 2006*

"It is so clearly written and well organized that even hesitant readers will be able to find the facts they need, whether for reports or personal information. . . . A succinct but complete resource."
— *School Library Journal, Sep '05*

Body Information for Teens

Health Tips about Maintaining Well-Being for a Lifetime

Including Facts about the Development and Functioning of the Body's Systems, Organs, and Structures and the Health Impact of Lifestyle Choices

Edited by Sandra Augustyn Lawton. 458 pages. 2007. 978-0-7808-0443-2.

Cancer Information for Teens

Health Tips about Cancer Awareness, Prevention, Diagnosis, and Treatment

Including Facts about Frequently Occurring Cancers, Cancer Risk Factors, and Coping Strategies for Teens Fighting Cancer or Dealing with Cancer in Friends or Family Members

Edited by Wilma R. Caldwell. 428 pages. 2004. 978-0-7808-0678-8.

"Recommended for school libraries, or consumer libraries that see a lot of use by teens."
— *E-Streams, May '05*

"A valuable educational tool."
— *American Reference Books Annual, 2005*

"Young adults and their parents alike will find this new addition to the *Teen Health Series* an important reference to cancer in teens."
— *Children's Bookwatch, Feb '05*

Complementary and Alternative Medicine Information for Teens

Health Tips about Non-Traditional and Non-Western Medical Practices

Including Information about Acupuncture, Chiropractic Medicine, Dietary and Herbal Supplements, Hypnosis, Massage Therapy, Prayer and Spirituality, Reflexology, Yoga, and More

Edited by Sandra Augustyn Lawton. 405 pages. 2006. 978-0-7808-0966-6.

Diabetes Information for Teens

Health Tips about Managing Diabetes and Preventing Related Complications

Including Information about Insulin, Glucose Control, Healthy Eating, Physical Activity, and Learning to Live with Diabetes

Edited by Sandra Augustyn Lawton. 410 pages. 2006. 978-0-7808-0811-9.

Diet Information for Teens, 2nd Edition

Health Tips about Diet and Nutrition

Including Facts about Dietary Guidelines, Food Groups, Nutrients, Healthy Meals, Snacks, Weight Control, Medical Concerns Related to Diet, and More

Edited by Karen Bellenir. 432 pages. 2006. 978-0-7808-0820-1.

"Full of helpful insights and facts throughout the book. . . . An excellent resource to be placed in public libraries or even in personal collections."
— *American Reference Books Annual, 2002*

"Recommended for middle and high school libraries and media centers as well as academic libraries that educate future teachers of teenagers. It is also a suitable addition to health science libraries that serve patrons who are interested in teen health promotion and education."
— *E-Streams, Oct '01*

"This comprehensive book would be beneficial to collections that need information about nutrition, dietary guidelines, meal planning, and weight control. . . . This reference is so easy to use that its purchase is recommended."
— *The Book Report, Sep-Oct '01*

"This book is written in an easy to understand format describing issues that many teens face every day, and then provides thoughtful explanations so that teens can make informed decisions. This is an interesting book that provides important facts and information for today's teens."
— *Doody's Health Sciences Book Review Journal, Jul-Aug '01*

"A comprehensive compendium of diet and nutrition. The information is presented in a straightforward, plain-spoken manner. This title will be useful to those working on reports on a variety of topics, as well as to general readers concerned about their dietary health."
— *School Library Journal, Jun '01*

Drug Information for Teens, 2nd Edition

Health Tips about the Physical and Mental Effects of Substance Abuse

Including Information about Marijuana, Inhalants, Club Drugs, Stimulants, Hallucinogens, Opiates, Prescription and Over-the-Counter Drugs, Herbal Products, Tobacco, Alcohol, and More

Edited by Sandra Augustyn Lawton. 468 pages. 2006. 978-0-7808-0862-1.

"A clearly written resource for general readers and researchers alike."
— *School Library Journal*

"This book is well-balanced. . . . a must for public and school libraries."
— *VOYA: Voice of Youth Advocates, Dec '03*

"The chapters are quick to make a connection to their teenage reading audience. The prose is straightforward and the book lends itself to spot reading. It should be useful both for practical information and for research, and it is suitable for public and school libraries."
— *American Reference Books Annual, 2003*

"Recommended reference source."
— *Booklist, American Library Association, Feb '03*

"This is an excellent resource for teens and their parents. Education about drugs and substances is key to discouraging teen drug abuse and this book provides this much needed information in a way that is interesting and factual."
— *Doody's Review Service, Dec '02*

Eating Disorders Information for Teens

Health Tips about Anorexia, Bulimia, Binge Eating, and Other Eating Disorders

Including Information on the Causes, Prevention, and Treatment of Eating Disorders, and Such Other Issues as Maintaining Healthy Eating and Exercise Habits

Edited by Sandra Augustyn Lawton. 337 pages. 2005. 978-0-7808-0783-9.

"An excellent resource for teens and those who work with them."
— *VOYA: Voice of Youth Advocates, Apr '06*

"A welcome addition to high school and undergraduate libraries." — *American Reference Books Annual, 2006*

"This book covers the topic in a lucid manner but delves deeper into every aspect of an eating disorder. A solid addition for any nonfiction or reference collection."
— *School Library Journal, Dec '05*

Fitness Information for Teens

Health Tips about Exercise, Physical Well-Being, and Health Maintenance

Including Facts about Aerobic and Anaerobic Conditioning, Stretching, Body Shape and Body Image, Sports Training, Nutrition, and Activities for Non-Athletes

Edited by Karen Bellenir. 425 pages. 2004. 978-0-7808-0679-5.

"Another excellent offering from Omnigraphics in their *Teen Health Series*. . . . This book will be a great addition to any public, junior high, senior high, or secondary school library."
— *American Reference Books Annual, 2005*

Learning Disabilities Information for Teens

Health Tips about Academic Skills Disorders and Other Disabilities That Affect Learning

Including Information about Common Signs of Learning Disabilities, School Issues, Learning to Live with a Learning Disability, and Other Related Issues

Edited by Sandra Augustyn Lawton. 337 pages. 2005. 978-0-7808-0796-9.

"This book provides a wealth of information for any reader interested in the signs, causes, and consequences

of learning disabilities, as well as related legal rights and educational interventions. . . . Public and academic libraries should want this title for both students and general readers."
— *American Reference Books Annual, 2006*

■

Mental Health Information for Teens, 2nd Edition
Health Tips about Mental Wellness and Mental Illness

Including Facts about Mental and Emotional Health, Depression and Other Mood Disorders, Anxiety Disorders, Behavior Disorders, Self-Injury, Psychosis, Schizophrenia, and More

Edited by Karen Bellenir. 400 pages. 2006. 978-0-7808-0863-8.

"In both language and approach, this user-friendly entry in the *Teen Health Series* is on target for teens needing information on mental health concerns."
— *Booklist, American Library Association, Jan '02*

"Readers will find the material accessible and informative, with the shaded notes, facts, and embedded glossary insets adding appropriately to the already interesting and succinct presentation."
— *School Library Journal, Jan '02*

"This title is highly recommended for any library that serves adolescents and parents/caregivers of adolescents."
— *E-Streams, Jan '02*

"Recommended for high school libraries and young adult collections in public libraries. Both health professionals and teenagers will find this book useful."
— *American Reference Books Annual, 2002*

"This is a nice book written to enlighten the society, primarily teenagers, about common teen mental health issues. It is highly recommended to teachers and parents as well as adolescents."
— *Doody's Review Service, Dec '01*

■

Sexual Health Information for Teens
Health Tips about Sexual Development, Human Reproduction, and Sexually Transmitted Diseases

Including Facts about Puberty, Reproductive Health, Chlamydia, Human Papillomavirus, Pelvic Inflammatory Disease, Herpes, AIDS, Contraception, Pregnancy, and More

Edited by Deborah A. Stanley. 391 pages. 2003. 978-0-7808-0445-6.

"This work should be included in all high school libraries and many larger public libraries. . . . highly recommended."
— *American Reference Books Annual, 2004*

"*Sexual Health* approaches its subject with appropriate seriousness and offers easily accessible advice and information."
— *School Library Journal, Feb '04*

Skin Health Information for Teens
Health Tips about Dermatological Concerns and Skin Cancer Risks

Including Facts about Acne, Warts, Hives, and Other Conditions and Lifestyle Choices, Such as Tanning, Tattooing, and Piercing, That Affect the Skin, Nails, Scalp, and Hair

Edited by Robert Aquinas McNally. 429 pages. 2003. 978-0-7808-0446-3.

"This volume, as with others in the series, will be a useful addition to school and public library collections."
— *American Reference Books Annual, 2004*

"There is no doubt that this reference tool is valuable."
— *VOYA: Voice of Youth Advocates, Feb '04*

"This volume serves as a one-stop source and should be a necessity for any health collection."
— *Library Media Connection*

■

Sports Injuries Information for Teens
Health Tips about Sports Injuries and Injury Protection

Including Facts about Specific Injuries, Emergency Treatment, Rehabilitation, Sports Safety, Competition Stress, Fitness, Sports Nutrition, Steroid Risks, and More

Edited by Joyce Brennfleck Shannon. 405 pages. 2003. 978-0-7808-0447-0.

"This work will be useful in the young adult collections of public libraries as well as high school libraries."
— *American Reference Books Annual, 2004*

■

Suicide Information for Teens
Health Tips about Suicide Causes and Prevention

Including Facts about Depression, Risk Factors, Getting Help, Survivor Support, and More

Edited by Joyce Brennfleck Shannon. 368 pages. 2005. 978-0-7808-0737-2.

■

Tobacco Information for Teens
Health Tips about the Hazards of Using Cigarettes, Smokeless Tobacco, and Other Nicotine Products

Including Facts about Nicotine Addiction, Immediate and Long-Term Health Effects of Tobacco Use, Related Cancers, Smoking Cessation, Tobacco Use Prevention, and Tobacco Use Statistics

Edited by Karen Bellenir. 440 pages. 2007. 978-0-7808-0976-5.

Health Reference Series